THE HEALING POWER OF

VITAMINS, MINERALS, AND HERBS

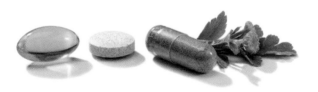

THE HEALING

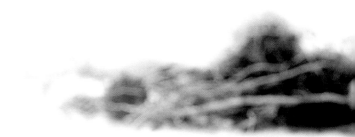

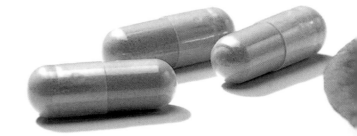

POWER OF
VITAMINS,
MINERALS,
AND HERBS

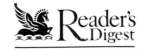

Reader's Digest

The Reader's Digest Association, Inc.
Pleasantville, New York / Montreal

THE HEALING POWER OF VITAMINS, MINERALS, AND HERBS

Project Staff

Editor
Wayne Kalyn

Designer
Susan Welt

Senior Development Editor
David Diefendorf

**Reader's Digest
Health and Science Books**

Group Editorial Director
Wayne Kalyn

Group Design Director
Barbara Rietschel

Reader's Digest General Books

**Editor-in-Chief,
U.S. General Books**
David Palmer

Executive Editor
Gayla Visalli

Managing Editor
Christopher Cavanaugh

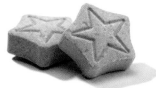

Note to Readers:
The information in this book should not be substituted for, or used to alter, medical therapy without your doctor's advice. For a specific health problem, consult your physician for guidance.

Address any comments about THE HEALING POWER OF VITAMINS, MINERALS, AND HERBS to Editor-in-Chief, U.S. General Books, Reader's Digest, Reader's Digest Road, Pleasantville, NY 10570.

To order additional copies of THE HEALING POWER OF VITAMINS, MINERALS, AND HERBS call 1–800–846–2100.

You can also visit us on the World Wide Web at http://www.readersdigest.com

Printed in the United States of America

Library of Congress Cataloging in Publication Data

The healing power of vitamins, minerals, and herbs : the a-z guide to enhancing your
    health and treating illness with nutritional supplements.
        p.   cm.
    Includes index.
    ISBN 0-7621-0132-6 (GB: alk. paper)
    1. Vitamin therapy.   2. Minerals—Therapeutic use.   3. Herbs—Therapeutic
use.   I. Reader's Digest Association.
RM259.H424 1999
615'.328—DC21   98-28049
                                                                              CIP

Created by Rebus, Inc.

Publisher
Rodney M. Friedman

Executive Editor
Sandra Wilmot

Editors
Toby Bilanow, Patricia A. Calvo

Managing Editor
Edward Petoniak

Assistant Editor
Jeremy D. Birch

Contributing Editors
Marya Dalrymple, Thomas Dickey

Chief of Information Services
Tom R. Damrauer

Researcher
Sylvia Taylor

Database Development Editor
Carney W. Mimms III

Database Support Technician
John Vasiliadis

Director, Design and Photography
Susan Darwin Ordahl

Design Assistant
Bree Rock

Photographer
Lisa Koenig

Photographer's Assistant
Christopher Lilly

Writers
Leslie Anders, Robert A. Barnett,
Jeanine Barone, Patrice Benneward,
Gloria Berlinsky, Colette Bouchez,
Lori Bernstein Davis, Edward Edelson,
Rowann Gilman, Evan Hansen,
Richard Holland, Joan Lippert,
Wendy Meyeroff, Natasha Raymond,
Sylvia Taylor, Gayle Turim, Carol Weeg

Copy Editors
Helen C. Dunn, Marsha Lloyd

Indexer
Patricia Woodruff

Medical Board of Advisors

Chief Consultant
David Edelberg, M.D.
Assistant Professor of Medicine,
  Rush Medical College, Chicago
Chairman and Founder,
  American WholeHealth, Inc.

Consultants
Keith Berndtson, M.D.
Roy R. Hall, M.D.
Tony V. Lu, M. D.
Mark Michaud, M.D.

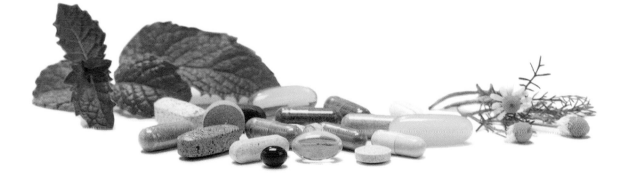

contents

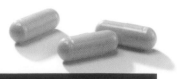

Introduction

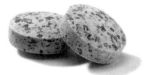

Part I Ailments

From acne to yeast infections, this section presents an alphabetical guide to some common disorders.

Part II Supplements

This color-coded section contains:

● vitamins ● minerals ● herbs ● nutritional supplements

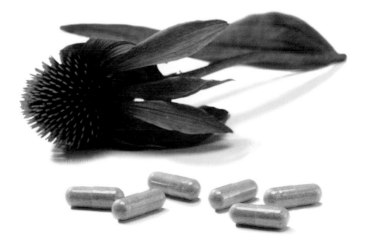

preface by David Edelberg, M.D.

Several years ago, I was your standard HMO primary-care gatekeeper: I saw one patient every 10 minutes, interrupted each one (if you believe the statistics) 14 seconds into the encounter, and then tossed off a prescription or two before moving quickly to the next examination room.

It didn't take long before I started to notice that many of my patients began their follow-up visits with a cheerless "I'm no better, Doc." This apparent lack of success, I knew, was nothing personal: Conventional medicine doesn't always fare well with chronic disease, the bread and butter of an internal medicine practice. I did find, however, that some hardy souls were actually getting better—but not as a result of my treatments. And when I asked to what they attributed their improvement, they'd mumble something about acupuncture or herbs from a nutritionist. Neither of these therapies was covered by health insurance plans, which meant the patients were paying for them out of their own pockets.

Common sense dictates that a doctor should never argue with patients who are getting better. So instead of informing them about the possible dangers of "unscientific" medicine, I began doing some research. By the time I'd left the HMO, I was making regular referrals to alternative practitioners, and in time began working with practitioners in various fields of alternative medicine, as well as with other primary-care physicians who shared my interest in complementary medicine. I have come to believe that our patients get better simply because, as doctors, we now have more tools at our disposal—two toolboxes, so to speak, offering conventional and alternative options. In addition, among us all, physicians and alternative practitioners alike, there is a mutual respect for one another's healing abilities.

Today, conventional medicine has fewer quarrels with alternative medicine than in the past. After years of speaking before medical groups, I find that the physicians I meet now are intellectually curious, mildly skeptical, and somewhat cautious, but always willing to learn about alternative treatments. As one medical school after another adds elective courses in alternative medicine, as residents and interns rotate through holistically oriented practices, the future of complementary therapies looks bright indeed.

This openness to exploring new methods of healing is especially relevant to what I see as the most significant trend in alternative medicine: the dramatic increase in the use of vitamins, minerals, herbs, and other nutritional supplements.

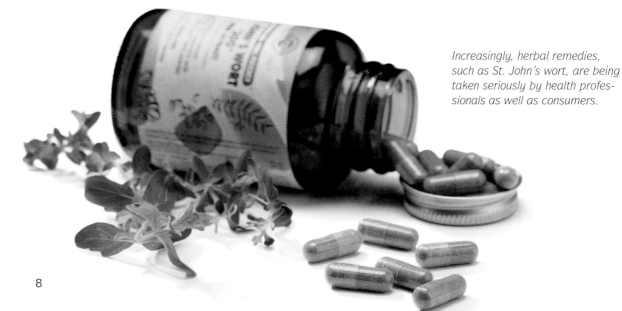

Increasingly, herbal remedies, such as St. John's wort, are being taken seriously by health professionals as well as consumers.

For many people, these supplements have come to play an important role in medical self-care, either as preventive medicine or as therapy for a variety of ailments. Behind this trend is a growing body of evidence—from researchers as well as practicing clinicians—that supplements promote good health. Furthermore, supplements are easy to obtain, and are often far less expensive than prescription drugs and many over-the-counter medications.

Yet the use of supplements is hotly debated among health experts, and sorting out claims and counterclaims can be difficult, even overwhelming. Indeed, a number of the benefits attributed to supplements remain unproved because the research is sketchy, lacking the exacting criteria that conventional medicine demands of any new therapy. Long-term risks aren't always known, and the marketing of supplements is regulated in such a way that what you read on a label is frequently of little value.

This book will help you better understand what the various supplements offer and how you can use them effectively and safely. The introductory section answers general questions about supplements, and also provides (on pages 32-35) basic supplement recommendations to help you maximize your health. For treating or preventing specific health problems, turn to the entries in the "Ailments" section, which begins on page 38; it features charts with supplement recommendations. You can find additional information on using many of these remedies in the "Supplements" section, beginning on page 228.

I do want to emphasize that even with all their proven benefits, nutritional supplements can't work miracles—and I'm not simply referring to the more outlandish claims made for some of them. It often takes more than just a pill to get results. But by combining supplements with a healthy diet and lifestyle changes (regular exercise, weight control, stress reduction), you may avoid standard medication.

With that in mind, this book can set you on a healing path, one where you take an active, more confident role in managing your own health.

David Edelberg, M.D.

David Edelberg, M.D., the chief consultant for this book, is a board-certified specialist in Internal Medicine, Section Chief of Holistic and Alternative Medicine at Illinois Masonic Medical Center (Chicago), and Assistant Professor of Medicine at Rush Medical College (Chicago). He is also founder and chairman of American WholeHealth, Inc., a health-care organization creating centers of integrated medicine throughout the United States.

About the recommendations

VITAMINS, MINERALS, HERBS, and other supplements offer a powerful resource for personal health and well-being. They can provide substantial benefits. At the same time, supplements—even if they are derived from plants and other natural sources—are chemical substances that can sometimes have marked side effects, and if used unwisely, they can be toxic.

The supplements and dosages recommended in this book are based on the findings of hundreds of research studies, as well as on the consulting doctors' clinical experience in treating patients with supplements. The dosages given in this book are averages. As with conventional drugs, you may find that a slightly higher or lower dose is appropriate for you, either to obtain the beneficial effects or to prevent any adverse reactions (which are relatively rare). For more information on using supplements safely and effectively, see pages 28-29.

Also, this book is not a substitute for face-to-face medical care from a doctor or other health-care professional. If you are undergoing medical treatment, or your doctor has prescribed a specific therapy for you, it's important that you follow through with this regimen.

Likewise, you should talk with your doctor before trying any of the remedies discussed in this book—particularly if you have a chronic health problem that warrants serious concern, such as heart disease or diabetes. The book's goal is to inform you about the numerous benefits that can come from taking supplements wisely—which means using them as a complement to, not a substitute for, responsible medical care.

The recommendations in this book do not apply to certain groups, specifically:

■ Pregnant women and nursing mothers. These women have special nutritional needs, and currently it's not known how most herbs and nutritional supplements will affect a baby.

■ Children age 16 or younger. Because a child's growth and development are so variable, even recommendations by age may not be appropriate for specific teenagers or younger children.

Individuals in the above groups can still benefit from supplements, but they should always consult a doctor before deciding what to take.

the new age of nutritional and herbal medicines

The substances and products that we think of as supplements are by no means entirely new. Vitamins in pill form have been available for more than 50 years. Herbs, also known as botanicals or phytomedicines (*phyto* means "plant" in Latin), have been staples in the sickroom and the kitchen for centuries, and were the primary form of medicine in the United States until this century. Yet only a decade ago, most vitamin pills were fairly uniform "one-a-day" formulas, and herbal remedies often had to be concocted at home or purchased in out-of-the-way health-food stores.

Today, in the United States, "dietary supplements," as they are officially called, encompass a dizzying array of vitamins, minerals, and herbs, as well as other compounds that have been extracted or created from natural sources. (These compounds carry names such as glucosamine, coenzyme Q_{10}, and—among those with recently substantiated disease-fighting potential—lycopene.)

Available without a prescription, supplements are sold in virtually every supermarket and drugstore. Many malls and shopping areas have stores devoted to marketing supplements, and you can also buy them through catalogs and over the Internet. Annual supplement sales now exceed $12 billion, and are expected to grow by at least 15% a year.

The public's interest in supplements can also be gauged by the mass media. Newspapers, TV, and radio regularly highlight their benefits—whether it's a review of 23 studies of St. John's wort for mild depression, a survey of the effects of ginkgo biloba on patients with dementia, or an article noting that the standard treatment for enlarged prostate in many European countries is not a conventional prescription drug, but the herb saw palmetto.

With all this attention and the rising sales of supplements, it isn't surprising that millions of Americans, including many doctors and scientists, have come to believe that substances such as garlic, echinacea, and grape seed extract, along with vitamins and minerals, are as beneficial to health as low-fat foods, exercise, and aspirin. According to a number of surveys, one-third to one-half of all Americans now regularly use various forms of supplements as preventive medicine or as therapies for a range of ailments—from common complaints such as colds and headaches to more serious health concerns, including arthritis, depression, and heart disease.

The changing view of supplements

The fact so many people are eager to try supplements, particularly when it is often hard to find reliable information about them, indicates that major changes in health care have brought herbal and nutritional remedies closer to mainstream medicine. Traditionally, the medical community has been skeptical of these remedies and of alternative medicine. But that is changing.

NEW RESEARCH

During the past decade, nutritional research has produced a flood of studies offering compelling evidence that specific foods and nutrients may help prevent, slow, or even reverse serious diseases. For example, several large-scale studies from Harvard University have provided strong evidence that vitamin E supplementation is linked to lower rates of heart disease in men and women. From these results, experts have concluded that a higher level of vitamin E than is found in the average American diet (or can possibly be obtained from food alone) very likely offers some protection against heart disease. These and similar studies cited throughout this book have convinced many scientists and other experts who formerly doubted that supplementation with reasonable amounts of vitamins and minerals could increase a person's chances of staving off disease and enjoying optimal health.

Though research into herbal remedies has lagged in the United States, in Europe herbs have been widely studied and scrutinized over the past 20 years, and standards have been established for their effectiveness and safety. In Germany, for example, a special body of scientists and health professionals, known as Commission E, has been investigating the usefulness and safety of herbal remedies since 1978, gathering information from scientific literature, clinical trials, and medical associations. It has issued reports on some 300 herbs—and has found about two-thirds of them to be safe and effective. New knowledge about the way herbs are used elsewhere has persuaded more American doctors and scientists to take a less dismissive view of herbal remedies.

Despite more extensive research, however, a number of benefits attributed to vitamins, minerals, and herbs remain unproved and controversial. Many doctors and researchers insist the studies on alternative remedies are not sufficiently rigorous. Furthermore, extreme claims of such benefits draw fire from critics either because they are without merit or because they leave the impression that anything "natural" is harmless, which is not always the case. Many of the studies have been small in scale, and most don't offer a long-term evaluation of benefits and side effects.

But as more studies are being conducted, some impressive evidence is accumulating. In the research on the herb St. John's wort and depression, for example, 15 studies have compared an extract of the herb to a placebo, or neutral pill, in order to test for a placebo effect (an improvement in symptoms that some people experience because they believe they are receiving treatment, even though the pill is inactive). In these studies, St. John's wort was found to be more effective than a placebo in treating mild to moderate depressive symptoms. Other studies have shown that the herb works as well as standard prescription medications for treating mild depression. Moreover, the side effects were said to be infrequent and relatively innocuous—a feature of many herbal remedies that is part of their appeal.

EMPHASIS ON PREVENTION

Increasingly, there is a greater emphasis—backed by growing numbers of medical experts—on lifestyle choices as a critical factor in staying well. This has led more people to pay attention to diet, exercise, and weight control. Many have also quit smoking and limited their alcohol intake. These actions can help prevent or relieve common complaints, including backache and constipation, and, more important, reduce the risk of serious ailments such as heart disease and cancer. (Researchers now think that three-quarters of all cancers occur mainly as a result of things people eat, drink, smoke, or encounter in the environment.)

Vitamins, minerals, and herbs can reinforce and enhance the benefit of these self-care measures, which are also essential for enjoying what might be termed optimal health—not simply the absence of illness, but the capacity to lead a full, vital, productive life.

Saw palmetto (shown as dried fruit and in capsules) is among the herbs that doctors in Europe often prescribe for prostate problems.

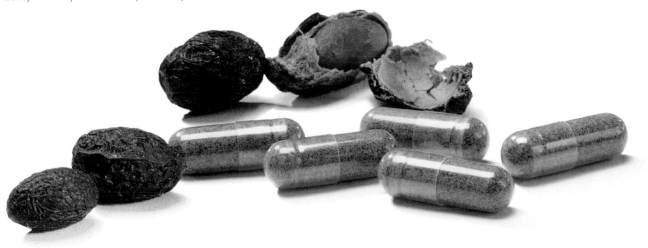

In 1994 the United States government passed a new set of regulations—the Dietary Supplement Health and Education Act—that loosened restrictions on the selling of vitamin, mineral, and herbal supplements. Reflecting and reinforcing the demands of consumers, the regulations have allowed supplement manufacturers to make certain claims about a product's health benefits without absolute proof of its therapeutic effects. The freedom to make these claims has been a key factor behind the enormous number and variety of supplements that have come on the market.

Integrative healing

In recent years, Americans—including many consumers and some doctors—have become increasingly aware of the limitations of conventional medicine. Though medical science has found cures for many troubling health problems (including some infectious diseases that caused sickness and premature death on a grand scale), it has been less successful in combating chronic illnesses such as heart disease, cancer, and diabetes. Likewise, drugs often offer potent treatments for numerous ailments, but they also pose the risk of powerful and distressing side effects. In addition, medications can be very expensive, and the cost—particularly if long-term therapy is required—may be prohibitive for many patients.

A good number of patients and doctors have also been frustrated by the growth of health maintenance organizations (HMOs) and similar managed-care health plans. Such plans have forced many Americans, often against their will, to change doctors, and, at the same time, have restricted their choice. Doctors, in turn, chafe because the time they spend with patients is limited. Surveys show that more people are now complaining that their doctors don't pay enough attention to them. Furthermore, many managed-care plans don't provide the same level of coverage that traditional insurers once did, so patients frequently have to pay more out of their own pockets for services rendered.

As awareness of these shortcomings of modern medicine has grown, consumers have become more enthusiastic about alternative approaches to treating ailments. Generally these methods—which include acupuncture, chiropractic medicine, massage therapy, and biofeedback, as well as herbal and nutritional therapies—are considered less invasive, safer, and more "holistic" (treating the whole person, rather than simply suppressing symptoms) than conventional treatments. As you read the entries in this book, you will see that supplements often act to enhance the body's own defenses. An herb you take to help treat an infection, for example, often doesn't directly kill bacteria (as an antibiotic would), but rather strengthens the immune system so your body can kill the bacteria.

Alternative therapies are also typically less expensive than conventional treatments; supplements, in particular, usually cost far less than prescription drugs, and may even be cheaper than some over-the-counter medications. Alternative therapies, such as acupuncture and chiropractic treatments, are now covered by some health-care plans.

Behind many of these alternative choices in healing is a common perspective: The body has remarkable powers of self-repair. According to this view, supplements, when used in a wise manner, can bolster the body's immune system to prevent disease. If a health problem does occur, they can also enhance and accelerate the self-healing process.

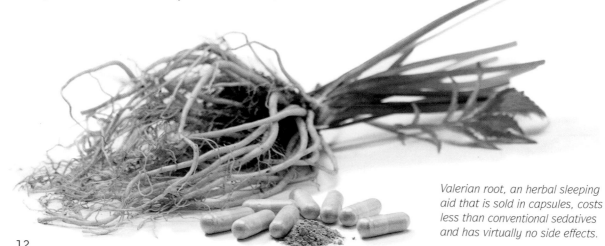

Valerian root, an herbal sleeping aid that is sold in capsules, costs less than conventional sedatives and has virtually no side effects.

Consumers have shown they want to try alternative approaches, and physicians are slowly responding to demands from patients. However, rather than thinking of supplements and other less-established remedies as "alternatives" that exclude conventional treatments, some doctors are attempting to integrate the two, so that alternative medicine options might be more appropriately viewed as "complementary," or "integrative," medicine, which can work hand-in-hand with Western medicine. (Recognizing this development, the federal government in 1992 established an Office of Alternative Medicine, which funds serious research at major medical centers to study complementary, and alternative, treatments.)

In an integrative approach, ideally, you and your doctor work together to reach a decision about which supplement or other therapy to use for treating your particular health problem (see page 14). On the other hand, many doctors and other members of the medical establishment are still resistant to complementary healing methods. Thus, there is no single reliable entity to supply advice about these remedies. In the end, consumers have to acquaint themselves with the various types of complementary therapies, including supplements.

Supplements—or drugs?

One reflection of the mainstream popularity of dietary supplements is that not only do most drugstores in the United States stock supplements, but they often shelve them near, if not next to, over-the-counter drugs. Both types of products make health-related claims, and both are supplied in dosage forms such as capsules, tablets, or powders. So a consumer may well ask, what's the difference?

NO SIMPLE ANSWER

Concerned about the marketing of supplements, legislators have made an effort to distinguish them from pharmaceutical drugs. By law, manufacturers of drugs (both over-the-counter and prescription) can make explicit claims about a product's ability to prevent or treat a recognized medical condition—for example, alleviating headaches or relieving heartburn. But such claims can be made only after a lengthy approval process by the Food and Drug Administration (FDA) that verifies the drug's safety and effectiveness.

According to the Dietary Supplement Health and Education Act, which regulates the marketing of such products, dietary supplements are intended to "supplement the diet" and contain one or more of the following: vitamins, minerals, herbs (also called botanicals), amino acids, and other nutritional substances. Supplements are not subjected to the rigorous testing and scrutiny that drugs receive, and therefore the labels on supplements cannot promise to cure or prevent diseases. But the labels can list potential benefits that affect bodily functions and general well-being, such as "promoting healthy cholesterol" or "aiding digestion."

Of course, such statements usually imply treatment for a health problem: People worried about high cholesterol levels and heart disease, for example, are likely to respond to anything promoting "healthy" cholesterol. Such links are frequently spelled out in manufacturers' brochures and sales materials as well as in news reports and other publications.

TRUTHFULNESS OF CLAIMS

Whether the assertions on supplement labels are always true is an issue that regulators have wrestled with but not solved. The law states that all claims must be "truthful and not misleading"—and in many cases, there is some scientific basis for them. But supplement manufacturers don't have to submit any data in advance of making a claim; they merely need to have the evidence on hand. Hence, labels must contain a statement that the claims "have not been evaluated by the Food and Drug Administration."

If many supplements do, in fact, act like drugs and are often used as drugs, why aren't they tested and marketed as drugs? Because vitamins, minerals, herbs, and other supplements can be derived directly from plants and other natural sources, they can't be patented. Thus there is little financial incentive for drug or supplement makers to spend millions on the research and approval process required for a nutrient to obtain the status of a drug. Once an herb or herb component receives FDA approval, any company can then sell the same product. (Compounds marketed as drugs have been chemically modified in laboratories to create unique products that can be patented.)

Government regulation of supplements will no doubt evolve as the use of supplements continues to grow and as more is learned about their effects. At some point, American regulations and practices may move closer to the systems of a number of European countries, where herbal remedies are examined and formulated with more rigor. For now, it is helpful to remember that the claims made on most supplement labels are not equivalent to—or as stringent as—those on most drug labels. A careful consumer should try to seek out additional, more detailed sources of information. This book is a good place to start that informative process.

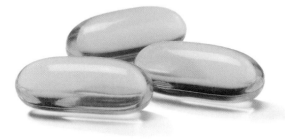

Extracted from natural sources, the fish oils in these capsules aren't patented or regulated like drugs.

You and your doctor

A GROWING NUMBER of doctors and patients are embracing an integrative, or complementary, approach to treating health problems. This entails carefully weighing both conventional and alternative methods in order to create a strategy best suited to a patient's needs. For example, a person with high blood pressure finds that the side effects from a prescription drug are distressing, and so he and his doctor decide on a course of therapy that combines supplements with other lifestyle adjustments to see if it can effectively lower the blood pressure with less distress.

Medical schools, however, teach their students very little about nutritional and herbal therapies. But because professional journals and postgraduate courses for physicians are giving these forms of treatment increasing attention, many doctors are becoming better acquainted with them. If your doctor is not sufficiently knowledgeable about nutritional or herbal medicine, he may well suggest that you work with a nutritionist or other health practitioner in this area (see page 30)—especially if he thinks you have a medical problem that normally responds well to supplement treatment.

If you find that your doctor is skeptical about an integrated approach to your problem, consider consulting a doctor who is more receptive. (Some of the organizations on page 31 can help you locate a qualified practitioner.) Such a doctor will probably have a better understanding of the effects of dietary supplements on the body than a conventional physician, an herbalist, or other nonphysician who isn't schooled in anatomy and physiology. No matter whom you work with, be sure to take these guidelines into account:

- **Don't diagnose yourself.** If you have symptoms that suggest an illness, see a doctor—either an M.D., a D.O. (doctor of osteopathic medicine), or a trained and licensed doctor of naturopathy.

- **Talk to your doctor.** Be sure to report all of your symptoms. Also, tell your doctor about any supplements that you are already taking, because some of them might not interact well with conventional drugs that you may be asked to try. Even if your doctor isn't receptive to herbal or nutritional remedies, you should still discuss any supplements you are taking or thinking about using, particularly if you have a chronic condition such as asthma, diabetes, heart disease, or high blood pressure.

- **Don't stop treatment.** Some supplements may complement, or even replace, conventional drugs. But you should never discontinue or alter the dosage of any prescribed medication without first consulting your doctor.

- **Recognize when conventional methods are best.** It can be foolish—and sometimes even dangerous—to seek alternative options for medical conditions that Western-trained doctors excel in treating or preventing. These include medical and surgical emergencies, physical injuries, acute infections such as pneumonia, sexually transmitted diseases, kidney infections, reconstructive surgery, and prevention of serious immunizable illnesses such as polio and diphtheria.

basic types of supplements

Anyone who has strolled down a dietary supplement aisle is aware of—and possibly overwhelmed by—the huge variety. Counting different brands and combinations of supplements, there are literally thousands of choices available. You'll hardly encounter this many in one location, but even a far more limited selection in your local supermarket can be confusing.

One reason for so much variety is that marketers are constantly trying to distinguish their own brands from others, and so they devise different dosages, new combinations, and creatively worded claims for their products. At the same time, scientists have found new and better ways of extracting nutritional components from plants and synthesizing nutrients in a laboratory—discoveries that have resulted in many new products.

To make informed decisions, it's essential to understand the terms used on supplement labels (see page 26), as well as the properties and characteristics of specific supplements (which you will find in Part II of the book, the "Supplements" section that starts on page 228). But to avoid feeling overwhelmed by all the choices facing you, it's useful first to learn the basic types of supplements that are available and the key functions they perform in helping to keep you healthy.

VITAMINS

A vitamin is a chemically organic substance (meaning it contains carbon) essential for regulating both the metabolic functions within the cells and the biochemical processes that release energy from food. In addition, evidence is accumulating that certain vitamins are antioxidants—substances that protect tissues from cell damage and may possibly help prevent a number of degenerative diseases (see page 17).

With a few exceptions (notably vitamins D and K), the body cannot manufacture vitamins, so they must be ingested in food or nutritional supplements. There are 13 known vitamins, and these can be categorized as either fat-soluble (A, D, E, and K) or water-soluble (eight B vitamins and C). The distinction is important because the body stores fat-soluble vitamins for relatively long periods (months or even years); water-soluble vitamins (except for vitamin B_{12}), on the other hand, remain in the body for a short time and must be replenished more frequently.

MINERALS

Minerals are present in your body in small amounts: All together, they add up to only 4% of body weight. Yet these inorganic substances, which are found in the earth's crust as well as in many foods, are essential for a wide range of vital processes, from basic bone

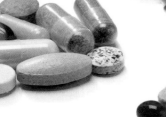

The pills shown here (clockwise from top) are minerals, herbal extracts, vitamins, and other nutritional supplements.

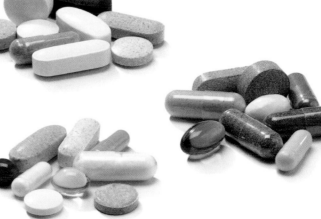

formation to the normal functioning of the heart and digestive system. A number of minerals have been linked to the prevention of cancer, osteoporosis, and other chronic illnesses.

As with vitamins, humans must replenish their mineral supply through food or with supplements. The body contains more than 60 different minerals, but only 22 are considered essential. Of these, seven —including calcium, chloride, magnesium, phosphorus, potassium, sodium, and sulfur—are usually designated macrominerals, or major minerals. The other 15 minerals are termed trace minerals, or microminerals, because the amount that the body requires each day for good health is tiny (usually it's measured in micrograms, or millionths of a gram).

HERBS

Herbal supplements are prepared from plants—often using the leaves, stems, roots, and/or bark, as well as the buds and flowers. Known for centuries as medicinal agents, many plant parts can be used in their natural form, or they can be refined into tablets, capsules, powders, tinctures, and other supplement formulations.

Many herbs have several active compounds that interact with one another to produce a therapeutic effect. An herbal supplement may contain all of the compounds found in a plant, or just one or two of the isolated compounds that have been successfully extracted. For some herbs, however, the active agents simply haven't been identified, so using the complete herb is necessary to obtain all its benefits.

Of the hundreds of remedies that are surfacing in the current rebirth of herbal medicines, the majority are being used to treat chronic or mild health problems. Increasingly, herbs are also being employed to attain or maintain good health—for example, to enhance the immune system, to help maintain low blood cholesterol levels, or to safeguard against fatigue. Less commonly, some herbs are now recommended as complementary therapy for acute or severe diseases.

NUTRITIONAL SUPPLEMENTS

These nutrients include a diverse group of products. Some, such as fish oils, are food substances that scientists have concluded possess disease-fighting potential. Flavonoids, soy isoflavones, and carotenoids are phytochemicals—compounds found in fruits and vegetables that work to lower the risk of disease and may alleviate symptoms of some ailments.

Other nutritional supplements, such as DHEA, melatonin, and coenzyme Q_{10}, are substances present in the body that can be re-created synthetically in a laboratory. A similar example is acidophilus, a "friendly" bacterium in the body that, taken as a supplement, may aid in the treatment of digestive disorders. Amino acids, which are building blocks for proteins and may play a role in strengthening the immune system and in other health-promoting activities, have been known to scientists for many years. Only recently, however, have they been marketed as individual dietary supplements.

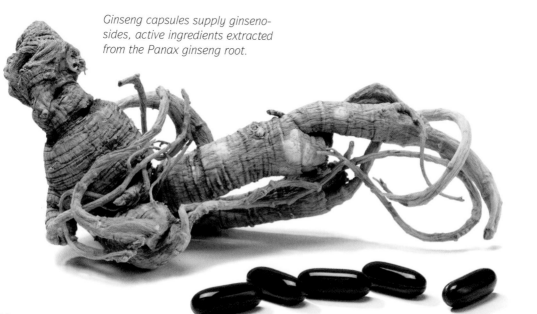

Ginseng capsules supply ginsenosides, active ingredients extracted from the Panax ginseng root.

how supplements
can benefit you

Many people take a multivitamin and mineral supplement as nutritional "insurance" against deficiencies. But recent research provides additional reasons for using a variety of supplements, including herbs, for both prevention and healing—and indicates that optimal levels may be higher than conventional wisdom has long dictated.

If you're basically healthy, is there any advantage to taking supplements on a regular basis? And if you develop a disorder or ailment, can you expect supplements to offer any help? What follows is a summary of the major benefits that, according to researchers, most people can expect if they use the supplements covered in this book. More detailed information about the therapeutic effects of specific supplements can be found in the entries in the "Supplements" section, beginning on page 228.

Enhancing your diet

Conventional wisdom has long held that as long as people who are healthy eat well enough to avoid specific nutritional deficiencies, they don't need to supplement their diet. The only thing they have to do is consume a diet that meets the RDAs—Recommended Dietary Allowances—and other guidelines for vitamin and mineral intakes developed by health agencies of the federal government (see page 21).

But even if one accepts the government's standards for vitamin and mineral intakes as adequate for good health, the evidence is overwhelming that most people don't come close to meeting those nutritional requirements. Surveys show that only 9% of Americans eat five daily servings of fresh fruits and vegetables—the amount recommended for obtaining the minimum level of nutrients believed necessary to prevent illness.

Average calcium consumption in the United States and Canada is estimated to be about 60% of the current suggested level of 1,000 mg for younger adults—and far below the 1,200 mg recommended for men and women ages 50 to 70.

According to a review of national data by experts at the University of California, Berkeley, people often make food choices that are nutritionally poor: For example, they are more likely to select french fries than broccoli as a vegetable serving, and will opt for a soft drink rather than a glass of skim milk as a beverage. Not only may these and other foods

The power of antioxidants

ALTHOUGH OXYGEN IS essential for life, it can have adverse effects on your body. In the normal process of using oxygen, chemical changes occur that create reactive unstable oxygen molecules called free radicals, which can damage cells and structures within cells, including genetic material (DNA). Free radicals also may form in response to external factors such as cigarette smoke and alcohol, pollutants such as nitrogen oxide and ozone, and ultraviolet light and other forms of radiation, including X rays. If the genetic material in cells is affected by free radicals and not repaired, it can be replicated in new cells, contributing to cancer and other health problems. Free radicals may also weaken artery walls, allowing fatty deposits that can lead to heart disease to collect.

However, cells have special agents for combating free radicals and repairing molecular damage. These free-radical fighters are called antioxidants. A great deal of recent research suggests that antioxidants may play important roles in preventing or delaying heart disease, cancer, and other ills, and may even halt the damage to cells, thereby slowing the effects of aging.

Vitamins C and E are perhaps the best-known antioxidants. The mineral selenium is also an antioxidant, as are carotenoids such as beta-carotene and lycopene. Enzymes and certain other compounds (such as glutathione) manufactured by the cells themselves also function as antioxidants. Some experts now think that a number of other substances, including certain herbs, may act as antioxidants as well. For example, green tea, grape seed extract, and ginkgo biloba (among others) are all thought to have antioxidant properties.

contribute too much fat and sugar to your diet, but they can also result in less-than-optimal intakes of vitamins, minerals, and disease-fighting phytochemicals. Many American diets, these experts point out, contain half the recommended amounts of magnesium and folic acid. Vitamins A, C, and B_6, as well as iron and zinc, are other nutrients that surveys show are at notably low levels in the American diet.

Even with the best nutritional planning, it is difficult to maintain a diet that meets the RDAs for all nutrients. For example, vegetarians, who as a group are healthier than meat eaters (and who tend to avoid junk foods lacking in vitamins and minerals), still may be deficient in some nutrients, such as iron, calcium, and vitamin B_{12}. And most people who want to maintain a healthy low-fat diet will have a problem obtaining the recommended amounts of vitamin E from their food alone, because so many of the food sources for

vitamin E are high in fat. Another complication is that a balanced diet may not contain the more specialized substances—fish oils, soy isoflavones, or alpha-lipoic acid—that researchers think may promote health. For generally healthy people who cannot always eat a well-balanced diet every day, a supplement can fill in these nutritional gaps or boost the nutrients they consume from adequate to optimal.

There are various other reasons why people who maintain good eating habits might benefit from a daily supplement. Some experts now believe that exposure to environmental pollutants—from car emissions to industrial chemicals and wastes—can cause damage in myriad ways inside the body at the cellular level, destroying tissues and depleting the body of nutrients. Many supplements, particularly

To get the antioxidant benefit of vitamin E, you could eat 18 ounces of sunflower seeds (a leading food source) or take one of these capsules.

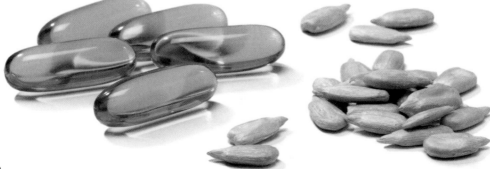

those that act as antioxidants, can help control the cell and tissue damage that follows toxic exposure (see "The Power of Antioxidants" on page 17). Recent evidence also indicates that certain medications, excess alcohol, smoking, and persistent stress may interfere with the absorption of certain key nutrients. And even an excellent diet would be unable to make up for such a shortfall.

As explained on pages 33-35, specific nutritional programs of vitamins, minerals, and other supplements can be designed that will take into account these and other environmental and lifestyle factors, which affect nutrient levels in the human body.

Preventing disease, slowing aging

For many years, it was thought that a lack of nutrients was linked only to specific deficiency diseases such as scurvy, a condition marked by soft gums and loose teeth that is caused by too little vitamin C. In the past three decades, however, thousands of scientific studies have all indicated that specific nutrients appear to play an important role in the prevention of a number of chronic, degenerative diseases common in contemporary Western societies.

Many recent studies highlighting the disease-fighting potential of different nutrients are mentioned throughout this book. What most of these studies reveal is that the level of nutrients associated with disease prevention is often significantly higher than the current RDAs. And to achieve these higher levels, the participants in these studies often had to depend on supplements.

In slowing or preventing the development of disease, some experts suggest that nutrients, particularly the antioxidants, can also delay the wear and tear of aging itself by reducing the damage done to cells. This idea doesn't mean vitamin E or coenzyme Q_{10}, for example, are "youth potions." But several recent studies, including work done at the Nutritional Immunological Laboratory at Tufts University, have found that supplementation with single nutrients, such as vitamin E, or with multivitamin and mineral supplements, appear to improve immune response among older people.

For example, a study of 11,178 elderly subjects, conducted by researchers at the National Institute on Aging, showed that the use of vitamin E was associated with a lowered risk of total mortality, and especially of death from heart disease. In fact,

vitamin E users were only half as likely to die of heart disease as those taking no supplements. In addition, there is evidence that antioxidant supplements are effective in lowering the risk of cataracts and macular degeneration, two age-related conditions in which vision slowly deteriorates.

Other supplements that serve as high-potency antioxidants against aging disorders include selenium, carotenoids, flavonoids, certain amino acids, and coenzyme Q_{10}. Some experts also believe that the herb ginkgo biloba may improve many age-related symptoms, especially those involving reduced blood flow, such as dizziness, impotence, and short-term memory loss. Substances found in echinacea and other herbs are reported to strengthen the immune system, and phytoestrogens such as soy isoflavones are thought to help delay or prevent some of the effects of menopause, as well as to help prevent cancer and heart disease. (A fuller discussion of aging can be found on pages 42-43).

Too many benefits: Too good to be true?

WHEN YOU SEE a supplement label that lists a variety of functions and benefits for a single herb or substance, you might wonder if this is more marketing hype than facts. You can't rely entirely on label claims, because they aren't scrutinized for accuracy by the government or any other agency. But as you will see in reading the entries in this book, some supplements do have multiple effects that are well documented.

Consider an herb such as green tea. According to many studies, its benefits may include helping control several cancers, including colon and pancreatic cancer; protecting against heart disease; inhibiting the action of bacteria; combating tooth decay; and acting as an antioxidant to bolster the immune system. All of these benefits aren't too surprising, given that researchers have identified various active components in green tea.

You should be aware that many common medications were initially developed for one purpose. As more people take the drugs and their effects are studied, new uses come to light. Imagine a drug that can cure headaches, relieve arthritis, help prevent heart disease, ease the pain of athletic injuries, and reduce the risk of colon cancer. It's aspirin, of course—and its precursor came from an herbal source, the bark of the white willow tree.

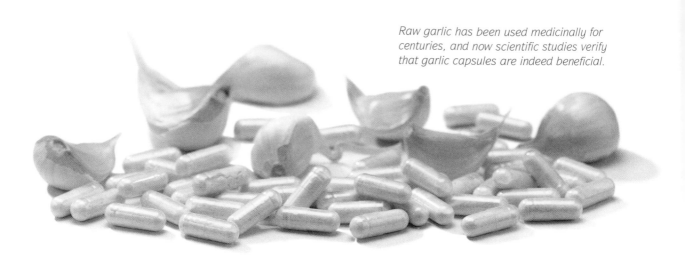

Raw garlic has been used medicinally for centuries, and now scientific studies verify that garlic capsules are indeed beneficial.

Alleviating and treating ailments

Many practitioners of complementary medicine recommend supplements for a wide range of health problems affecting virtually every body system. For most of these conditions, conventional physicians would be more likely to prescribe drugs, though they might treat some disorders with supplements. For example, iron may be prescribed for some types of anemia, vitamin A (in the drug isotretinoin, or Accutane) for severe acne, and high doses of the B vitamin niacin for reducing high cholesterol levels.

In this book, certain vitamins and minerals are suggested for the treatment of specific ailments. However, the use of nutritional supplements as remedies, especially for serious conditions, is controversial. Most doctors practicing conventional medicine are skeptical of their efficacy and believe it is sometimes dangerous to rely on them. But based on published data and their clinical observations, nutritionally oriented physicians and practitioners think the use of these supplements is justified—and that to wait years for unequivocal proof to appear would be wasting valuable time. Until there is clearer, more consistent evidence available, you should be careful about depending on nutritional supplements alone to treat an ailment or injury.

For thousands of years, however, various cultures have employed herbs for soothing, relieving, or even curing many common health problems, a fact not ignored by medical science. The pharmaceutical industry, after all, arose as a consequence of people using herbs as medicine. Recent studies suggest that a number of the claims made for herbs have validity, and the pharmacological actions of the herbs covered in this book are often well documented by clinical studies as well as historical practice. In Europe, a number of herbal remedies, including St. John's wort, ginkgo biloba, and saw palmetto, now are accepted and prescribed as medications for treating disorders such as allergies, depression, impotence, and even heart disease. Of course, even herbs and other supplements with proven therapeutic effects should be used judiciously for treating an ailment (pages 28-29 offer guidelines for utilizing these remedies safely and effectively).

What supplements won't do

Despite the many promising benefits that supplements offer, it's important to note their limits—and to question some of the extravagant claims currently being made for them.

■ As the word itself suggests, supplements are not meant to replace the nutrients available from foods. Supplements will never make up for a poor diet: They can't counteract a high intake of saturated fat (which is linked to an increased risk of heart disease and cancer), and they can't replace every nutrient found in food groups that you ignore. Also, although scientists have isolated and extracted a number of disease-fighting phytochemical compounds from fruits, vegetables, and other foods, there may be many others that are undiscovered—and ones you can get only from foods. In addition, some of the known compounds may work only in combination with others in various foods, rather than as single isolated ingredients in supplement form.

■ Supplements won't compensate for habits known to contribute to ill health, such as smoking or a lack

RDAs, DVs, RDIs: What do those numbers mean?

OVER THE YEARS, government-sponsored committees of nutritional experts, including those in the National Academy of Sciences and the Food and Drug Administration, have established various guidelines for the amounts of vitamins and minerals needed by most individuals to achieve and maintain good health. Understanding what these different standards signify can be confusing. All of them, however, represent similar values based on the "gold standard" of vitamin and mineral intake: the RDAs, or Recommended Dietary Allowances.

THE FIRST RDAS

The first RDAs were developed in 1941 and have been revised periodically by the Food and Nutrition Board of the National Research Council. The RDAs are different for men, women, and children, for different age groups, and for pregnant or lactating women. Some years ago, a new standard, the Reference Daily Intake, or RDI, was created for each nutrient. The RDIs are intended to represent nutrient needs of an average healthy person. In most cases they are the highest levels of adult RDAs, though they also take into account other guidelines.

On many labels of vitamin and mineral supplements (as well as on food labels), you will see a set of figures under the heading "% Daily Value," or DV. The Daily Value is simply a percentage of the RDI. It tells you how much of a particular nutrient is supplied by a dose of the supplement (or, in the case of food labels, by a serving of food). The sample label on page 26 shows how the DV typically appears.

The RDIs replace an older value called the U.S. RDA. Though this value is no longer used for foods, some supplement labels continue to state nutrient values as a percentage of the U.S. RDA.

SLIGHTLY REVISED GUIDELINES

Recently, the Food and Nutrition Board introduced a new set of values called Dietary Reference Intakes (DRIs). These include RDAs as well as Adequate Intakes for certain nutrients for which there is not enough evidence to establish an RDA. In releasing new recommendations, the board raised some RDA levels to take into account the prevention of disorders other than deficiency diseases. For example, the latest recommendation for folic acid for women age 18 and older has been raised from 180 mcg to 400 mcg—a level thought to protect against certain birth defects and heart disease.

In the "Supplements" section of this book (under "How Much You Need"), each of the vitamin and mineral entries notes the RDA or Adequate Intake for that nutrient. Deficiencies from getting too little of a nutrient, and any adverse effects from getting too much, are also indicated when they are known.

ARE THEY ENOUGH?

It's important to remember that the RDAs, RDIs, and DRIs are recommendations, not requirements, for large groups of people. The values are at a level assumed to supply the nutrient needs of most people, plus a generous margin of safety. Many experts, however, think RDAs (especially those for vitamins) are still much too low for maintaining optimal health or for treating certain diseases. Also, the values don't take into account such variables as smoking, alcohol consumption, exposure to pollutants, and medication use, all of which can interfere with nutrient absorption. The basic daily formula on page 33 generally provides higher levels of nutrients than the RDAs. Additional nutrients to meet specific needs are suggested as well (see page 34-35).

---

of exercise. Optimal health requires a wholesome lifestyle (see page 18)—particularly if, as people get older, they are intent on aging well.

■ Although some of the benefits ascribed to supplements are unproved but plausible, other claims are far-fetched. Weight-loss preparations are the leading example. Though they're extremely popular, it's questionable whether any of them can help you shed pounds without the right food choices and regular exercise. Products that claim to "burn fat" won't burn enough on their own for significant weight loss.

■ Similarly, claims of boosting performance, whether physical or mental, are difficult to prove—and any "enhancement" will be a limited one at best in a healthy person. Though a supplement may improve mental functioning in someone experiencing mild to severe episodes of memory loss, it may have a negligible effect on the memory or concentration of most adults. Likewise, a supplement shown to combat fatigue isn't going to turn the average jogger into an endurance athlete. Nor is it clear that "aphrodisiac" supplements are effective for enhancing sexual performance if you aren't suffering from some form of sexual dysfunction.

■ No supplements have been found to cure any serious diseases—including cancer, heart disease, diabetes, or AIDS. The right supplement, however, may help improve a chronic condition and relieve symptoms such as pain or inflammation. But first you need to consult a health professional for treatment.

buying supplements:
preparations and forms

The many choices available allow you to find supplements that are safe, effective, and convenient. But some of these "special" formulations appear to provide little additional benefit, and they are frequently not worth the extra expense.

Supplements come in a variety of forms that affect both their ease of use and, in some cases, their rate of absorption. (Each supplement entry lists the available forms for that supplement.)

Common forms

For most people, tablets and capsules are the most convenient form of supplement to take, but there are other options as well.

TABLETS Easily stored, tablets will generally keep longer than other supplement forms. In addition to the vitamin itself, tablets often contain generally inert additives known as excipients. These compounds bind, preserve, or give bulk to the supplement, and help tablets break down more quickly in the stomach. Increasingly, supplements are available in capsule-shaped, easy-to-swallow tablets called "caplets."

CAPSULES The fat-soluble vitamins A, D, and E are typically packaged in "softgel" capsules. Other vitamins and minerals are processed into powders or liquids and then encapsulated. Like tablets, capsules are easy to use and store. They also tend to have fewer additives than tablets, and there is some evidence that they dissolve more readily (though this doesn't mean they are better absorbed by the body—just that they may be absorbed more quickly).

POWDERS People who find pills hard to swallow can use powders, which can be mixed into juice or water, or stirred into food. (Ground seeds such as psyllium and flaxseed often come in powdered form.) Powders also allow dosages to be adjusted easily. Because they may have fewer binders or additives than tablets or capsules, powders are useful for individuals who are allergic to certain substances. In addition, powders are often cheaper than tablets or capsules.

LIQUIDS Liquid formulas for oral use are easy to swallow and can be flavored. Many children's formulas are in liquid form. Some supplements (such as vitamin E) also come in liquids for applying topically to the skin. Eyedrops are another type of liquid.

About the label claims

ADVERTISING CLAIMS IMPLY that the vitamins derived from "natural" sources (such as vitamin E from soybeans) are better than "synthetic" vitamins created chemically in a laboratory. They may state that their natural products are more potent or more efficiently absorbed—and manufacturers generally charge more for natural products. But what is "natural"?

Actually, most supplements, no matter what their source, undergo processing with chemicals in laboratories. Some products labeled "natural" are really synthetic vitamins with plant extracts or minute amounts of naturally derived vitamins mixed in. Hence, "vitamin C from rose hips" may be mostly synthetic. And even the most natural products are refined and processed, and contain some additives. In any case, there's no difference chemically between natural and synthetic vitamins—nor can your body distinguish between the two.

Some researchers consider natural sources of vitamin E more effective than synthetic versions. But the International Units (IUs) used to measure vitamin E's potency take this into account, so a capsule designated to provide 400 IUs will have that potency no matter what its source.

Generally, there's no reason to pay more for supplements advertised as "natural." The cheapest synthetic vitamin or mineral supplement will give you the same benefit. Of course, the cheapest supplement isn't always the best. You should check the excipients, or additives, in a supplement to be sure that you aren't allergic to any—and you may have to pay more for a supplement with fewer of these inert filler ingredients.

CHEWABLES Such supplements—usually packaged as flavored wafers—are particularly recommended for those who have trouble getting pills down. In this book, the most common wafer form is DGL, a licorice preparation. DGL is activated by saliva, so the wafers must be chewed, not simply swallowed.

LOZENGES A number of supplements are available as lozenges or drops that are intended to dissolve gradually in the mouth, either for ease of use or, in the case of zinc lozenges, to help in the treatment of colds and the flu.

SUBLINGUAL TABLETS A few supplements, such as vitamin B_{12}, are formulated to dissolve under the tongue, providing quick absorption into the bloodstream without interference from stomach acids and digestive enzymes.

Special formulations

You will usually pay more for a supplement if the label says "timed-release" or "chelated." Does it provide extra benefits? Hardly ever, according to available data, and so paying more for this type of product is generally a waste of money.

TIMED-RELEASE FORMULAS

These formulas contain microcapsules that gradually break down to release the vitamin steadily into the bloodstream over roughly 2 to 10 hours, depending on the product. ("Sustained-release" is another term that describes the same process.)

There are no reliable studies showing that timed-release formulas are more efficiently utilized by the body than conventional capsules or tablets—in fact, the gel-like substance that acts to delay the release may actually interfere with the absorption of fat-soluble vitamins. And although timed-release versions of niacin may help prevent unpleasant side effects, this formulation (which is commonly used to lower cholesterol) can be harmful, so is not recommended.

CHELATED MINERALS

Chelation is a process in which a mineral is bonded to another substance, or "chelator"—usually an amino acid. This attached substance is supposed to enhance the body's absorption of the mineral. In most cases, there's no proof that chelated minerals are absorbed any better or any quicker than nonchelated minerals.

In fact, there is no solid information that any process or added ingredients improve the absorption of vitamins or most minerals. It's more important that supplements meet standards for dissolving within a set period of time—indicated by the designation "USP" on the label (see page 27).

Herbal remedies

You can purchase whole herbs and make up your own formulations. But for ease of use, tablets, capsules, and the other prepackaged forms described here (including forms for external use) are readily available in drugstores, supermarkets, and health-food stores.

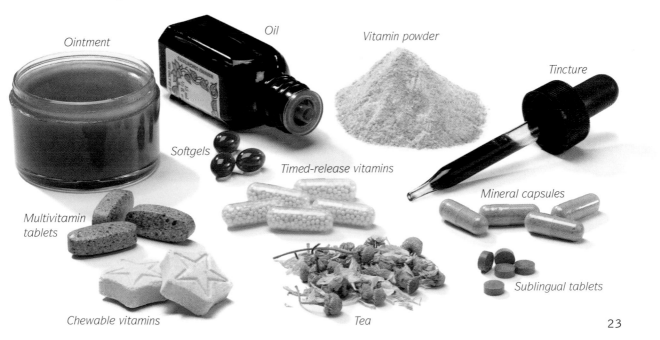

Ointment

Oil

Vitamin powder

Tincture

Softgels

Timed-release vitamins

Mineral capsules

Multivitamin tablets

Chewable vitamins

Tea

Sublingual tablets

TABLETS AND CAPSULES

You can avoid the taste of the herb if you take it in tablet or capsule form. Both tablets and capsules are prepared using either a whole herb or an extract containing a high concentration of the herb's active components. In either form, the constituents are ground into a powder that can be pressed into tablets or encapsulated. Some herbs are available in enteric-coated capsules, which pass through the stomach to the small intestine before dissolving, minimizing potential gastrointestinal discomfort and, for some herbs, enhancing absorption into the bloodstream.

TINCTURES   These concentrated liquids are made by soaking the whole herb or parts of it in water and ethyl alcohol. The alcohol extracts and concentrates the herb's active components. (Nonalcoholic concentrations can be made using glycerin.) Tinctures are usually taken in small doses—say 20 drops, or 1 ml, three times daily—diluted with water or juice.

TEAS, INFUSIONS, DECOCTIONS

Less concentrated than tinctures, teas and infusions are brewed from fresh or dried flowers, leaves, or roots of an herb; these can be purchased in bulk or in tea bags. Although tea is generally made with boiling water, the herbal teas recommended in this book are prepared as infusions, using hot water on the verge of boiling, which preserves the beneficial oils that can be dissipated by the steam of boiling water. As for decoctions, the tougher parts of an herb (stems or bark) are generally simmered for at least half an hour.

Use these liquid remedies as soon as possible after brewing them, because they start to lose their potency within a few hours of exposure to air. Store them in tightly sealed glass jars in the refrigerator, and they'll retain some strength for up to three days.

OILS   Oils extracted from herbs can be commercially distilled to form potent concentrations for external use. These so-called essential oils are usually placed in a neutral "carrier" oil, such as almond oil, before use on the skin. (Milder "infused" oils can be prepared at home.) Essential herbal oils should never be ingested. The exception is peppermint oil. A few drops on the tongue are recommended for bad breath, and capsules are beneficial for irritable colon.

GELS, OINTMENTS, AND CREAMS

Gels and ointments, which are made from fats or oils of aromatic herbs, are applied to the skin to soothe

When you buy standardized extracts

THE AMOUNT OF an active or main ingredient in a standardized herbal extract is often expressed as a percentage: Milk thistle "standardized to contain 80% silymarin" means that 80% of the extract contains that ingredient. Accordingly, recommendations in this book for most standardized products are given as percentages. For example, a 150 mg dose of milk thistle standardized to contain 80% silymarin contains 120 mg silymarin (150 x .80 = 120). Sometimes, though, a standardized extract product will simply state the actual amount of active ingredient you're getting (e.g., 120 mg silymarin) rather than listing a percentage.

rashes, heal bruises or wounds, and serve other therapeutic purposes. Creams are light oil-and-water mixtures that are partly absorbed by the skin, allowing it to breathe while also keeping in moisture. Creams can be used for moisturizing dry skin, for cleansing, and for relieving rashes, insect bites, or sunburn.

Standardized extracts

When herbs are recommended in this book, we often suggest you look for "standardized extracts." Herbalists and manufacturers use this term to describe the consistency of a product. When creating an herbal supplement, manufacturers can extract the active components from the whole herb. These active ingredients—say, the allicin in garlic or the ginsenosides in ginseng—are then concentrated and made into a supplement (tablets, capsules, or tinctures). They are standardized to supply you with a precise amount in each dose.

Sometimes, instead of standardized extracts, manufacturers process the whole, or crude, herb. In this case, the whole herb is simply air- or freeze-dried, made into a powder, and then packaged into a supplement—again a capsule, tablet, tincture, or other form.

Whether a standardized extract or the crude herb is better is an ongoing controversy among herbalists. Supporters of crude herb supplements contend that the whole herb may contain still unidentified active ingredients, and that only through ingesting the entire herb can all the benefits be obtained. On the other hand, advocates of standardized extracts argue that the active ingredients in whole herbs can vary greatly depending on where they're grown and how the herbs are harvested and processed. Standardization

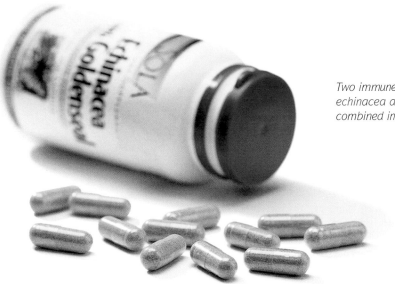

Two immune-system boosters, echinacea and goldenseal, are combined in this formula.

proponents say the only way to be sure you're receiving a consistent amount of active ingredients is by taking standardized extracts.

Although standardized products are indeed more consistent from batch to batch, this fact doesn't guarantee that they are more effective than whole-herb products. But in many cases, you would have to use a much greater amount of a whole herb to achieve a similar therapeutic effect. More to the point, reliability and consistency can be of great value, particularly when a product proves to be beneficial for a specific disorder.

Multisupplements

Multivitamin and mineral formulas are not new products, and many herbs have traditionally been paired with others to enhance their benefits. The most straightforward pairings combine herbs with similar effects, such as valerian and chamomile, which both act as sedatives. Other formulas include herbs that address different symptoms of an ailment, not unlike a combination cold remedy that has one ingredient for congestion, another for sore throat. Still others feature an array of substances touted as antioxidant "cocktails." And supplement manufacturers have also marketed herbs with vitamins and other nutritional supplements such as amino acids.

Some of these combinations can promote health and may also save you money. In addition, you may find that fewer pills are needed to obtain the desired effect. For example, liver detoxifying products called lipotropic combinations often include the nutrients choline, inositol, and methionine and the herb milk

thistle—all of which, in a blend, assist liver function. These formulas cost less and are more convenient to take than individual supplements.

In some combination products, however, certain ingredients are present in such small quantities that they can't have any therapeutic effect. They are there simply to promote the product. So it pays to check the label to determine the amount of each ingredient.

The hype factor

IN AN EFFORT to distinguish one brand from another, supplement manufacturers have come up with their own jargon in promoting their products. The following terms commonly appear on supplement labels and in advertisements. Each term implies a superior product, but none has a standard definition agreed upon by experts or by the regulations governing the manufacture and sale of supplements. Pay attention to the specific ingredients and directions on a label rather than the hype of these terms:

- Clinically Proven
- Essential
- Guaranteed Potency
- Highly Concentrated
- Maximum Absorption
- Natural (or Naturally Occurring)
- Nutritionally Comprehensive
- Pure
- Quality Extract
- Scientifically Standardized

buying supplements:
how to read a label

Ideally, a label should tell you everything you need to know before buying and using a supplement. Until recently, many labels on dietary supplements provided very little information. Fortunately, a ruling by the Food and Drug Administration (FDA) will help to make labeling more consistent.

The FDA has stipulated that by March 1999, vitamins, minerals, herbs, and other dietary supplements must carry a "Supplement Facts" panel listing ingredients by weight and giving the percentage of the Reference Daily Intake (RDI), expressed as Percent Daily Value (DV), for those nutrients with an established RDI. The ruling also specifies the meaning of such terms as "high potency" (opposite). In the case of herbs, the part of the plant—the leaf or root, for example—used in the product must be identified.

The key terms that you will find on revamped supplement labels are summarized on these two pages. This kind of detailed information doesn't guarantee a superior product. But it is a step toward enabling consumers to make a more informed decision about which supplement to buy.

What the terms mean

STATEMENT OF IDENTITY   A description of the type of supplement, typically appearing above or below the brand name. The statement of identity must include either the words "dietary supplement" or "supplement" preceded by the name of the dietary ingredient (such as "magnesium supplement") or the type of ingredient (such as "antioxidant supplement" or "herbal supplement").

STRUCTURE-FUNCTION CLAIM   A statement clarifying the beneficial effect of the product on a structure or function of the body (or its effect on general

---

Understanding Supplement Facts

SERVING SIZE An amount suggested by the manufacturer, expressed in the form (such as capsules or tablets) the supplement is packaged in. The values in the panel are keyed to the serving size.

MEASUREMENTS Standard units of measurement. The most common measurements are milligram, or mg (one-thousandth of a gram), and microgram, or mcg (one-millionth of a gram). Vitamins A and E are measured in international units (IU), which is a measure of the activity of fat-soluble vitamins. (Vitamin D and beta-carotene are also usually measured in IU.)

Supplement Facts
Serving Size 1 tablet

Amount per tablet		% Daily Value
Vitamin A	10,000 IU	200%
Vitamin C	500 mg	834%
Vitamin E	400 IU	1334%
Selenium	200 mcg	285%
Goldenseal powdered (root)	250 mg	*

*Daily Value not established

PERCENT DAILY VALUE (DV) Percentage of FDA-recommended Reference Daily Intake (RDI) supplied by specific nutrients (turn to page 21 for more information). An asterisk (*) under the heading "% Daily Value" indicates that a daily value has not been established for that ingredient.

well-being). "A tonic for your digestive system" and "an aid to joint mobility" are examples of structure-function claims. Such a claim also must be accompanied on the product label by a disclaimer indicating that the statement has not been evaluated by the Food and Drug Administration, and that the product is not intended to diagnose, treat, cure, or prevent any disease.

DISEASE CLAIM   A statement showing a link between a supplement and a disease or health-related condition. Only a few supplements are eligible to carry these claims, which must be authorized by the FDA or based on evidence from certain scientific bodies showing a supplement/health link. An example is the claim that calcium is linked to a lower risk of osteoporosis, assuming the supplement contains sufficient amounts of calcium.

"HIGH POTENCY"   A term that can be used only if a single-nutrient supplement contains 100% or more of the Daily Value, or DV. In multi-ingredient products, two-thirds of the nutrients for which the DV is known must supply 100% of the DV—and these nutrients must be identified.

DIRECTIONS   Instructions on the amount of the supplement the manufacturer suggests as the appropriate dosage, and when and how best to take it (with meals or a glass of water, for example).

INGREDIENTS   A list of everything included in the supplement, arranged in decreasing order by weight. Ingredients include binders, fillers, coatings, preservatives, coloring agents, and other inert substances. If an ingredient is cited in the "Supplement Facts" panel (such as ascorbic acid for vitamin C), it does not have to be included in the ingredients list.

CHILD WARNING   A precautionary statement that all supplements should be kept in a place where children can't reach them. (Youngsters have been known to ingest toxic amounts of some supplements accidentally.) Products containing iron must carry a specific warning about the dangers of accidental iron overdose in children.

STORAGE ADVICE   Advice on how best to store the product. Most dietary supplements should be kept in a cool, dry place, which means they shouldn't be stored in either the bathroom or the refrigerator, where moisture can damage them. (There are, however, some products that should be refrigerated after opening; if this is the case, the label will tell you so.)

The USP designation

TO HELP CONSUMERS, the United States Pharmacopeia (USP), an independent body of experts that sets standards of purity and potency for conventional drugs, has established comparable standards for vitamins, minerals, and some herbs. A USP designation on a supplement label indicates that the product, according to the manufacturer, meets USP standards for purity, strength, and disintegration (how efficiently the supplement dissolves in the digestive tract).

Compliance with USP standards is left up to manufacturers, and the absence of "USP" on a label doesn't mean that a brand has failed to meet these standards (the manufacturer may choose not to do the test, and for some supplements, there are no standards). Keep in mind, too, that there is as yet no independent verification that a supplement with the "USP" mark does in fact meet those standards. But on a product from a nationally known manufacturer, the presence of "USP" means that it is very likely the standards have been met.

NAME AND PLACE OF BUSINESS   The name and address of the manufacturer, packer, or distributor. This is the address you can write to for more product information. There may also be a telephone number on the label that you can call.

EXPIRATION DATE   A date when the supplement may start to lose its full potency. An expiration date (which may appear on the bottom of the bottle) is not required by law; in effect, it is a pledge from the manufacturer that the product will remain "fresh" up to that point. However, companies are under no legal obligation to base this promise on laboratory testing, as is the case with conventional drugs. Supplements that don't carry an expiration date may retain their full potency for months after you buy them. But because you don't know how long the product has been on the store shelf, you are generally better off buying a product that has an expiration date. And it's always best to finish the product before the expiration date.

using supplements
safely and effectively

Although supplement manufacturers are prohibited from making direct claims about curing or treating diseases, the Food and Drug Administration (FDA) has otherwise given them great leeway, and the safety or effectiveness of a supplement doesn't have to be demonstrated.

Responsible manufacturers are careful to print instructions about proper use on their labels, but you may encounter many brands that do not supply them. The entries in this book provide detailed information about the benefits, uses, side effects, and forms of supplements, as well as the doses that are considered safe and effective. In the back of the book, you will find a section listing interactions between supplements and commonly prescribed medications. Here are some general guidelines to keep in mind.

The proper balance

All nutrients influence one another, and researchers have discovered a number of links that affect how well the body absorbs or utilizes them. For example, fat-soluble vitamins (A, D, E, and K) require some dietary fat to facilitate absorption, so it's important to take these vitamins with food. Iron taken with meals is best absorbed with small amounts of meat and foods containing vitamin C. Calcium absorption is improved by taking supplements with meals, and the effect of calcium on building healthy bones is enhanced when it is taken with magnesium. Other nutrients, when taken in combination, likewise enhance one another's individual benefits. For example, biotin and other B vitamins, taken with a mixed amino acid complex and vitamin C, all work to help the body build proteins needed for strong nails.

The proper amounts

Dietary supplements are generally safe when consumed in the appropriate dosages. But it's important to remember that more isn't necessarily better—and sometimes it can be worse. For example, the mineral selenium is recommended for many disorders, from cataracts to cancer prevention. But taking doses even slightly higher than those recommended can cause loss of hair and other toxic reactions. When using supplements, it's a good idea to avoid high doses, particularly extremely high ones ("megadoses").

VITAMINS AND MINERALS

Most vitamins can be taken in significantly higher doses than their RDAs without producing adverse reactions. However, some fat-soluble vitamins, which are stored in the body rather than excreted, may be toxic at high doses. In particular, overloading on vitamin A or D is dangerous. Although very high doses of some other vitamins—such as vitamin C—are not toxic, certain individuals may experience side effects. Reducing the dosage can usually remedy the situation.

Some minerals, taken in large doses or over time, can block the absorption of other minerals. Zinc, for instance, can hamper copper absorption. Also, large amounts of certain minerals are linked to disease— several studies show that too much iron in men, for example, increases their risk of heart disease. For these reasons, even doctors who believe the RDAs for many vitamins are too low think the levels for minerals are generally adequate for optimal health.

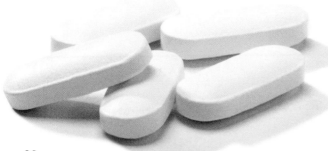

Calcium and magnesium, here blended in one pill, should be taken together to maximize calcium's bone-building benefit.

According to reviews by experts in pharmacology and toxicology, serious side effects or toxic reactions associated with herbal medicines are rare. Still, some once-popular medicinal herbs, such as foxglove and chaparral, are now recognized as toxic. Occasionally, some people exhibit serious allergic reactions to an herb, which may include hives or difficulty breathing.

Furthermore, because no uniform quality control for herbal preparations exists, the chemical composition of an herbal remedy can vary greatly from batch to batch. And it may contain potentially toxic contaminants and other ingredients that influence side effects or effectiveness. Products that contain standardized extracts may be more reliable than those that don't in terms of getting a proper dose of a particular supplement. But whenever you buy a supplement—whether it is a standardized extract or a whole herb in a pill, tincture, or other form—you are still dependent on the manufacturer's integrity.

In addition, using some herbs for medicinal purposes can be risky for people with certain health conditions or for those on particular medications. Garlic, for example, may intensify the effects of anticoagulant drugs, while licorice—which aids digestive problems and enhances the immune system—can raise blood pressure. Some herbs may have no immediate adverse effects but may cause side effects or prove harmful when taken over the long term. When using supplements, always follow dosage recommendations closely. In addition, notify your doctor at once if your condition worsens or if any serious adverse reactions develop.

The issue of quality control

How do you know what a product actually contains? The Food and Drug Administration (FDA) requires that manufacturers list all of the active ingredients on each label. But monitoring of the contents of supplements is sporadic, so no one is sure about the degree of compliance.

Established manufacturers of supplements presumably have a reputation to protect, and so take measures to ensure that their products contain what is stated on the labels. But herbal supplements can be problematic. A study published in *The Lancet*, a leading British medical journal, reported that some ginseng supplements contained no active ingredient; other tests found that the amount of active ginsenosides in different brands varied widely. And in a survey sponsored by the Good Housekeeping Institute, the levels of an active ingredient in St. John's wort were inconsistent among brands.

One step you can take as an educated consumer is to call the manufacturer of a particular supplement to find out how long the company has been in business and how the supplement's potency is assured. You can also ask your doctor or other health professionals who make use of supplements for their recommendations of reliable products.

Safety guidelines

BECAUSE SUPPLEMENTS, especially herbs, can have potent primary effects and side effects, keep these points in mind when using them:

- **Shop carefully.** Because there is no independent guarantee of purity or potency, it's your responsibility to select brands with a reputation for quality.

- **Take the recommended dosages.** As with conventional drugs, overdosing with a supplement can have serious consequences. With herbs and nutritional supplements, start with the lowest dose when a dosage range is given.

- **Monitor your reactions.** At the first sign of an adverse reaction, discontinue using the supplement. Also stop if the herb doesn't seem to be working for you (though give it time—some herbs may take a month or more to have a noticeable effect).

- **Take a break.** Doctors using conventional medications typically recommend "drug holidays" for certain non-life-threatening conditions such as a persistent headache, eczema, or mild depression. The same wisdom applies to supplements: It's best to take them for specified periods (which are suggested in the "Ailments" entries), then stop temporarily to see if the condition has improved. If the problem returns, you may need to take the supplement long term as a "maintenance" medication.

- **Avoid risks.** If you have symptoms that indicate a serious problem, don't self-treat it with supplements: See a doctor or other trained health professional. Very young or elderly people, and pregnant or lactating women, should also consult a doctor before using supplements. And always ask your doctor or pharmacist about possible interactions with any drugs you are taking.

practitioners
and organizations

A number of different health practitioners are knowledgeable about vitamin, mineral, and herbal supplements and may be able to give you general information, as well as advice based on an assessment of your specific needs.

One of the strengths of conventional medicine is the teaching of diagnostic skills, so you should consider seeing a physician for a proper diagnosis of an ailment, particularly if you have symptoms with which you are not familiar. Naturopathic doctors, herbalists, and some chiropractors, all of whom are practitioners of alternative medicine, are generally more knowledgeable about the use of herbs and nutritional supplements than most conventional doctors or other practitioners, but they have less training in making diagnoses. Therefore, you are best served when pursuing alternative medical options for a specific disorder if you have consulted a conventionally trained doctor beforehand.

To find an alternative practitioner, initially talk to your regular doctor. However, many conventional doctors are reluctant to make referrals to alternative practitioners, so you may have to turn elsewhere for suggestions. Speak with family and friends; they may have suggestions based on their personal experiences. Also, your health insurer may have a list of practitioners for referral. Some of the organizations listed on the opposite page can also provide referrals.

Inquire about certification and licensing requirements, which vary from state to state; this information can help protect a consumer. When you consult an alternative practitioner, ask about his or her background and experience working with nutritional and herbal remedies. Be wary of anyone who promises cures that seem too quick or easy, or who wants to put you on a regimen that will cost a lot of money.

COMPLEMENTARY PHYSICIAN (M.D.)

A doctor with an M.D. degree has completed four years of medical school, and has received additional training in a hospital as an intern and a resident. An M.D. must also pass demanding National Board Examinations to obtain a state medical license.

A growing number of doctors with backgrounds in conventional medicine are utilizing nutritional and herbal supplements in their work. Often these complementary physicians are family practitioners or internists specializing in common medical problems. If you can't locate a complementary physician in your area, two organizations may prove helpful: the American Holistic Medical Association and the American College for Advancement in Medicine (addresses are listed on the opposite page). Be aware, though, that many complementary physicians are not members of these organizations.

NATUROPATHIC DOCTOR (N.D.)

Physicians who practice naturopathic medicine believe in the healing power of nature—including the human body's innate resources—for treating health problems. A naturopathic physician and patient work together to help the body promote its own well-being. To achieve this, the practitioner assesses a patient's lifestyle and provides recommendations on diet, exercise, and other habits. Prevention of illness is the primary goal of naturopathic doctors, who may use nutritional and herbal supplements as preventive "tonics." These physicians also treat health problems using a range of therapies that include acupuncture and massage as well as herbal remedies.

Most N.D.s now receive a degree from a school of naturopathy, where students take four years of graduate training, which involves extensive courses in nutrition and herbal medicine. However, only a handful of states license naturopathic doctors. Some other states allow them to practice under certain restrictions. It's a good idea to see a naturopathic doctor who has graduated from an accredited school (listed opposite).

HERBALIST

Unlike a licensed naturopathic physician, who must undergo rigorous training that meets established criteria, anyone can hang out a sign saying "herbalist." You can obtain a referral to an herbalist who has completed programs at an herbal school through the American Herbalists Guild. Another association, the American Botanical Council, answers questions about herbs and conducts research. A qualified professional herbalist will take a medical history and assess your lifestyle and any other factors affecting your health—including any allergies you have and any medications you are taking—before recommending a remedy for a specific complaint.

NUTRITIONIST   A good nutritionist will review your medical history and then consult with you about your eating and exercise habits, as well as your general lifestyle, in order to suggest adjustments. Nutritionists should also be familiar with supplements, but opinions often vary among them as to the importance of supplementation. As with herbalists, there are no licensing requirements for nutritionists. Many nutritionists are registered dietitians (R.D.s), which means they are certified by the American Dietetic Association; they have at least a bachelor's degree in nutrition or a related science; and they have completed an internship and passed a comprehensive examination.

There are also competent nutritionists who aren't R.D.s. Ask for a referral from your doctor, local hospital, the department of nutrition at the nearest university, or the American Dietetic Association.

PHARMACIST   For many people, a licensed pharmacist is the most accessible health professional. A pharmacist's training—four years of postgraduate education at an accredited school of pharmacy that offers a Doctor of Pharmacy (a Pharm. D. degree)—is in the use of conventional medications, but pharmaceutical journals and professional associations are increasingly addressing the use of supplements. As a result, your pharmacist may be able to answer many of your questions about herbal and nutritional therapies and offer advice about the potential benefits, limitations, and side effects of specific supplements you may be thinking of taking. A good pharmacist will ascertain your state of health before suggesting any supplement, and may decide to refer you to a physician for additional evaluation. (Pharmacists must be registered with a state pharmaceutical board; a certificate should be displayed in the drugstore where they work.)

For more information

You can contact the following organizations for information about nutritional and herbal therapies. Some can also help you find a practitioner.

American Association of Naturopathic Physicians
601 Valley Street, Suite 105
Seattle, WA 98109
(206) 298-0126 (office)
(206) 298-0125 (referral line)
http://www.naturopathic.org

American Botanical Council
P.O. Box 144345
Austin, TX 78714
(512) 926-4900
http://www.herbalgram.org

American College for Advancement in Medicine
23121 Verdugo Drive, Suite 204
Laguna Hills, CA 92653
(949) 583-7666
Internet: http://www.acam.org

American Dietetic Association
216 West Jackson Boulevard
Chicago, IL 60606
(312) 899-0040
http://www.eatright.org

American Herbalists Guild
P.O. Box 70
Roosevelt, UT 84066
(435) 722-8434
http://www.healthy.net/herbalists

American Holistic Medical Association
6728 Old McLean Village Drive
McLean, VA 22101-3906
(703) 556-9728
http://www.ahmaholistic.com

Ask Dr. Weil's Local Practitioners Database
http://cgi.pathfinder.com/drweil/practitioner/search/

★ **Bastyr University**
14500 Juanita Drive, NE
Bothell, WA 98011
(425) 823-1300
http://www.bastyr.edu

★ **National College of Naturopathic Medicine**
11231 SE Market Street
Portland, OR 97216
(503) 255-4860
http://www.ncnm.edu

The government's Office of Alternative Medicine (OAM)—a division of the National Institutes of Health (NIH)—sponsors research and evaluation of unconventional medical practices and disseminates this information to the public. For fact sheets, information packages, and publications, contact:

OAM Clearinghouse
P.O. Box 8218
Silver Spring, MD 20907-8218
(888) 644-6226
Fax: (301) 495-4957
http://altmed.od.nih.gov

★ *Accredited schools of naturopathic medicine. (Additional schools are awaiting accreditation.)*

a basic formula
for optimal health

One of the principal benefits that vitamins, minerals, and other nutrients provide is to safeguard health on a long-term basis—by helping to protect the human body against chronic, debilitating diseases that pose the most serious threat to longevity. But what is the best way to obtain this key preventive benefit? The advisory board for this book, headed by Dr. David Edelberg, suggests that everyone will profit by taking a daily high-potency supplement that contains approximately the amounts of the nutrients listed in the chart opposite.

This basic supplement formula contains vitamins and minerals in higher potencies than those found in typical "one-a-day" type formulas, which generally supply no more than the Recommended Dietary Allowance, or RDA, for each nutrient. (Levels that meet the highest RDA values are indicated on supplement labels by "100%" under the heading "% Daily Value" or "% U.S. RDA." Those with an asterisk * have no RDA.) Think of RDA levels as the nutritional counterpart of accommodations in a budget motel: They are sufficient to prevent vitamin-deficiency diseases (they provide basic shelter), but won't necessarily help against other types of disease (they don't offer cable TV).

Because a high-potency combination, by contrast, contains relatively high levels of nutrients—in particular the antioxidant nutrients—it's thought to combat tissue damage at the cellular level. Studies indicate that such levels are associated with preventing cancer, heart disease, osteoporosis, and other chronic illnesses that can hamper, and shorten, your life.

Choosing a brand

If you're accustomed to taking a "one-a-day" type of supplement, you may be surprised to learn that a high-potency formula (with vitamins and minerals at higher levels) may require taking more than one pill a day. In fact, with some brands, you'll need to consume anywhere from two to six tablets or capsules daily. *Be sure to read the ingredients and serving size on any label carefully* to calculate how many tablets are necessary to obtain the nutrient levels that are right for you.

When you are evaluating different brands, *don't worry if you can't find a supplement that exactly matches the amounts shown in the chart,* which are indicated in ranges. Unlike drug dosages, where

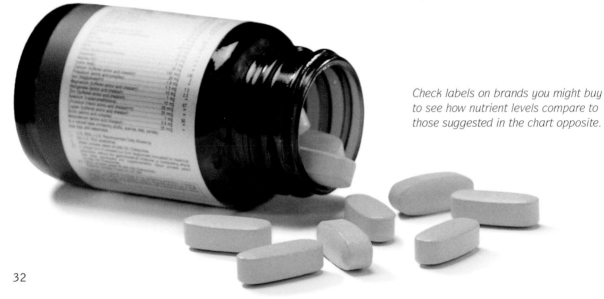

Check labels on brands you might buy to see how nutrient levels compare to those suggested in the chart opposite.

THIS CHART SHOWS the nutrients that a daily multivitamin and mineral should contain, the RDA for each nutrient, and the optimal levels for obtaining preventive benefits, which depend on your diet. The more nutrients you get from foods, the fewer you need from a supplement (see "How Much to Take" below to help decide which column applies to you). Because supplements vary greatly, just try to stay within the flexible ranges given here for each nutrient.

VITAMINS	RDA	A (EXCELLENT DIET)	B (SOUND DIET)	C (POOR DIET)
B$_1$ (Thiamin)	1.2 mg	1.5-30 mg	30-60 mg	60-100 mg
B$_2$ (Riboflavin)	1.3 mg	1.7-30 mg	30-60 mg	60-100 mg
B$_3$ (Niacin)	16 mg	20-30 mg	30-50 mg	50-100 mg
B$_5$ (Pantothenic acid)	*	10-60 mg	60-100 mg	100-200 mg
B$_6$	1.7 mg	2-25 mg	25-60 mg	60-100 mg
B$_{12}$	2.4 mcg	6-100 mcg	100-400 mcg	400-800 mcg
Beta-carotene	*	5,000-10,000 IU	10,000-15,000 IU	15,000-25,000 IU
Biotin	*	30-100 mcg	100-400 mcg	400-600 mcg
Folic acid	400 mcg	400 mcg	400-600 mcg	600-800 mcg
Vitamin A	5,000 IU	2,500 IU	2,500 IU	2,500 IU
Vitamin C	60 mg	60-300 mg	300-600 mg	600-900 mg
Vitamin D	400 IU	400 IU	400 IU	400 IU
Vitamin E	15 IU	30-200 IU	200-300 IU	300-400 IU

MINERALS				
Boron	*	100 mcg-1 mg	1-2 mg	2-4 mg
Calcium	1,200 mg	50-150 mg	150-200 mg	200-300 mg
Chromium	*	50-65 mcg	65-100 mcg	100-200 mcg
Copper	*	1 mg	1-1.5 mg	1.5-2 mg
Iron **	10 mg	5-10 mg	10-18 mg	18 mg
Magnesium	350 mg	100 mg	100-200 mg	200-300 mg
Manganese	5 mg	3-5 mg	5-10 mg	10-20 mg
Molybdenum	*	25-65 mcg	65-100 mcg	100-200 mcg
Potassium	*	30-80 mg	80-100 mg	100 mg
Selenium	70 mcg	20-100 mcg	100-200 mcg	200 mcg
Vanadium	*	10-50 mcg	50-100 mcg	100 mcg
Zinc	15 mg	15 mg	15-20 mg	20-30 mg

* No RDA is established for these nutrients.

** Iron recommendations apply only to younger women; men and postmenopausal women should not choose a supplement containing iron.

exactness can be crucial, vitamin and mineral intakes need not be precise, because nutrients work far more gradually than drugs do. Also, these supplemental nutrients are interacting with, and building upon, the nutrients you obtain from food. Simply try to choose a supplement with dosages close to those that the chart recommends.

One other point: Some high-potency vitamin and mineral formulas have herbs and other nutrients added as general preventive "tonics." If you choose this type of supplement, check the entries on those ingredients (beginning on page 228) to be sure that the levels don't exceed recommended ranges.

How much to take

Use the chart above with these guidelines in mind:

■ If your diet is nutritionally excellent, take the amounts recommended in column A. These levels are sufficient if you regularly eat foods low in fat, get five to six generous servings of fruit and vegetables every day, and have meat, chicken, or fish several times a week in small portions.

■ If your diet is basically sound, take the amounts recommended in column B. They are intended for someone who usually eats three meals a day, with at least one or two servings of fruits and vegetables, and who doesn't gorge on fatty foods—but who skips a lunch or breakfast in an average week and may grab one or two "fast food" meals.

■ If your diet is poor, take the amounts recommended in column C. These levels are intended for someone who routinely skips meals, who skimps on fruits, vegetables, and grains (the foods that are considered the richest sources of vitamins and minerals), and who normally eats a slice of pizza or a deli sandwich and a diet cola for lunch.

Special considerations

Another reason to increase your supplement intake may be your personal health history. For example, taking folic acid, vitamin B_6, and vitamin B_{12} may help you prevent heart disease (see the entry "Heart Disease Prevention" on page 134).

Similarly, if you have a family history of high blood pressure, cancer, or another chronic ailment, additional supplements are recommended for preventive purposes (see the ailment entries for specifics).

And while you may not be suffering from—or at risk for—a specific disorder, you may still have nutrient needs that can benefit from increased supplementation. If you fit into one of the categories listed on this and the opposite page, you should consider taking the suggested nutrient(s). The basic daily multivitamin and mineral formula you choose may supply part or even all of this additional supplementation. But in most cases, you will probably have to purchase individual supplements to take in addition to your basic daily formula.

If you are a woman

Beginning in their mid-20s, humans gradually lose bone mass—and in women, this process accelerates after menopause. If bone loss advances sufficiently, osteoporosis develops. To slow the loss of bone, adult women of all ages should include extra calcium in their daily supplement program.

RECOMMENDATION Total daily calcium intake, from both diet and supplements, should total at least 1,200 mg and can safely be as high as 2,500 mg. (For additional recommendations on how to prevent osteoporosis, see page 182.)

If you are a man over age 50

One condition common in older men is BPH, or benign prostatic hyperplasia, an enlargement of the prostate (a walnut-size gland just below the bladder that produces seminal fluid). If this occurs, it can interfere with urination.

RECOMMENDATION Consider adding saw palmetto—160 mg twice a day—for prostate health. This herb helps relieve inflammation and affects prostate-related hormone levels (see page 350).

If you are a vegetarian

Strict vegetarians—those who avoid all animal foods, including dairy and egg products—can eat a balanced diet if they consume a variety of fruits, vegetables, and grains. But one nutrient not supplied by these foods is vitamin B_{12}, found in eggs, meats, poultry, fish, and dairy products. Over time, therefore, strict vegetarians can develop B_{12}-deficiency anemia (see page 376).

RECOMMENDATION Be sure your basic daily formula supplement includes 100 mcg of vitamin B_{12}.

If you exercise frequently

Regular exercise or athletic activity, especially if it is prolonged or intense, breaks down muscle fiber. This wear and tear, which can be accompanied by a loss of flexibility, gets worse as a person ages.

RECOMMENDATION Consider adding creatine monohydrate—1 teaspoon (5 grams) a day—to help in muscle repair. Additional magnesium—200 mg daily—is also helpful, because this mineral plays a key role in muscle contractions.

Other supplements that contribute to muscle endurance and energy are the amino acid-like substance carnitine (500 mg twice a day) and the nutritional supplement coenzyme Q_{10} (50 mg daily).

If you're over age 50 and feeling a slow decline in energy levels despite exercising regularly, you can also add the herb Siberian ginseng (100 mg a day) or talk to your doctor about the hormone DHEA (25 mg daily). You'll need to have your blood DHEA levels measured before taking the supplement.

If you are on a weight-loss diet

Dieting to lose weight can trigger hunger pangs and cause blood sugar levels to vacillate.

RECOMMENDATION Add chromium (200 mcg twice a day) to your basic formula; it can assist the body in using fat and prevent swings in blood sugar. The supplement 5-HTP (100 mg three times a day) can help stem urges to overeat (see page 184).

If you smoke

Nutritional supplements will not appreciably reduce your risk of developing heart disease, lung disease, or cancer. But you may be able to combat some of the effects of smoking with extra antioxidants.

RECOMMENDATION Try taking grape seed extract (100 mg twice a day) or green tea extract (250 mg twice a day). See pages 204-205 for advice on how to quit smoking.

If you consume alcohol

Drinking alcohol in moderation—no more than two drinks a day for men, one for women—can actually be good for you, because it helps lower the risk of heart disease. But drinking more heavily—three or more drinks a day for men, two or more for women—can deplete certain nutrients. Excess alcohol is also associated with an increased risk of liver disease, as well as other health problems.

RECOMMENDATION Help protect your liver with milk thistle (150 mg twice a day). Extra vitamin C (1,000 mg a day) and extra B vitamins (a single B-50 complex capsule, plus an extra 100 mg of thiamin) can also be beneficial.

For extra antioxidant protection, consider taking additional supplements, such as the vitamin C tablets shown here.

Claim for antioxidants

ANTIOXIDANTS ARE AN important component of a daily formula, so it is useful to know what claims can be made for them on a supplement bottle. As part of a new labeling law that manufacturers must adhere to by March 1999, the Food and Drug Administration (FDA) has declared that a product claiming to be a "good source of antioxidants" must have at least 10% of the daily value (DV) of one or more established antioxidants; for a claim of "high in antioxidants" there must be at least 20% of the DV.

However, these percentages apply just to the vitamins C, E, and beta-carotene—the only antioxidant nutrients for which a recommended daily value exists. Other recognized antioxidants, such as flavonoids and selenium, have no recommended daily amounts, so manufacturers won't be able to make content claims for them. But they are allowed to identify these nutrients as antioxidants.

Of course, to determine the antioxidant content, you should check the actual amounts listed on the label, and not simply depend on the promotional claims made by the manufacturer.

how to use this book

What exactly is dong quai? How does vitamin E help protect your heart? Which herbal remedies are most effective for combating allergies? How do you obtain selenium's antioxidant benefits?

These or similar questions may have occurred to you if you take—or have considered using—nutritional or herbal supplements. Whether you want to know how a particular supplement works, what dose is safe and effective, or if a certain supplement can cause any side effects, you can find the latest information in *The Healing Power of Vitamins, Minerals, and Herbs.* In addition, the book offers practical advice that will help take the confusion out of buying supplements, whether you shop in a health-food store, drugstore, catalog, or even over the Internet.

The book is divided into two major parts. Part I, **Ailments,** starts on page 38 and is an A-to-Z compendium of 94 common health concerns that you can help alleviate or possibly prevent with the aid of supplements. Each entry reviews the symptoms, provides a clear explanation of the condition, and highlights a chart of recommended supplements and dosages. The entry also explains how the supplements work within your body to improve the condition, and presents recent research findings on treating the problem, as well as additional steps you can take toward better health.

Part II, **Supplements,** contains detailed information on 81 vitamins, minerals, herbs, and other types of nutritional supplements: how they work, the latest scientific findings on their benefits, and safe and effective dosage levels. These entries include a wealth of tips and precautions for choosing and using supplements—ranging from advice on increasing vitamin and mineral absorption to shopping hints that will save you money. As explained on page 228, each entry is color-coded to indicate at a glance the type of supplement being covered.

The introduction on the preceding pages provides an overview of current knowledge about supplements, along with information on the various forms of supplements available in stores and mail-order catalogs (pages 15-16), what to look for when buying supplements (pages 22-27), and advice on safely using supplements safely (pages 28-29). There is also a basic daily vitamin and mineral formula that the board of consultants for this book recommends to protect your body more effectively against disease (page 33).

In the back of the book there is a section listing potential interactions between supplements and commonly used conventional medications. If you are taking a medication, check to see if it is in this section. You will also find a glossary with definitions of key terms and an appendix that details supplements recommended for specific ailments that don't have their own entries in the "Supplements" section.

Throughout the book, photographs illustrate different supplement forms, as well as natural sources of vitamins, minerals, and herbs—such as the flaxseeds shown here, which can be pressed into oil. The oil is also sold in capsule form.

PART I: AILMENTS

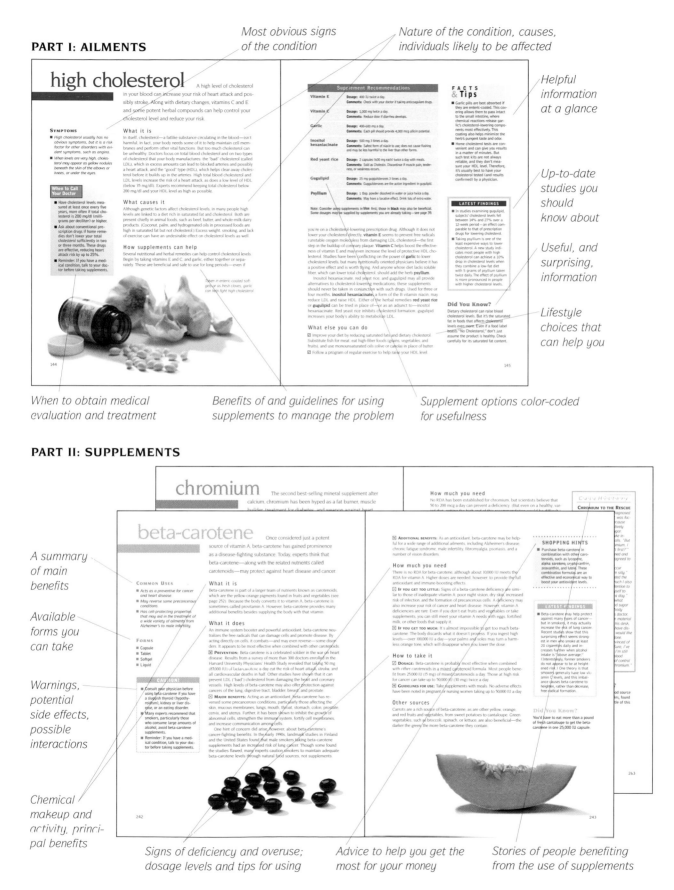

Most obvious signs of the condition

Nature of the condition, causes, individuals likely to be affected

Helpful information at a glance

Up-to-date studies you should know about

Useful, and surprising, information

Lifestyle choices that can help you

When to obtain medical evaluation and treatment

Benefits of and guidelines for using supplements to manage the problem

Supplement options color-coded for usefulness

PART II: SUPPLEMENTS

A summary of main benefits

Available forms you can take

Warnings, potential side effects, possible interactions

Chemical makeup and activity, principal benefits

Signs of deficiency and overuse; dosage levels and tips for using

Advice to help you get the most for your money

Stories of people benefiting from the use of supplements

PART I

ailments

THIS SECTION COVERS more than 90 disorders, listed in alphabetical order, from acne to yeast infections. Each entry features a chart with recommendations for vitamins, minerals, herbs, and other nutritional supplements. These are the remedies for the ailment that the consultants for this book have found to be most helpful and most readily available. Supplements shown in blue in the chart are generally the most effective for a broad range of people, so consider starting with one or more of them. Supplements in black may also be beneficial or may work better for you. In addition, there may be other therapies or supplements that are useful as well.

It's strongly recommended that before taking any supplement, you turn to Part II, the "Supplements" section of this book, and read about it in detail. Please be sure to observe any warnings and precautions prior to using a supplement—and always consult a doctor or other health-care professional if your illness hasn't been previously diagnosed or if your condition worsens.

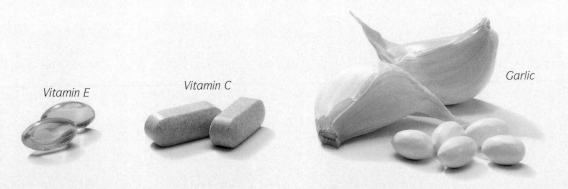

Vitamin E

Vitamin C

Garlic

About the recommendations

SPECIFIC DOSAGE SUGGESTIONS are listed in each of the profiles that follow. These numbers are the total daily amount of a particular nutrient or herb you'll need to treat that disorder. In practical terms, this means you may have to adjust the numbers to factor in the amount of these same supplements you may already be getting in your daily multivitamin or in individual supplements you're using for other health reasons.

For example, we suggest taking 400 IU of vitamin E a day for cancer prevention. If your daily multivitamin supplies 400 IU, you won't need to take any additional vitamin E to meet the recommendation. If you also suffer from angina (which calls for 800 IU of vitamin E) you will have to take only 400 IU more to meet that requirement as well.

The dosages here are meant to be informative, but each person is different. If you have a serious medical condition, check with your doctor about your own case and the appropriate dose for you. Always read the label and never exceed the recommended dosage for a supplement, even though you may be treating several ailments.

A final word: Though we've made every effort to include widely available dosages, the strengths of supplement products vary greatly. Many qualified people—health professionals, pharmacists, health-store staff—can help you determine an equivalent dose.

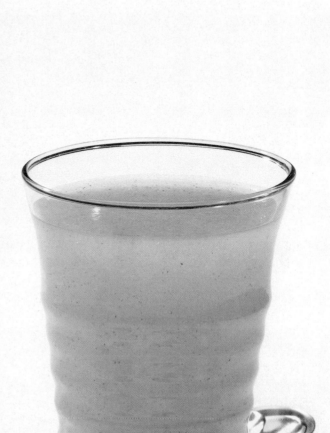

Natural remedies for treating high cholesterol—one of the more than 90 ailments covered here—include vitamins, herbs, and nutritional supplements.

Psyllium

Red yeast rice

Inositol hexaniacinate

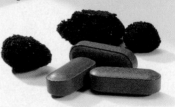
Gugulipid

acne

Although most people associate acne with the trying teen years, it can actually erupt at any age. Indeed, up to 8% of those who had clear skin in their youth develop acne as adults. Fortunately, there are a variety of ways to control outbreaks—no matter how old you are when they occur.

SYMPTOMS

- *Hard red bumps or pus-filled lesions on the skin.*
- *Red, inflamed skin with fluid-filled lumps or cysts.*

When to Call Your Doctor

- If acne doesn't respond to self-care within three months.
- If severe acne develops: fluid-filled lumps, red or purple inflammation, cysts, or hard nodules under the skin.
- If skin is continually red and flushed, even if no pimples actually appear.
- Reminder: If you have a medical condition, talk to your doctor before taking supplements.

What it is

Pimples and other skin eruptions are the hallmark of acne, a sometimes chronic condition of the face, back, chest, neck, shoulders, and other areas of the body. The most common form (acne vulgaris) encompasses blackheads, whiteheads, and raised red blemishes with semisolid centers. In severe cases (cystic acne), clusters of painful, fluid-filled cysts or firm, painless lumps appear beneath the skin's surface; both can lead to unsightly permanent pitting and scarring. For teenagers especially, acne can be an embarrassing and emotionally difficult condition.

What causes it

Acne occurs when the sebaceous glands at the base of the hair follicles of the skin secrete too much sebum. This thick, oily substance is normally released from the pores to keep the skin lubricated and healthy. If the sebum backs up, it can form hard plugs that block the pores and cause pimples. Should one of these oil plugs rupture beneath the skin's surface, a localized bacterial infection can develop.

Hormonal imbalances can lead to an overproduction of sebum—a common problem during adolescence, especially in boys. In women, menstrual periods or pregnancy can also create acne-producing hormonal disturbances. Other acne triggers include emotional stress, the friction or rubbing of clothing against the skin, and certain medications, particularly steroids, contraceptives, or drugs that affect hormone levels. Heredity may play a role as well.

Contrary to popular belief, acne probably isn't caused by eating chocolate, shellfish, nuts, or fatty snacks or by drinking colas. However, some doctors—and patients—contend that acne can be brought on or aggravated by certain foods or food allergies.

Many people find liquid drops a convenient way to get acne-fighting doses of vitamin A.

Supplement Recommendations

Vitamin A	**Dosage:** 25,000 IU a day; reduce dose to 10,000 IU a day when healing is noticed or after 1 month. Use pills or drops. **Comments:** Women who are pregnant or considering pregnancy should not exceed 5,000 IU a day.
Vitamin B$_6$	**Dosage:** 50 mg each morning. **Comments:** Long-term doses of more than 200 mg a day for chronic acne can cause nerve damage.
Vitamin C	**Dosage:** 1,000 mg twice a day. **Comments:** Reduce dose if diarrhea develops.
Zinc/Copper	**Dosage:** 30 mg zinc and 2 mg copper a day. **Comments:** Add copper only when using zinc longer than 1 month.
Flaxseed oil	**Dosage:** 1 tbsp. (14 grams) a day. **Comments:** Can be mixed with food; take in the morning.
Evening primrose oil	**Dosage:** 1,000 mg 3 times a day. **Comments:** Can substitute 1,000 mg borage oil once a day.

Some dosages may be supplied by supplements you are already taking—see page 39.

How supplements can help

Most people will benefit from trying all of the supplements that are recommended in the chart; they can be safely combined. It often takes three to four weeks, or longer, to notice results. All can be used long term, as well as with conventional acne medications.

Vitamin A is important because it plays a role in controlling overproduction of sebum, the root cause of acne. Because it aids in balancing levels of acne-related hormones, **vitamin B$_6$** may be useful for acne aggravated by menstrual cycles or menopause. And **vitamin C** promotes immune system health, helping to keep acne-causing bacteria in check. Taken with any or all of these vitamins, **zinc** enhances immune function, reduces inflammation, and promotes healthy hormone levels. Because long-term use of zinc inhibits **copper** absorption, it should be taken with that mineral. It may also help to take zinc along with essential fatty acids: Two excellent sources are **flaxseed oil** and **evening primrose oil.** Essential fatty acids aid in diluting the oily sebum, reducing the likelihood of clogged pores.

What else you can do

☑ Wash daily, using ordinary soap and water.

☑ Eat a balanced diet; avoid foods you feel may act as acne triggers.

☑ Choose cosmetics labeled "noncomedogenic" or "oil-free."

☑ Avoid picking pimples; it increases inflammation and can cause scarring.

aging

Many people live well into their 80s—and beyond. As the body ages, however, various systems slow down, and the risk of disease increases. Even though you can't stop time, you can forestall some of the negative effects of aging with a healthy lifestyle and well-chosen supplements.

SYMPTOMS

- *Slowing of cognitive processes: difficulty accessing memory and learning and remembering new people and events.*
- *Sensory decline: delay in refocusing eyes and impaired ability to hear high-pitched sounds.*
- *Weakened immune system: increased susceptibility to colds, the flu, and other illnesses.*
- *Decline in muscle and bone mass.*
- *Increased risk of developing heart disease and cancer.*

When to Call Your Doctor

- You need a complete physical every year after age 50. See your doctor right away, however, if you are concerned about the risk of age-related diseases.
- Reminder: If you have a medical condition, talk to your doctor before taking supplements.

What it is

Put simply, aging is the process of growing old. Every part of the body is affected: Among other changes, hair turns gray, skin wrinkles, joints and muscles lose flexibility, bones become weak, memory declines, eyesight diminishes, and immunity is impaired.

What causes it

Cells in the body divide a set number of times; then they die and are replaced by new cells. With age, this process slows, and a progressive deterioration of all body systems begins. Though some of this decline is normal and inevitable, many researchers believe that unstable oxygen molecules called free radicals accelerate the process, making us old before our time. Some damage is unavoidable because free radicals are produced during the normal course of cell activity. But you may be able to slow aging by avoiding outside factors that foster free-radical formation—cigarette smoke, pollution, excessive alcohol, and radiation from X rays or the sun—and by enhancing your body's own antioxidant defenses. Manufactured by the cells and obtained through diet, antioxidants are powerful weapons that can disarm free radicals.

How supplements can help

Some supplements should be used daily by everyone concerned about the effects of aging. **Vitamin C** and **vitamin E** are antioxidants that fight free radicals. Vitamin C and **flavonoids** work within the cell's watery interior. Vitamin E protects the fatty membranes that surround cells; in addition, it improves immune function in older people and reduces the risk of some age-related conditions, including heart disease, some forms of cancer, and possibly Alzheimer's. **Green tea extract,** long prized for its longevity-promoting properties, and grape seed extract (100 mg twice a day) are other antioxidants that may be more potent than vitamins C and E.

   Folic acid, a B vitamin, maintains red blood cells and promotes the healthy functioning of nerves. Moreover, it protects the heart by helping

People over age 50 may need to take extra folic acid and vitamin B$_{12}$.

Supplement Recommendations

Vitamin C/ Flavonoids	**Dosage:** 1,000 mg vitamin C and 500 mg flavonoids twice a day. **Comments:** Reduce vitamin C dose if diarrhea develops.
Vitamin E	**Dosage:** 400 IU a day. **Comments:** Check with your doctor if taking anticoagulant drugs.
Green tea extract	**Dosage:** 250 mg twice a day. **Comments:** Standardized to contain at least 50% polyphenols.
Folic acid/ Vitamin B$_{12}$	**Dosage:** 400 mcg folic acid and 1,000 mcg vitamin B$_{12}$ once a day. **Comments:** Take sublingual form for best absorption.
Carnitine	**Dosage:** 500 mg L-carnitine twice a day. **Comments:** If using longer than 1 month, add mixed amino acids.
Evening primrose oil	**Dosage:** 1,000 mg 3 times a day. **Comments:** Can substitute 1,000 mg borage oil once a day.
Glucosamine	**Dosage:** 500 mg glucosamine sulfate twice a day. **Comments:** Increase to 3 times a day if you have osteoarthritis. Take with food to minimize digestive upset.
Ginkgo biloba	**Dosage:** 40 mg 3 times a day. **Comments:** Standardized to have at least 24% flavone glycosides.

Note: Consider using supplements in blue first; those in black may also be beneficial. Some dosages may be supplied by supplements you are already taking—see page 39.

the body process homocysteine, an amino acid-like compound that may raise the risk of heart disease. Folic acid is assisted by **vitamin B$_{12}$,** which fosters healthy brain functioning. Taking this vitamin is important because many older people lose the ability to absorb it from food, and low B$_{12}$ levels can cause nerve damage and dementia. The amino acid-like substance **carnitine** contributes to a healthy heart because it helps transport oxygen to the cells and produces energy. **Evening primrose oil** contains gamma-linolenic acid (GLA), which is essential to a number of body processes. As it ages, the body loses its ability to convert the fats present in foods to GLA.

In addition, certain supplements are vital to specific concerns. **Glucosamine** helps maintain joint cartilage and eases the pain of arthritis. Because it enhances blood flow, the herb **ginkgo biloba** may improve such age-related conditions as dizziness, impotence, and memory loss.

What else you can do

☑ Protect yourself from excessive sun. Ultraviolet rays make skin age faster.

☑ If you smoke, quit. Smoking speeds bone and lung deterioration.

☑ Build and maintain bone and muscle mass with weight-bearing exercise, such as walking and weight training.

☑ Eat a variety of fruits and vegetables—they're rich in antioxidants.

FACTS & Tips

■ Although more research is needed, some experts recommend people over age 50 take a coenzyme Q$_{10}$ supplement to minimize the effects of aging. This substance helps transport energy throughout the body and acts as an antioxidant, but the body's own production declines with age. If you want to add coenzyme Q$_{10}$ to your regimen, take 50 mg twice a day (food enhances its absorption).

LATEST FINDINGS

■ Though there is no magic bullet for longevity, vitamin E may add years to your life. In a recent study from the National Institute on Aging, people who took vitamin E supplements were about half as likely to die of heart disease—the nation's leading killer—as those not using vitamin E.

■ There's more good news about vitamin E. According to a recent study by researchers at Tufts University in Boston, the vitamin strengthened the immune system in people age 65 and older. Those who took 200 IU of vitamin E daily over a four-month period showed significant immune system improvement compared with people who were given other doses of the vitamin or a placebo.

■ A recent Swiss study found a connection between high levels of antioxidants (such as beta-carotene and vitamin C) in the blood and better memory skills in older people.

Did You Know?

By age 75, the average person has 30% fewer cells in the body than he or she once had.

alcoholism

Abstinence is the best course for those who can't control their drinking. Although not a cure, various supplements may help heavy drinkers overcome their craving for alcohol, support them during the taxing withdrawal process, and set them on the road to recovery.

SYMPTOMS

- Constantly seeking opportunities to drink; being unable to cut intake; putting alcohol before family, friends, and work.
- Needing more and more alcohol to achieve the same effect.
- Reacting indignantly to criticism of drinking; adamantly denying the problem.
- Experiencing withdrawal signs (tremors, seizures, and hallucinations) if drinking is stopped.

When to Call Your Doctor

- If you drink before breakfast.
- If binges last 48 hours or more.
- If you have blackouts or falls.
- If you routinely turn to alcohol to relieve stress or pain.
- If your drinking is ruining your personal relationships.
- Reminder: If you have a medical condition, talk to your doctor before taking supplements.

What it is

An intense physical and psychological dependence on alcohol is the hallmark of alcoholism—which many consider a chronic disease, like diabetes or hypertension. Though alcohol appears to protect the heart when taken in moderation, excessive drinking over time can damage the liver, pancreas, intestine, brain, and other organs. It can also cause malnutrition when empty alcohol calories replace a nourishing diet.

What causes it

Drinking has a social component: It makes most people feel talkative and relaxed. Precisely why some people pursue alcohol to excess remains a mystery; psychosocial factors play a role, but there seems to be a strong genetic component as well. Indeed, children of alcoholics are at high risk for the disease, even when raised in nondrinking households.

How supplements can help

The recommended supplements, all of which can be taken together, can play several important roles in weaning problem drinkers from alcohol and helping them through the initial recovery period, which may last for weeks or even months. In addition to supplements, prescription drugs are usually needed to help weather withdrawal symptoms.

Most heavy drinkers are deficient in important nutrients, including B vitamins, vitamin C, and amino acids (protein), because they do not consume a healthy diet and because alcohol has toxic effects; it may be beneficial to continue therapy for several months, or longer, to help restore depleted nutrients. **Vitamin C** can help to strengthen the body

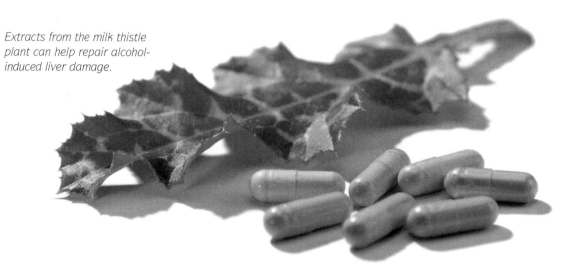

Extracts from the milk thistle plant can help repair alcohol-induced liver damage.

Supplement Recommendations

Vitamin C/ Vitamin E	**Dosage:** 1,000 mg vitamin C 3 times a day; 400 IU vitamin E daily. **Comments:** Vitamin C helps boost the effects of vitamin E.
Vitamin B complex	**Dosage:** 1 pill, plus extra 100 mg thiamin, each morning with food. **Comments:** Look for a B-50 complex with 50 mcg vitamin B_{12} and biotin; 400 mcg folic acid; and 50 mg all other B vitamins.
Amino acids	**Dosage:** Mixed amino acid complex (see label for dosage amount), plus L-glutamine (500 mg twice a day), NAC (500 mg twice a day), and GABA (750 mg twice a day). **Comments:** For best absorption, take on an empty stomach.
Kudzu	**Dosage:** 150 mg 3 times a day. **Comments:** Standardized to contain at least 0.95% daidzen.
Milk thistle	**Dosage:** 250 mg 3 times a day between meals. **Comments:** Standardized to contain at least 70% silymarin.
Chromium	**Dosage:** 200 mcg twice a day. **Comments:** Take with food or a full glass of water.
Evening primrose oil	**Dosage:** 1,000 mg 3 times a day. **Comments:** Can substitute 1,000 mg borage oil once a day.
Kava	**Dosage:** 250 mg 3 times a day. **Comments:** Standardized to contain at least 30% kavalactones.

Note: Consider using supplements in **blue** first; those in **black** may also be beneficial. Some dosages may be supplied by supplements you are already taking—see page 39.

during this difficult period, clearing alcohol from the tissues and reducing mild withdrawal symptoms; it is most useful when taken with **vitamin E.** The **B-complex vitamins,** the **amino acid glutamine,** and extracts from the **kudzu** vine appear to reduce the craving. Be sure to take extra thiamin as well to help ease withdrawal symptoms. The herb **milk thistle,** the **amino acid NAC** (N-acetylcysteine), and phosphatidylcholine (500 mg three times a day) strengthen the liver, helping it rid the body of toxins.

The mineral **chromium** should be taken to prevent fatigue caused by low blood sugar (hypoglycemia), a common problem in alcoholics. **Evening primrose oil** provides the fatty acid GLA (gamma-linolenic acid); this substance stimulates production of a brain chemical called prostaglandin E, which works to prevent withdrawal symptoms such as seizures and depression. It also assists in protecting the liver and nervous system. The herb **kava** and the **amino acid GABA** (gamma-amino-butyric acid) are both natural sedatives that can aid sleep.

What else you can do

☑ Join a support group, such as Alcoholics Anonymous (AA).
☑ Try acupuncture. It may reduce the craving for alcohol.

allergies

For millions of people, the simple act of petting a cat, dusting the end tables, or opening a window invites sniffles and sneezes. But it's not the cat, dust, or pollen that's actually responsible for your symptoms—it's the overreaction of your own immune system.

SYMPTOMS

- *Red, itchy, or puffy eyes, sometimes with "allergic shiners"— dark circles around the eyes.*
- *Sneezing.*
- *Swollen nasal passages.*
- *Runny nose with a clear discharge.*
- *Irritated throat.*
- *Fatigue.*

When to Call Your Doctor

- If you experience wheezing or difficulty breathing—it may be a sign of an asthma attack, requiring immediate treatment.
- If you develop a headache or fever that gets worse when you bend forward, or your nasal discharge turns yellow or green— it may be a sinus infection.
- If allergy symptoms interfere with daily activities and natural supplements don't help.
- Reminder: If you have a medical condition, talk to your doctor before taking supplements.

What it is

"Allergic rhinitis" is the medical term for the nasal symptoms caused by allergies to a variety of airborne particles. The condition can be an occasional inconvenience or a problem so severe that it interferes with almost every aspect of daily life. If you notice symptoms in warm weather, you may have seasonal allergies, commonly called hay fever, triggered by tree or grass pollen in spring and by ragweed in the fall. If you have symptoms year-round—called perennial allergies—the most likely culprits are mites in household dust, mold, or animal dander. You may be allergic to one or more of these irritants. For either type of allergy, the symptoms are the same. People with allergic rhinitis may have a decreased resistance to colds, flu, sinus infections, and other respiratory illnesses.

What causes it

When bacteria, viruses, or other substances enter the body, the immune system sets out to destroy those that can cause illness, but ignores such harmless particles as pollen. In some individuals, however, the immune system can't tell the difference between threatening and benign material. As a result, innocuous particles can trigger the release of a naturally occurring substance called histamine and other inflammatory compounds in the area where the irritant entered the body—the nose, throat, or eyes.

No one knows why the immune system overreacts this way, but some experts think that poor nutrition and pollutants in the air may weaken the system. Allergic rhinitis also runs in some families.

Nettle supplements help reduce nasal inflammation and may ease allergy symptoms.

Supplement Recommendations

Quercetin	**Dosage:** 500 mg twice a day. **Comments:** Use 20 minutes before meals; often sold with vitamin C.
Nettle	**Dosage:** 250 mg 3 times a day on an empty stomach. **Comments:** Standardized to contain at least 1% plant silica.
Vitamin A	**Dosage:** 10,000 IU a day. **Comments:** Women who are pregnant or considering pregnancy should not exceed 5,000 IU a day.
Vitamin C	**Dosage:** 1,000 mg 3 times a day. **Comments:** Reduce dose if diarrhea develops.
Pantothenic acid	**Dosage:** 500 mg 3 times a day. **Comments:** Take with meals.
Ephedra	**Dosage:** 130 mg standardized extract 3 times a day. **Comments:** May cause insomnia. Don't use if you have high blood pressure, heart disease, or anxiety or take an MAO inhibitor.

Note: Consider using supplements in **blue** first; those in **black** may also be beneficial. Some dosages may be supplied by supplements you are already taking—see page 39.

How supplements can help

For seasonal allergies, take all supplements in the chart from early spring through the first frost. In place of prescription or over-the-counter drugs, try **quercetin.** Whereas drugs simply block the effect of histamine, this flavonoid inhibits its release—without any side effects. Combining it with the herb **nettle** can combat sneezing, itching, and swollen nasal passages.

Vitamin A and **vitamin C** support the immune system; vitamin C, the main antioxidant in the cells of the respiratory passages, may also have anti-inflammatory and antihistamine effects. The B vitamin **pantothenic acid** may reduce nasal congestion. You may want to take these three nutrients during allergy season, even if you opt for traditional drugs for specific symptom relief.

And, for severe cases of hay fever, **ephedra** *(Ma huang)* may be useful because it opens the respiratory passages. You can use ephedra with quercetin and nettle, but not with prescription or over-the-counter antihistamines or decongestants.

What else you can do

☑ Stay indoors with the windows closed when pollen counts are high. Use an air-conditioner even in the car and clean the filter regularly.

☑ Eliminate carpets and use furniture slipcovers that can be washed. Encase mattresses and pillows in allergy-proof covers and wash bedding weekly in very hot water. Dust mites collect in these areas.

☑ Clean damp areas to prevent the growth of mold.

alzheimer's disease

This slowly progressive brain disorder—marked by increasing memory loss and disorientation—is a wrenching experience for patients and caregivers. Early treatment may help to slow or temporarily reverse the course of this devastating illness.

SYMPTOMS

- *Memory loss, including an inability to recall recent events and difficulty finding appropriate words or solving basic problems.*
- *Disorientation, including getting lost in a familiar place—such as a home or neighborhood.*
- *Personality changes, marked by agitation, anxiety, combativeness, indifference to others, social withdrawal, or poor judgment.*
- *Language impairment, such as rambling speech, long pauses, and thought repetition.*

When to Call Your Doctor

- If you or a loved one experiences serious disorientation or a change in behavior—get a full medical exam, including an assessment for dementia.
- Reminder: If you have a medical condition, talk to your doctor before taking supplements.

What it is

Alzheimer's disease, a degenerative brain disorder, impairs memory and mental functioning. The onset is typically very slow. Initially, Alzheimer's sufferers have short-term memory loss and difficulty making decisions; they may forget how to perform simple tasks. Advanced stages bring loss of memory and speech, loss of bladder and bowel control, and changes in temperament, such as excessive hostility or withdrawal. Alzheimer's affects about 6% of people over age 65, and 20% of those over 85.

What causes it

Experts still aren't sure what causes Alzheimer's disease. They do know it is marked by a major loss of nerve cells in the brain, particularly in areas controlling memory and thinking. The disease is also characterized by reduced levels of brain chemicals important for memory. Decreased blood flow in the brain or a series of small strokes may contribute to memory loss as well. A family history of the disease can increase the risk of developing Alzheimer's; other possible causes include serious head injury, cardiovascular disease, and slow-acting viruses. Studies indicate that aluminum (such as from cookware) is an unlikely cause of Alzheimer's.

How supplements can help

Though there's no cure for Alzheimer's, scientists continue to make strides in treating the symptoms. A number of supplements may help restore mental functioning during the earlier stages of the disease and even delay the onset of advanced symptoms. Begin taking supplements as soon as possible; take them individually or together. It may be at least eight weeks before you notice any results. The supplements can also be used with prescription drugs, such as tacrine or donepezil, but always check with your doctor first.

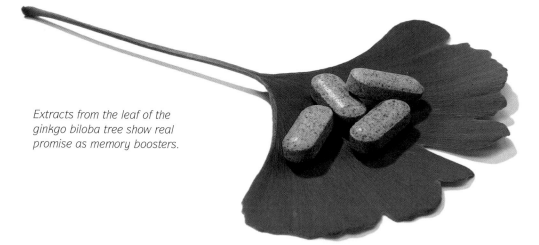

Extracts from the leaf of the ginkgo biloba tree show real promise as memory boosters.

Supplement Recommendations

Ginkgo biloba	**Dosage:** 80 mg 3 times a day. **Comments:** Standardized to have at least 24% flavone glycosides.
Antioxidants	**Dosage:** 2,000 mg vitamin C, 400 IU vitamin E, and mixed carotenoids providing 25,000 IU vitamin A activity a day. **Comments:** These may be sold in a single supplement.
Coenzyme Q$_{10}$	**Dosage:** 100 mg twice a day. **Comments:** For best absorption, take with food.
Vitamin B complex	**Dosage:** 1 pill, plus extra 50 mg vitamin B$_6$, a day with food. **Comments:** Look for a B-100 complex with 100 mcg vitamin B$_{12}$ and biotin; 400 mcg folic acid; and 100 mg all other B vitamins.
Evening primrose oil	**Dosage:** 1,000 mg 3 times a day. **Comments:** Can substitute 1,000 mg borage oil once a day.
Gotu kola	**Dosage:** 200 mg extract or 400-500 mg crude herb 3 times a day. **Comments:** Extract standardized to have 10% asiaticosides. May reduce fatigue and depression and stimulate central nervous system.
Siberian ginseng	**Dosage:** 100-300 mg 3 times a day. **Comments:** Standardized to contain at least 0.8% eleutherosides.

Note: Consider using supplements in **blue** first; those in **black** may also be beneficial. Some dosages may be supplied by supplements you are already taking—see page 39.

One promising supplement is the herb **ginkgo biloba.** Controlled trials have shown that ginkgo, which increases the brain's blood supply, may improve memory in some patients. It may have antioxidant properties as well, playing a key role in maintaining healthy nerve cells. Other **antioxidants** that may be beneficial include vitamin C, vitamin E, mixed carotenoids, and **coenzyme Q$_{10}$;** these are often combined in convenient and economical commercial preparations.

In addition, be sure to get enough B vitamins—low levels have been associated with Alzheimer's. Include **vitamin B complex,** as well as extra vitamin B$_6$. Also worth trying are **evening primrose oil** and the herbs **gotu kola** and **Siberian ginseng;** all may improve memory by improving the transmission of nerve impulses. Two other nutrients may help by boosting memory-enhancing brain chemicals: the amino acid-like substances acetyl L-carnitine (500 mg three times a day) or phosphatidylserine (100 mg three times a day). See which one works best for you.

What else you can do

☑ Exercise. Even a short daily walk may help improve mental abilities.

☑ Keep your mind active by reading or practicing memory exercises.

☑ Stay relaxed to improve memory and concentration.

anemia

Looking pale? Feeling weak and tired? There's a quick blood test available to assess whether anemia is to blame—and if so, whether it's caused by iron-poor blood or something else. Your doctor is the best person to ask about whether certain supplements might be right for you.

What it is

Anemia is a condition in which there is a shortage of red cells in the blood or a deficiency of hemoglobin (the oxygen-carrying pigment) in these cells. When anemia occurs, the body doesn't get enough oxygen, and weakness and fatigue result. Although symptoms may not appear—or may be very mild—for a long time, the condition can be life-threatening if it is left undiagnosed and untreated. Should you suspect you are anemic, it's essential that you see your doctor promptly to ascertain the underlying cause. Treatment will vary, depending on the diagnosis.

What causes it

Iron deficiency, the most common cause of anemia, usually results from a gradual, prolonged blood loss, which depletes the body's iron stores. Without enough iron, hemoglobin levels fall. Menstruating women, particularly those with heavy periods, are prone to iron-deficiency anemia. However, men and women can develop iron deficiency from any condition that causes slow bleeding—including long-term hemorrhoids, rectal polyps, or ulcers; stomach or colon cancer; or prolonged use of aspirin or other nonsteroidal anti-inflammatory drugs (NSAIDs), such as ibuprofen. Because so many foods are fortified with iron, iron-deficiency anemia can rarely be attributed to a lack of this mineral in the diet.

Less common is anemia that results from a deficiency of vitamin B_{12} (in which case it's called pernicious anemia) or folic acid. Both nutrients are essential to red blood cell production. Alcoholics, smokers, people with certain digestive disorders, vegetarians, those over age 50, and pregnant or lactating women are the most likely to be at risk, either because of poor nutrition or an inability to absorb these nutrients properly. Other forms of anemia can be traced to chronic illnesses (for example, cancer, lupus, or rheumatoid arthritis); hereditary disorders such as sickle-cell anemia; or exposure to toxic drugs, chemicals, or radiation.

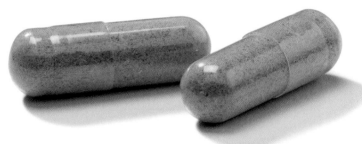

Iron supplements for so-called tired blood can be dangerous if you don't have an iron deficiency.

Supplement Recommendations

Iron	**Dosage:** 30 mg 3 times a day with meals.
	Comments: Your doctor may prescribe a higher dosage.
Vitamin C	**Dosage:** 500 mg 3 times a day.
	Comments: Take with meals to enhance iron absorption from foods.
Vitamin B$_{12}$/ Folic acid	**Dosage:** 1,000 mcg B$_{12}$ and 400 mcg folic acid in sublingual form twice a day for 1 month.
	Comments: Always take B$_{12}$ and folic acid together. If still anemic after oral B$_{12}$ supplements, you may need B$_{12}$ injections.
Yellow dock	**Dosage:** 1,000 mg each morning.
	Comments: Or take ½ tsp. tincture twice a day.
Dandelion	**Dosage:** 1 tsp. fresh juice or tincture with water twice a day.
	Comments: Take with yellow dock to enhance iron absorption.

Note: Consider using supplements in **blue** first; those in **black** may also be beneficial. Some dosages may be supplied by supplements you are already taking—see page 39.

How supplements can help

Before taking supplements, you need to determine the underlying cause of your anemia. It's especially important to see a doctor about iron-deficiency anemia, which may be caused by internal bleeding. If you're advised to take supplements, have blood work every month to see if they are worthwhile.

If iron-deficiency anemia is diagnosed, the mineral **iron** combined with **vitamin C** may be of value. Iron is a key component of hemoglobin, and vitamin C helps the body absorb the mineral. Take iron only under your doctor's supervision, because too much can be dangerous.

Various herbs may also be useful. **Yellow dock** has modest amounts of iron, but it's well absorbed and can raise blood iron levels. Other iron-rich herbs include seaweed and dulse. Taken as a tincture, juice, or tea, some herbs (**dandelion,** burdock, mint, and linden flowers) may enhance the body's ability to absorb iron from foods or supplements.

Vitamin C may be beneficial if you have anemia caused by a deficiency of vitamin B$_{12}$ or folic acid as well; it aids the body in absorbing these nutrients. **Vitamin B$_{12}$** and **folic acid** should always be taken in tandem, and under a doctor's supervision, because a high intake of one can mask a deficiency of the other. Together they work to boost production of red blood cells. Once anemia is corrected and a problem with absorption has been ruled out as a cause, the amount of B$_{12}$ and folic acid in your daily multivitamin may be sufficient to prevent a recurrence.

What else you can do

☑ Eat foods rich in iron (dried beans, liver, red meat, dried fruits, nuts, shellfish); in folic acid (citrus fruits, asparagus, spinach, mushrooms, liver, soybeans, wheat germ); and in vitamin B$_{12}$ (liver, shellfish, lamb, beef, cheese, fish, eggs).

angina

Although conventional medications for angina may help relieve the intense chest pain of this heart disorder, they do very little to halt the physiological mechanisms behind it. Vitamins, minerals, and natural remedies may actually improve the condition—or at least keep it from worsening.

SYMPTOMS

- *Crushing or squeezing chest pain.*
- *Weakness.*
- *Sweating.*
- *Shortness of breath.*
- *Palpitations.*
- *Nausea.*
- *Light-headedness.*

When to Call Your Doctor

- If you have any of the above symptoms for the first time.
- If there is any change in the normal pattern of your angina attacks—for example, if they increase in frequency, intensity, or duration, or if they are brought on by new activities.
- If an angina attack lasts more than 15 minutes, which may be a heart attack—call for an ambulance immediately.
- Reminder: If you have a medical condition, talk to your doctor before taking supplements.

What it is

When your heart isn't getting enough blood and oxygen, the crushing, squeezing pain of angina is typically the result. Usually the pain begins below the breastbone and radiates to the shoulder, arm, or jaw, increasing in intensity until it reaches a plateau and then diminishes. The attack can last up to 15 minutes.

What causes it

Angina is a direct result of the buildup of plaque (atherosclerosis) in the arteries that supply the heart with blood. Like any other muscle in the body, the heart needs blood and oxygen to do its work of pumping blood throughout the circulatory system.

With atherosclerosis, arteries may be wide enough to provide sufficient blood flow during rest, but they can't supply enough oxygen-rich blood when physical activity increases the demand on the heart. Any exertion—climbing stairs, running for the bus, shoveling snow, even having sex—can trigger some angina attacks. Other cases of angina are not related to physical activity but occur when a small blood clot forms on the surface of a blood vessel's plaque and temporarily blocks a coronary artery. Angina may also result if a coronary artery goes into spasm.

How supplements can help

The supplements listed in the chart can all be used together or alone. They can also complement your prescription angina medications; never stop your heart medication without first consulting your doctor, however.

The antioxidant effect of vitamins C and E can help prevent cell damage: **Vitamin C** aids in the repair of the arteries injured by plaque, and **vitamin E** blocks the oxidation of LDL ("bad") cholesterol, the initial step in the formation of plaque. In addition, some people with heart disease have low levels of vitamin E as well as the mineral **magnesium,** which may inhibit spasms of the coronary arteries.

Derived from berries or other parts of the plant, hawthorn is a good heart-protective herbal treatment.

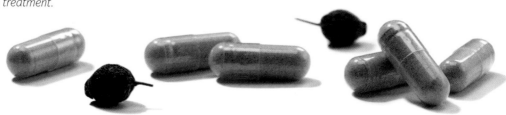

Supplement Recommendations

Vitamin C	**Dosage:** 1,000 mg 3 times a day.
	Comments: Reduce dose if diarrhea develops.
Vitamin E	**Dosage:** 400 IU twice a day.
	Comments: Check with your doctor if taking anticoagulant drugs.
Magnesium	**Dosage:** 200 mg twice a day.
	Comments: Do not take if you have kidney disease.
Arginine	**Dosage:** 500 mg L-arginine 3 times a day on an empty stomach.
	Comments: If using longer than 1 month, add mixed amino acids.
Carnitine	**Dosage:** 500 mg L-carnitine 3 times a day on an empty stomach.
	Comments: If using longer than 1 month, add mixed amino acids.
Taurine	**Dosage:** 500 mg L-taurine 3 times a day on an empty stomach.
	Comments: If using longer than 1 month, add mixed amino acids.
Coenzyme Q$_{10}$	**Dosage:** 100 mg twice a day.
	Comments: For best absorption, take with food.
Hawthorn	**Dosage:** 100-150 mg 3 times a day.
	Comments: Standardized to contain at least 1.8% vitexin.
Essential fatty acids	**Dosage:** 1 tbsp. flaxseed oil a day; 2,000 mg fish oils 3 times a day.
	Comments: Take fish oils if you don't eat fish at least twice a week.

Some dosages may be supplied by supplements you are already taking—see page **39**.

Amino acids can benefit the heart in several ways. **Arginine** plays a role in forming nitric oxide, which relaxes artery walls. One study found that taking this amino acid three times a day increased the amount of time individuals with angina could exercise at moderate intensity without having to stop because of chest pain. **Carnitine,** an amino acid-like substance, allows heart muscle cells to use energy more efficiently, and another amino acid, **taurine,** may temper heart rhythm abnormalities.

Like carnitine, the nutritional supplement **coenzyme Q$_{10}$** enhances the heart muscle, reducing its workload, and the herb **hawthorn** improves blood flow to the heart. **Essential fatty acids** may be effective in lowering triglyceride levels and keeping arteries flexible.

What else you can do

☑ Eat a low-fat, fiber-rich diet; use canola or olive oil instead of butter.

☑ Don't smoke and avoid smoky places.

☑ Learn to relax. Meditation, t'ai chi, and yoga may reduce angina attacks.

☑ Join a support group. Determine what brought you to this point in your life and what you can do to begin reversing the disease.

anxiety and panic

Everyone feels anxious from time to time, but some people are uneasy so often—or have scary episodes called panic attacks—that anxiety interferes with their normal life. Taking B vitamins, certain minerals, and calming herbs may help.

SYMPTOMS

Acute anxiety
- *Extreme fear.*
- *Rapid heartbeat and breathing.*
- *Excessive perspiration, chills, or hot flashes.*
- *Dry mouth.*
- *Dizziness.*

Chronic anxiety
- *Muscle tension, headaches, and back pain.*
- *Insomnia.*
- *Depression.*
- *Low sex drive.*
- *Inability to relax.*

When to Call Your Doctor

- Do not replace prescription anti-anxiety medications, such as alprazolam, lorazepam, or diazepam, with herbs or supplements without talking to your doctor. Cutting back suddenly can be dangerous.
- Anxiety symptoms can mimic those of a serious illness, or may be caused by certain medical conditions or drugs. See your doctor to rule out these as possibilities.
- Reminder: If you have a medical or psychiatric condition, talk to your doctor before taking supplements.

What it is

When faced with a potentially dangerous situation—a large barking dog, for example—anxiety is a healthy response. Your brain, sensing the danger, signals for the release of hormones to prepare your body to defend itself. Muscles tense, heartbeat and breathing rate increase, and the blood even becomes more likely to clot (in the event of injury). In some individuals, this response is set in motion even when there is no obvious threat. Such a reaction can be bad for your health, causing exhaustion, poor concentration, a sense of detachment from yourself or your surroundings, headaches, stomach problems, and an increase in blood pressure.

Anxiety disorders come in two basic forms. Generalized anxiety disorder (GAD) is a chronic condition that involves a recurring sense of foreboding and worry accompanied by mild physical symptoms. A panic attack, on the other hand, comes on suddenly and unexpectedly, with symptoms so violent that the episodes are often mistaken for a heart attack or another life-threatening condition.

What causes it

Some scientists think that the central nervous systems of people with anxiety disorders may overreact to stress and take a longer time than most to return to a calmer state. Anxiety may begin with an upsetting event—an accident, divorce, or death—or it may have no identifiable root.

There may also be a biochemical basis for anxiety. Studies have shown that people who are prone to panic attacks have higher blood levels of lactic acid, a chemical produced when muscles metabolize

Kava's root supplies its active ingredients. These are processed into standardized extracts and sold as tinctures, pills, and teas.

Kava	**Dosage:** 250 mg 2 or 3 times a day as needed. **Comments:** Look for standardized extracts in pill or tincture form that contain at least 30% kavalactones.
Calcium/ Magnesium	**Dosage:** 600 mg of each a day. **Comments:** Take with food; sometimes sold in a single supplement.
Vitamin B complex	**Dosage:** 1 pill, plus extra 100 mg thiamin, each morning with food. **Comments:** Look for a B-50 complex with 50 mcg vitamin B_{12} and biotin; 400 mcg folic acid; and 50 mg all other B vitamins.
Valerian	**Dosage:** 250 mg twice a day. **Comments:** Should be standardized to contain 0.8% valerenic acid. May cause drowsiness; take at bedtime for insomnia.
St. John's wort	**Dosage:** 300 mg 3 times a day. **Comments:** Should be standardized to contain 0.3% hypericin.

Note: Consider using supplements in **blue** first; those in **black** may also be beneficial. Some dosages may be supplied by supplements you are already taking—see page 39.

see page 39

sugar without enough oxygen. Other research suggests that anxiety may be the result of an overproduction of stress hormones by the brain and adrenal glands.

How supplements can help

In many cases, herbal and nutritional remedies for anxiety can be used in place of prescription drugs, which may be addictive and have other unpleasant side effects. Several studies have shown that the herb **kava** is very useful for anxiety—perhaps as effective as prescription drugs; it reduces symptoms such as nervousness, dizziness, and heart palpitations. In addition, people with anxiety should add **calcium, magnesium,** and a **vitamin B complex** supplement, plus extra thiamin. These nutrients are important for the healthy functioning of the nervous system, especially for the production of the key chemical messengers in the brain called neurotransmitters.

Valerian, known as a sleep aid, can be used at low doses throughout the day for a calming effect. Try this herb if kava doesn't work for you. Even if you're taking kava during the day, you can have a nighttime dose (250 to 500 mg) of valerian if you have trouble falling asleep. **St. John's wort** can be added to kava or valerian if you are depressed as well as anxious. At least a month is needed before the full effect of St. John's wort will be felt; the other supplements begin working immediately.

What else you can do

☑ Cut out caffeine, alcohol, and excess sugar, which may trigger anxiety.

☑ Do aerobic exercises regularly. They burn lactic acid, produce natural feel-good chemicals (endorphins), and enhance your use of oxygen

☑ See a therapist to develop more positive ways of coping.

arrhythmias

The heart, workhorse of the body, beats more than 100,000 times a day, pumping life-giving blood through thousands of miles of arteries, capillaries, and veins. Irregular heart rhythms—or arrhythmias—can disrupt this process and require careful medical evaluation.

What it is

Arrhythmias are abnormal rhythms of the heart. They may be as fleeting as a single missed beat, or they may be more serious, causing the heart to beat irregularly or unusually fast or slowly for extended periods.

What causes it

For many people with arrhythmias, the cause is unclear. However, some cases can be traced to a heart condition, such as coronary artery disease, a heart valve defect, or in rare cases, an infection of the heart. Thyroid or kidney disease, certain drugs, and imbalances of magnesium or potassium in the body can contribute to arrhythmias. Abnormal rhythms may also be induced by a high intake of caffeine or alcohol, heavy smoking, and stress.

How supplements can help

It's important to remember that some arrhythmias can be serious. The supplements listed in the chart are meant to complement—not to replace—standard treatments. Never discontinue a heart drug without consulting your doctor first. All the supplements can be used together, but your doctor should determine which ones you should take and in what order. They may work within a week, but often need to be used long term.

Magnesium supplements often benefit people with heart-rhythm disorders, many of whom are deficient in this mineral. Magnesium is vital for coordinating the activity of nerves (including those that initiate heartbeats) and muscles (including the heart). Also valuable is **hawthorn,** an herb that has been used as a heart tonic for centuries: It increases blood flow to the heart, making it beat more strongly and restoring rhythm. **Coenzyme Q$_{10}$** also helps steady heart rhythm and may be particularly

The amino acid taurine may be helpful for people with heart-rhythm disorders.

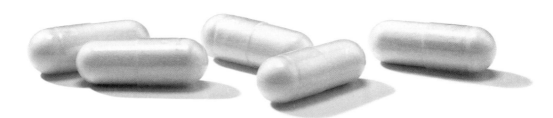

Supplement Recommendations

Magnesium	**Dosage:** 400 mg twice a day.	
	Comments: Do not take if you have kidney disease.	
Hawthorn	**Dosage:** 100-150 mg 3 times a day.	
	Comments: Standardized to contain at least 1.8% vitexin.	
Coenzyme Q$_{10}$	**Dosage:** 50 mg twice a day.	
	Comments: For best absorption, take with food.	
Fish oils	**Dosage:** 1,000 mg 3 times a day.	
	Comments: Take only if you don't eat fish at least twice a week.	
Cactus grandiflorus	**Dosage:** 25 drops tincture 3 times a day.	
	Comments: Known as night-blooming cereus; may cause diarrhea.	
Manganese	**Dosage:** 20 mg every morning.	
	Comments: Often included in multivitamin and mineral formulas.	
Amino acids	**Dosage:** 1,500 mg L-taurine twice a day; 500 mg L-carnitine 3 times a day.	
	Comments: For long-term use, try a mixed amino acid complex.	
Astragalus	**Dosage:** 400 mg twice a day or 3 cups of tea a day.	
	Comments: Supplying 0.5% glucosides and 70% polysaccharides.	

Note: Consider using supplements in **blue** first; those in **black** may also be beneficial. Some dosages may be supplied by supplements you are already taking—see page 39.

see page 39

useful for people who have previously suffered a heart attack or have another form of heart disease. In addition, **fish oils** are being extensively studied for treating heart ailments; early results strongly suggest that they are effective at relieving arrhythmias.

Other supplements may stabilize heart rhythm as well. Some recommend the herb **cactus grandiflorus;** it is often used with hawthorn. The trace mineral **manganese,** which promotes healthy nerves, and the **amino acids** taurine and carnitine increase oxygen supply to the heart. Taken as a tea, pill, or tincture (30 drops three times a day), the herb **astragalus** has been found to contain various substances that stabilize heart rhythm. Doctors also occasionally prescribe potassium supplements to prevent arrhythmias, though for most people, eating fresh fruits and vegetables is a better way to get adequate supplies of this mineral.

What else you can do

☑ Reduce or eliminate caffeine and alcohol.

☑ If you smoke, quit. No supplement can compensate for the long-term cardiac damage caused by smoking.

☑ Exercise regularly. Aerobic exercise strengthens the heart.

☑ Reduce stress. Relaxation techniques such as biofeedback may help.

FACTS & Tips

- Sipping astragalus tea may help—but don't drink it all day long. Herbal teas can be potent medicine, so limit your intake to three cups a day.

- If you don't like the taste of astragalus, try other herbal teas or tinctures. The herb barberry and its cousin Oregon grape both contain compounds known as berberines, which have been shown to reduce arrhythmias; angelica contains a mixture of substances that combat arrhythmias; and ginkgo biloba, like hawthorn, improves blood flow to the heart.

- Many doctors recommend eating salmon, mackerel, herring, or sardines at least twice a week to help reduce the risk of fatal arrhythmias. It's a good idea: Cold-water fish may be an even better source of healing omega-3 fatty acids than fish oil capsules.

LATEST FINDINGS

- In a recent study from Denmark, 55 heart attack survivors were given capsules of either fish oils or olive oil (placebo). After three months, those receiving the fish oils did significantly better on heart tests, indicating that they were less likely to suffer from serious arrhythmias.

- According to a study in the *Journal of the American College of Cardiology,* 232 people who had frequent arrhythmias significantly reduced their likelihood of abnormal heart rhythms after just three weeks by increasing their intake of magnesium and potassium.

arthritis

Probably the most common age-related disease, osteoarthritis affects the joints of 16 million Americans, most over age 50. But pain and stiffness are not inevitable: Supplements may greatly relieve symptoms and slow the cartilage degeneration that's at the root of this disorder.

SYMPTOMS

- *The onset of osteoarthritis is often gradual, marked by mild joint stiffness and pain—especially in the morning and after exercise— that are relieved by rest.*

- *Bone growths, or spurs, may develop at affected joints, causing pain, a gnarled appearance, and decreased mobility.*

When to Call Your Doctor

- If joint pain is accompanied by fever, which may signal infectious arthritis and require immediate medical attention.
- If pain and stiffness develop quickly, which may be a sign of rheumatoid arthritis.
- If you self-diagnose mild osteoarthritis, which should be confirmed by your doctor.
- Reminder: If you have a medical condition, talk to your doctor before taking supplements.

What it is

With osteoarthritis, your joints gradually lose their cartilage—the smooth, gel-like, shock-absorbing material that prevents adjacent bones from touching. Most commonly affected are the fingers, knees, hips, neck, and spine. As cartilage loss continues, the friction of bone rubbing against bone can cause pain and joint instability.

What causes it

Osteoarthritis may be the result of decades of joint wear and tear, though genetic factors, excess weight, and impairments in the body's ability to repair cartilage may also play a role. Some cases are linked to a specific cause, such as a previous injury to a joint; the overuse of a joint occupationally or athletically; or a congenital defect in joint structure.

How supplements can help

There is no sure cure for osteoarthritis, but **glucosamine,** a cartilage-building sugar compound, is one of the most helpful remedies for relieving arthritis pain. It appears to slow joint damage over time, though whether it can actually reverse the disease is unknown. To enhance its effectiveness, try glucosamine along with one other supplement listed in the chart. Allow at least a month to judge results; then, if necessary, substitute another supplement to use with glucosamine to see if it works better for you. These supplements can be used long term, as well as with conventional pain relievers, such as aspirin and acetaminophen.

Several large studies are assessing the impact of glucosamine when it's combined with another cartilage-building compound, **chondroitin**

Used topically, cayenne cream is one of the most effective pain relievers for arthritis.

Supplement Recommendations

Glucosamine
Dosage: 500 mg glucosamine sulfate 3 times a day.
Comments: Take with food to minimize digestive upset.

Chondroitin
Dosage: 400 mg chondroitin sulfate 3 times a day.
Comments: Often sold in combination with glucosamine.

Niacinamide
Dosage: 1,000 mg 3 times a day.
Comments: High doses can cause liver damage and other serious side effects; physician monitoring is necessary during treatment.

Cayenne cream
Dosage: Apply topical cream to affected joints several times a day.
Comments: Standardized to contain 0.025%-0.075% capsaicin.

Boswellia
Dosage: 1 pill 3 times a day.
Comments: Each pill standardized to have 150 mg boswellic acid.

Sea cucumber
Dosage: 1,000 mg a day.
Comments: Also known as bêche-de-mer.

SAM
Dosage: 400 mg twice a day for 2 weeks, then 200 mg twice a day as a maintenance dose.
Comments: May have mild gastrointestinal side effects. Should not be taken by people with manic-depressive illness.

Note: Consider using supplements in **blue** first; those in **black** may also be beneficial. Some dosages may be supplied by supplements you are already taking—see page 39.

see page 39

FACTS & Tips

- By age 40, nine out of ten people have X-ray evidence of arthritic changes; many later develop joint pain and stiffness. Natural supplements may slow this degenerative process.
- Veterinarians have been using glucosamine and other supplements to treat arthritic pets for years, with great success.
- The stiffer your joints, the less you're inclined to exercise. Fight that response: Inactivity weakens nearby muscles, further destabilizing joints and increasing pain.

LATEST FINDINGS

- One recent study showed that glucosamine may be particularly useful against arthritis in the knee. And two earlier studies found that glucosamine was as effective as or more effective than ibuprofen for relief of many different types of arthritis symptoms.
- Taking 400 IU or more of vitamin D a day may help slow or halt the progression of osteoarthritis of the knee, according to the results of a new study. However, more is not always better: In high doses (taking more than 1,000 IU a day), vitamin D can be toxic.

(some experts believe this compound is poorly absorbed and of limited effectiveness). Other supplements that can be taken with glucosamine include **niacinamide,** which may be particularly effective in relieving knee pain; **boswellia,** a gummy tree resin that may inhibit inflammation and build cartilage; and **sea cucumber,** a Chinese remedy that may, through unknown mechanisms, reduce pain and stiffness and boost grip strength. One form of the amino acid methionine called **SAM** (S-adenosylmethionine) has anti-inflammatory effects similar to ibuprofen and has been shown to rebuild cartilage. Gelatin, containing the amino acids glycine and proline and other joint-building nutrients, may also be worth trying if other measures fail; little is known about its effectiveness.

Any of these therapies can be used along with topically applied **cayenne cream** for pain relief. The capsaicin in cayenne inhibits production of substance P, a chemical involved in sending pain messages to the brain. Initial applications, however, may cause a burning sensation.

What else you can do

☑ Engage in moderate low-impact exercise such as walking or swimming to strengthen muscles and improve overall joint condition.

☑ Apply heat or ice to joints for 20 minutes three times a day to help reduce pain.

Did You Know?

Glucosamine supplements cost the same as many prescription arthritis medications—about $30 for a month's supply—but have few of the serious side effects, such as gastrointestinal bleeding, that the drugs commonly do.

asthma

Between 12 and 15 million Americans have asthma—often a lifetime condition—and these numbers increase each year. Although this lung disease always requires medical management, there are several steps you can take on your own to minimize the frequency and severity of asthma attacks.

What it is

Asthma is a disease in which the airways of the lungs swell and tighten, restricting airflow and making it hard to breathe. During an asthma attack, the smallest airways (the bronchioles) constrict. This causes the release of chemicals such as histamine that increase inflammation and swelling and produce excess mucus. Though many asthma attacks are mild and easily controlled at home, severe ones can cause sufferers to begin to suffocate. And for 5,000 Americans each year, an asthma attack is fatal.

What causes it

External or internal factors can provoke asthma attacks, and some people are sensitive to both. Outside triggers usually involve an allergen, such as pet dander, a food, dust and dust mites, insects (including cockroaches), pollen, and many environmental pollutants. Internal triggers, which are usually less obvious and can be harder to avoid, include stress, anxiety, temperature changes, exercise, and respiratory infections such as bronchitis.

How supplements can help

The supplements in the chart are meant to complement conventional asthma therapy. Never stop taking medication prescribed for asthma without consulting your doctor. People with asthma are often deficient in key nutrients, especially vitamin C, magnesium, and vitamin B_6. **Vitamin C,** the major antioxidant present in the lining of the respiratory tract, appears to act immediately to combat inhaled oxidants. In addition,

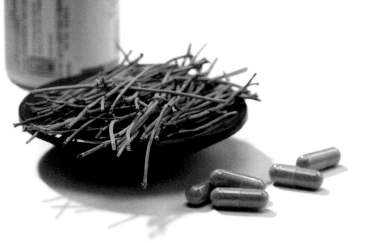

Ephedra, made from twigs of a shrub, is sometimes used in moderate doses to treat the symptoms of asthma.

Supplement Recommendations

Vitamin C	**Dosage:** 1,000 mg 3 times a day. **Comments:** Reduce dose if diarrhea develops.
Magnesium	**Dosage:** 400 mg twice a day. **Comments:** Take for 6 weeks to achieve adequate levels.
Vitamin B$_6$	**Dosage:** 50 mg twice a day. **Comments:** Especially important if you take the prescription asthma drug theophylline.
Quercetin	**Dosage:** 500 mg 3 times a day. **Comments:** Use 20 minutes before meals; often sold with vitamin C.
Ephedra	**Dosage:** 130 mg standardized extract 3 times a day. **Comments:** May cause insomnia. Don't use if you have high blood pressure, heart disease, or anxiety or take an MAO inhibitor.
Licorice	**Dosage:** 200 mg standardized extract 3 times a day. **Comments:** Can raise blood pressure; see your doctor before taking.

Some dosages may be supplied by supplements you are already taking—see page 39.

it may halt an allergic reaction by preventing the cells from releasing histamine. Furthermore, Vitamin C is very effective for exercise-induced asthma; according to various studies, taking 2,000 mg before a workout may even thwart an asthma attack. As for the mineral **magnesium,** it can prevent attacks by inhibiting the contraction of the bronchial muscles. Other studies have shown that **vitamin B$_6$** supplements reduce wheezing and other asthma symptoms.

it may halt an allergic reaction by preventing the cells from releasing histamine. Furthermore, Vitamin C is very effective for exercise-induced asthma; according to various studies, taking 2,000 mg before a workout may even thwart an asthma attack. As for the mineral **magnesium,** it can prevent attacks by inhibiting the contraction of the bronchial muscles. Other studies have shown that **vitamin B$_6$** supplements reduce wheezing and other asthma symptoms.

The flavonoid **quercetin** has two main effects: It inhibits the release of histamine, and as an antioxidant, it neutralizes unstable oxygen molecules, which can cause bronchial inflammation. The herb **ephedra** (also called *Ma huang*) can widen respiratory passages. It appears to work best when used with herbal products that bring up phlegm, such as **licorice** or horehound. (Don't use licorice for longer than a month.) But ephedra has many side effects; for asthma, it is best taken under a doctor's care.

What else you can do

☑ Keep your home clear of dust and pollen. Avoid cigarette smoke.

☑ Stay away from cats; their dander is highly allergenic.

☑ Remain calm. Managing stress helps fight asthma.

☑ Treat colds and the flu promptly to reduce the chances of an attack.

☑ Wear a scarf over your mouth and nose to warm the cold winter air.

☑ Keep an asthma diary to help you determine your asthma triggers.

☑ Drink at least eight glasses of water a day to keep mucus loose.

FACTS & Tips

■ Substances in green tea can help reduce the airway inflammation that accompanies an asthma attack. Taking time for a cup of tea can be soothing and calming as well. You can safely drink several cups of green tea a day in combination with other nutritional and herbal remedies.

■ Yoga is an excellent activity for people with asthma. Not only does it enhance breathing, it is also relaxing.

■ An inexpensive device, called a peak-flow meter, measures how fast and how hard you can exhale air from your lungs. Its results, compared to levels set by your doctor or to previous readings, can often predict an asthma attack, even a day or two in advance.

Did You Know?

Eating lots of onions may help asthma sufferers. The mustard oils (isothiocyanates) they contain seem to promote healthy lungs.

athlete's foot

The most common fungal infection of the skin, athlete's foot typically begins between the toes, causing itching, scaling, and sometimes painful breaks in the skin. This generally harmless but unusually pesky condition may be relieved with various natural remedies.

SYMPTOMS

- *Scaling and peeling between the toes. In severe cases, there may be cracks between the toes.*
- *Redness, itching, scaling, and tiny blisters along the sides and soles of the feet.*
- *Soft and painful skin.*
- *Infected toenails that can become thickened, discolored, or crumbly.*

When to Call Your Doctor

- If there's no improvement in a week to 10 days after starting treatment with supplements.
- If home treatment does not provide a complete cure within four weeks.
- If any area becomes red and swollen, a sign of a more serious bacterial infection.
- Reminder: If you have a medical condition, talk to your doctor before taking supplements.

What it is

"Athlete's foot" is the common term for a fungal infection called *tinea pedis*. The fungi that cause it are tiny, plantlike cells found on the skin of all humans. They can multiply out of control under certain conditions. The fungi thrive in cramped, damp places, such as inside shoes and socks. In some people, athlete's foot occurs entirely between the toes, where the skin cracks, peels, and becomes scaly. In others, the infection appears on the soles and sides of the feet or affects the toenails.

What causes it

The most common fungi causing athlete's foot are called *Trichophytons*. Though poorly ventilated shoes and sweaty socks provide an excellent breeding ground for the fungi, athlete's foot is not highly contagious, so walking barefoot in a locker room does not increase your risk.

How supplements can help

Many doctors prescribe conventional antifungal medications for persistent cases of athlete's foot. These drugs can be very effective—and very costly. For milder cases, supplements can be an inexpensive way to combat this infection; symptoms should begin to clear up within a week.

Tea tree oil can be a cost-effective way to battle a case of athlete's foot.

Supplement Recommendations

Vitamin C	**Dosage:** 1,000 mg twice a day. **Comments:** Long-term use may prevent recurrences; reduce dose if diarrhea develops.
Tea tree oil	**Dosage:** Apply to affected areas of skin twice a day. **Comments:** Never ingest tea tree oil.
Garlic oil	**Dosage:** Apply oil to affected areas of skin twice a day. **Comments:** Can be used in place of tea tree oil.
Calendula	**Dosage:** Apply cream or lotion to affected areas twice a day. **Comments:** Standardized to contain at least 2% calendula. Use with caution if you're allergic to daisylike flowers.

Note: Consider using supplements in **blue** first; those in **black** may also be beneficial. Some dosages may be supplied by supplements you are already taking—see page 39.

Vitamin C, an antioxidant, promotes immune function and aids the body in fighting fungal infections. It can be taken while using any of the topical supplements listed in the chart.

Tea tree oil, a powerful natural antifungal agent, alters the chemical environment of the skin, making it inhospitable to fungal growth. Effective topical preparations include creams or lotions containing tea tree oil; look for products that contain tea tree oil as one of the top ingredients, or make your own by adding two parts tea tree oil to three parts of a neutral oil, such as almond oil. For an antifungal foot bath, add 20 drops of tea tree oil to a small tub of warm water; soak your feet for 15 minutes two or three times a day. Dry the feet well and dab a few drops of undiluted tea tree oil on the affected areas. If pure tea tree oil irritates your skin, use one of the topical preparations described below.

Rub **garlic oil** directly onto the affected areas. Garlic contains a natural fungus-fighting substance called allicin that can help to clear up athlete's foot. You can also try dusting your feet with garlic powder. Derived from a golden daisylike flower, **calendula** is another useful option. Widely available in health-food stores, this herb relieves inflammation and soothes the skin, which promotes healing.

What else you can do

☑ Keep your feet clean and dry. With a hair dryer set on low, dry your feet. If you prefer to use a towel, launder it after each use.

☑ Wear clean, dry socks. Air your shoes after each use, and don't wear the same pair every day.

☑ Go barefoot when you can, or opt for sandals or other well-ventilated shoes that allow your feet to breathe.

☑ Try over-the-counter antifungal lotions and powders; but avoid those that contain cornstarch, which can encourage fungal growth.

☑ Cut your toenails straight across to help prevent fungal infection.

FACTS & Tips

- Supplements may be useful for other types of fungal skin infections as well. Jock itch, for example, is caused by the same type of fungus responsible for most cases of athlete's foot, and the two conditions often occur together. Topical treatments can be applied to the groin area twice a day.

- Try using supplements along with over-the-counter or prescription antifungal creams and lotions. Creams are good for the soles of the feet. But between the toes, apply a lotion: It is absorbed faster than a cream and won't trap moisture, which could prolong the problem.

LATEST FINDINGS

- For stubborn cases of athlete's foot, particularly those affecting the nails, prescription drugs work remarkably well. But they can be very expensive and have dangerous side effects. For example, recent studies have found the new oral prescription drug itraconazole to be effective against persistent fungal infections. But it's costly: $700 or more for a three-month treatment. It can also cause liver damage, so patients taking it must visit a doctor to have periodic blood tests to monitor their liver function.

Did You Know?

Athlete's foot does not often occur in children under age 12. If a child shows symptoms similar to those of athlete's foot, odds are it's another skin condition, and you may need to consult a pediatrician about it.

back pain

Because humans defy gravity by standing upright, the spine is often under stress. This condition frequently leads to back pain, the most common ailment affecting Americans today. The secret to relief is to strengthen both the vertebrae and the surrounding tissues.

SYMPTOMS

- *Aching or stiffness along spine, especially during movement.*
- *Sharp pain in the upper or lower back, or down the leg.*
- *Debilitating pain after exercise, strenuous activity, or exertion.*
- *Aching and discomfort after long periods of sitting or standing.*

When to Call Your Doctor

- If pain is disabling or accompanied by fever or vomiting.
- If tingling or numbness appears in the arms or legs, or intense pain extends down the back of the leg (sciatica).
- If pain and stiffness affect one area of the spine upon waking.
- If pain follows a fall or car accident.
- Reminder: If you have a medical condition, talk to your doctor before taking supplements.

What it is

Though frequently quite uncomfortable, most backaches are not serious. Typically, the lower back, which supports almost all of the body's weight, is the area most affected. But inflammation of or even a minor injury to any of the bones in the spine (vertebrae) or the muscles, cartilage, nerves, or other tissues connected to the spine can bring on pain.

What causes it

Most back pain is the result of muscle strain. Poor posture, weakened bones or cartilage, a slipped disk, a pinched nerve, or stress and emotional upset can also cause the discomfort. A disease such as arthritis or osteoporosis can predispose a person to chronic back pain.

How supplements can help

Before beginning a therapeutic supplement program, check with your doctor to determine whether medical or surgical treatment is warranted. Supplements are aimed at building stronger bones and muscles, reducing inflammation, and treating pain. Effects may be felt within a week.

People prone to back problems should start with vitamins and minerals that strengthen bones and cartilage, such as **calcium, magnesium, vitamins C** and **D,** and **manganese.** In addition, various other supplements are worth trying, either singly or in combination. Some hospitals have had success using **bromelain,** an enzyme found in pineapple, to reduce inflammation and pain from surgery, trauma, sports injuries, and arthritis. The nutritional supplement **glucosamine** builds cartilage,

Called "nature's aspirin," white willow bark reduces the inflammation that often accompanies pain.

Supplement Recommendations

Calcium/ Magnesium	**Dosage:** 600 mg calcium and 250 mg magnesium a day. **Comments:** Can be purchased as part of a bone-building formula.
Bromelain	**Dosage:** 500 mg 3 times a day on an empty stomach. **Comments:** Should provide 6,000 GDU or 9,000 MCU daily.
Glucosamine	**Dosage:** 500 mg glucosamine sulfate 3 times a day. **Comments:** Take with food to minimize digestive upset.
White willow bark	**Dosage:** 1 or 2 pills 3 times a day (follow package directions). **Comments:** Should be standardized to contain 15% salicin.
Vitamin C	**Dosage:** 1,000 mg 3 times a day. **Comments:** Reduce dose if diarrhea develops.
Vitamin D	**Dosage:** 400 IU a day. **Comments:** Avoid doses above 1,000 IU a day, which may be toxic.
Manganese	**Dosage:** 60 mg a day for 2 weeks. **Comments:** After 2 weeks, reduce dose to 20 mg a day.
Flaxseed oil	**Dosage:** 1 tbsp. (14 grams) a day. **Comments:** Can be mixed with food; take in the morning.

Note: Consider using supplements in **blue** first; those in **black** may also be beneficial. Some dosages may be supplied by supplements you are already taking—see page 39.

including the tissue supporting the spinal disks. And the herb **white willow bark** has pain-relieving characteristics similar to aspirin, but with fewer side effects. Rich in omega-3 fatty acids, **flaxseed oil** may also have healing analgesic and anti-inflammatory properties. All these supplements may reduce the need for conventional pain relievers and, except for white willow bark, can be taken along with them.

Other beneficial supplements include S-adenosylmethionine, or SAM (200 mg three times a day), a form of the muscle-strengthening, collagen-building amino acid methionine; boswellia (150 mg boswellic acid three times a day), an herbal remedy from India with anti-inflammatory properties; and niacinamide (500 mg three times a day), a form of niacin that may be effective against arthritic back pain. The herb devil's claw (400 mg three times a day) may be particularly useful for inflammatory pain from arthritis or degenerative spine disease (spondylosis).

What else you can do

☑ To improve posture, wear comfortable footwear; consider orthotics.

☑ Try therapeutic massage, chiropractic (spinal alignment), acupuncture, or TENS (transcutaneous electrical nerve stimulation) for pain relief.

☑ Don't bend from the waist without bending your knees when lifting.

☑ Sit in a chair with lower-back support; take frequent breaks to stretch.

FACTS & Tips

■ Over-the-counter pain relievers may be very effective against back and neck pain—but they can have dangerous side effects, such as stomach or intestinal bleeding. Natural supplements are a safer alternative and may reduce—or even eliminate—your need for conventional drugs.

LATEST FINDINGS

■ A German study of 109 people who had low back pain for at least six months suggests that the herb devil's claw (named for its large, claw-shaped fruit) may be a valuable complement to conventional medication. Half received devil's claw and half were given a placebo; all patients were also free to take prescription painkillers as needed. After one month, nine in the devil's claw group, but only one in the placebo group, were pain-free.

■ Strengthening stomach muscles helps prevent back injuries. A recent study shows that partial sit-ups (or crunches), done by lifting the torso halfway up while the knees are bent at a 90° angle, are the best way to strengthen stomach muscles because they place the least stress on lower back muscles. Full sit-ups or "cross-the-knee" crunches can injure your back.

Did You Know?

Doctors sometimes recommend a week or two of bed rest for back pain. But new research shows that unless you have a slipped disk (an intensely painful condition), just one or two days of rest can be more beneficial.

bad breath

This bothersome complaint affects literally millions of Americans and has fueled a billion-dollar-a-year industry. Strict oral hygiene and natural remedies can provide relief. And if bad breath persists, careful dental or medical detective work often uncovers a correctable underlying cause.

SYMPTOMS

- *Regularly experiencing a disagreeable taste is a sign that the breath leaving your mouth probably has an unpleasant odor.*
- *Many people with bad breath don't taste or smell it themselves, so look for possible clues from others: They step back when you speak, for instance. If you suspect a problem, ask someone you trust for an honest opinion.*
- *Bleeding gums signal gingivitis, an inflammation of the gums that can sometimes cause bad breath.*

When to Call Your Doctor

- If bad breath does not improve despite self-care measures— your dentist or doctor can check for an underlying medical cause, such as gum disease or a chronic sinus infection.
- Reminder: If you have a medical condition, talk to your doctor before taking supplements.

What it is

Whether it's called bad breath or halitosis, nobody wants an unpleasant odor emanating from his mouth. In the simplest cases, this problem can be traced back to smoking, drinking alcohol, or eating foods notorious for their lingering odors, including garlic, onions, and anchovies. But sometimes, the condition can become chronic, caused by an underlying medical condition.

What causes it

Bad breath usually results from the multiplication of odor-causing bacteria in the mouth. The drier your mouth, the more bacteria thrive. Any condition that reduces saliva production can contribute to bad breath—including advancing age, breathing through the mouth, crash diets (the less food you chew, the less your salivary flow), certain medications, even the time of day ("morning breath" occurs because salivation is considerably reduced during sleep). Bacteria may also collect on the tongue, in food debris that accumulates on dentures, and on the teeth—especially when plaque or cavities are present. If bad breath persists, underlying gum disease or a chronic sinus infection is often the cause.

How supplements can help

Natural strategies for bad breath work best in combination with regular and thorough oral hygiene, including flossing and brushing the teeth, as well as brushing the tongue (especially the back part), where odor-causing bacteria are likely to flourish.

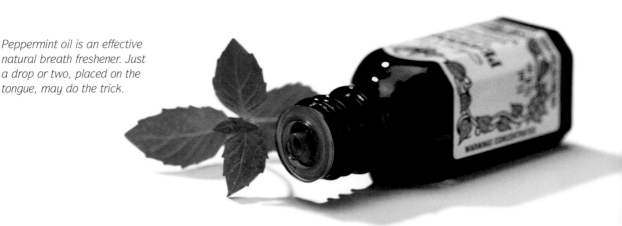

Peppermint oil is an effective natural breath freshener. Just a drop or two, placed on the tongue, may do the trick.

Supplement Recommendations

Peppermint	**Dosage:** 1 or 2 drops essential oil of peppermint, placed on tongue.
	Comments: Larger amounts of peppermint oil can cause heartburn. Drinking peppermint tea may also be helpful.
Fennel	**Dosage:** Chew a pinch of fennel seeds after meals or as needed.
	Comments: Chew thoroughly for best effect. Anise seeds or cloves can also be used.
Parsley	**Dosage:** Chew on a fresh parsley sprig after meals or as needed.
	Comments: Some natural breath fresheners contain parsley oil as a key ingredient.
Spirulina	**Dosage:** Rinse the mouth with a commercial chlorophyll-rich "green" drink (follow package instructions).
	Comments: Alternatively, tablets can be chewed.

Some dosages may be supplied by supplements you are already taking—see page 39.

Place just a drop or two of **peppermint** oil on the tongue a couple of times a day—larger amounts of the pure oil may cause digestive upset. Beyond its pleasant taste and aroma, peppermint oil is effective in killing bacteria. Drinking peppermint or spearmint teas, as well as plenty of plain water, may also help to fight bad breath by keeping the mouth moist.

Another approach is to chew on several **fennel** seeds, anise seeds, or cloves to freshen the breath; they can be conveniently carried in a small, sealed container. Fresh **parsley** has a similar effect; it's also high in chlorophyll (the chemical that gives plants their green color), which has long been recognized as a powerful breath freshener. Chlorophyll is also found in commercially available "green" drinks containing **spirulina,** wheat grass, chlorella, or other herbs. These chlorophyll-rich liquids are best swished around the mouth, then swallowed. Alternatively, try spirulina tablets, which should be chewed thoroughly.

What else you can do

☑ Brush your teeth after each meal and floss at least once a day. When you can't brush, rinse your mouth out with some water.

☑ Use a moist toothbrush, a tongue scraper (available at some pharmacies and health-food stores), or a metal spoon held upside down to scrape off any coating on the back of the tongue and cleanse that area.

☑ Avoid strong-smelling foods and alcohol; don't smoke.

☑ If a chronic sinus infection or postnasal drip is contributing to bad breath, consider using a sinus irrigator—a device found in most health-food stores that delivers a saltwater solution into the nostrils—to clean sinuses regularly.

FACTS & Tips

- Licorice-flavored anise seeds can easily be made into a breath-freshening mouthwash or beverage. Boil several teaspoons of seeds in one cup of water for a few minutes, then strain and cool.

- Ensure that your toothbrush remains bacteria-free by storing it in grapefruit seed extract or hydrogen peroxide; rinse it well before brushing. An electric toothbrush sanitizer may also be effective.

- Commercially available mouthwashes may reduce bacteria in the mouth, but they have only a temporary effect and are not a substitute for regular flossing and brushing.

- Some practitioners believe that poor digestion may contribute to some cases of bad breath. They advise adding extra fluid and fiber (such as psyllium) to the diet to avoid constipation. Colon-cleansing herbal formulas, available at health-food stores, may also be recommended.

Did You Know?

In many ancient Asian societies, subjects were required to chew several cloves to freshen their breath before they were allowed to have an audience with the king.

bronchitis

This generally temporary illness often develops after a cold or the flu. However, for about 5% of Americans (mostly smokers), bronchitis is a serious, recurring disease. Acute and chronic symptoms are similar and may be effectively relieved with the use of certain supplements.

SYMPTOMS

Acute bronchitis
- *Cough that produces white, yellow, or green phlegm.*
- *Low fever (100°F or less).*
- *Coarse breath sounds (called rhonchi) that change or disappear when coughing.*
- *Chest muscle pain from coughing.*

Chronic bronchitis
- *Persistent cough producing yellow, white, or green phlegm for at least three months of the year for two consecutive years.*
- *Wheezing, breathlessness.*
- *Coughing during exertion, no matter how slight.*

When to Call Your Doctor

- If a persistent cough interferes with your sleep or compromises your daily activities.
- If mucus becomes darker or thicker or increases significantly in volume.
- If your fever is above 100°F.
- If your breathing becomes increasingly difficult or if you cough up blood.
- If your symptoms last more than 48 hours.
- Reminder: If you have a medical condition, talk to your doctor before taking supplements.

What it is

Bronchitis is an inflammation of the windpipe and bronchial tubes, the large airways that lead to the lungs. These airways swell and thicken, paralyzing the cilia, the tiny hairs that line the respiratory tract and sweep away dust and germs. Mucus builds up, resulting in a cough.

There are two types of bronchitis: acute and chronic. Acute is marked by a slight fever that lasts for a few days and a cough that goes away after several weeks. In chronic bronchitis, a hacking cough along with discolored phlegm persists for several months and may disappear and recur.

What causes it

Acute bronchitis frequently follows a cold or the flu, though it can also result from a bacterial infection or exposure to chemical fumes. Chronic bronchitis occurs when the lungs have been irritated for a long time. The primary cause of chronic bronchitis is cigarette smoking. People with long-term exposure to secondhand smoke, workers routinely exposed to chemical fumes, and individuals with chronic allergies are also susceptible.

How supplements can help

Supplements can help strengthen your body's immune response and also stimulate its normal process of loosening and bringing up phlegm. The supplements for acute bronchitis should be taken only while you are ill. Those for chronic bronchitis require long-term use.

Astragalus root helps fight off the viral or bacterial infections that can lead to bronchitis.

Supplement Recommendations

Vitamin C/ Flavonoids	**Dosage:** 1,000 mg vitamin C and 500 mg flavonoids 3 times a day. **Comments:** Reduce vitamin C dose if diarrhea develops.
Vitamin A	**Dosage:** 25,000 IU a day for 1 month. **Comments:** Women who are pregnant or considering pregnancy should not exceed 5,000 IU a day.
Horehound	**Dosage:** As a tea, 3 or 4 cups a day. **Comments:** Use 1 or 2 tsp. per cup of hot water; add honey to taste.
NAC	**Dosage:** 500 mg (acute) or 250 mg (chronic) 3 times a day. **Comments:** Take between meals. For long-term use, add 30 mg zinc and 2 mg copper daily.
Echinacea	**Dosage:** 200 mg 4 times daily (acute) or twice a day (chronic). **Comments:** Standardized to contain 3.5% echinacosides.
Astragalus	**Dosage:** 200 mg 4 times daily (acute) or twice a day (chronic). **Comments:** Supplying 0.5% glucosides and 70% polysaccharides.

Note: Consider using supplements in **blue** first; those in **black** may also be beneficial. Some dosages may be supplied by supplements you are already taking—see page 39.

see page 39

The following vitamins should be used daily. **Vitamin C** is particularly helpful in fighting off viruses that attack the respiratory system. Take it coupled with powerful antioxidants called **flavonoids** (or bioflavonoids), which are natural antivirals and anti-inflammatories. **Vitamin A** is also important for immune health. In chronic bronchitis, both vitamins assist in the healing of damaged lung tissue.

For an acute attack, drink **horehound** tea to help thin mucus secretions. Or use the herb slippery elm in place of horehound if you prefer. The amino acid-like substance **NAC** (N-acetylcysteine) also thins mucus and has been reported to reduce the recurrence rate of bronchitis.

The herbs **echinacea** and **astragalus** have antibacterial, antiviral, and immune-strengthening properties. At the higher doses, they can be used to fight off acute bronchitis. For chronic or seasonal bronchitis, try taking the following herbs in rotation: echinacea (200 mg twice a day), astragalus (200 mg twice a day), pau d'arco (250 mg twice a day), and 1,500 mg of reishi or 600 mg of maitake mushrooms a day. Use one herb for one week, then switch to another; continue this cycle as long as needed.

What else you can do

☑ Quit smoking—and avoid situations where others smoke.

☑ Drink plenty of fluids, such as diluted fruit juices and herbal teas. Dehydration can cause mucus to become thick and difficult to cough up.

☑ Eliminate the use of aerosol products (hair sprays, deodorants, and insecticides), which can irritate airway passages.

☑ Stay indoors when the air quality is poor if you have chronic bronchitis.

FACTS & Tips

■ When suffering from bronchitis, people often have difficulty breathing while they're eating. So try to avoid foods that are hard to chew, such as meats and raw vegetables.

■ Antihistamines and decongestants won't help alleviate lung symptoms—and they may actually make your condition worse. That's because these drugs can dry up and thicken mucus, making it more difficult for you to cough up.

Did You Know?

Only 10% of bronchitis cases are the result of a bacterial infection, so don't automatically assume you need antibiotics for this condition. Such drugs can reduce the body's levels of "good" bacteria, and they can also make individual bacterial strains more resistant to the antibiotics themselves.

burns

Most burns are not serious and can be managed with simple care at home. Soothing herbal ointments such as aloe vera or calendula can be applied to mild burns. In addition, a number of vitamins, minerals, and other supplements can be taken orally to help promote healing and prevent infection.

SYMPTOMS

First-degree burns
- *Tenderness, redness.*
- *Possible swelling.*

Second-degree burns
- *Pain, redness, blisters.*
- *Mild to moderate swelling.*

Third-degree burns
- *No immediate pain or bleeding because nerves are damaged.*
- *Charred skin or black, white, or red skin.*
- *No blisters, but serious swelling.*

When to Call Your Doctor

- If a first-degree burn covers a large area or is very painful.
- If a second-degree burn occurs on your face or hands, or covers two or more inches of skin.
- If you have a third-degree, chemical, or electrical burn— go to the hospital.
- If you have fever, vomiting, chills, or swollen glands; if pus forms in blisters; or if an unpleasant odor emanates from the burn—these may be signs of infection.
- If you are in doubt about the severity of a burn.
- Reminder: If you have a medical condition, talk to your doctor before taking supplements.

What it is

A burn is damage to the skin caused by heat, chemicals, or electricity. Most burns occur at home, and occasionally they require hospitalization. Varying in depth and size, burns are classified as first, second, or third degree. Most sunburns, for example, are considered first-degree burns because they involve only the outer layer of skin, whereas second-degree burns injure part of the underlying skin layer. Affecting all the skin layers, third-degree burns cause harm to the muscles, bones, nerves, and blood vessels below. They are always a medical emergency and require timely treatment, such as skin grafting, to aid recovery and minimize scarring.

What causes it

Burns are commonly caused by scalding water, hot oil or grease, hot foods, or overexposure to sun. More serious injuries may result from fire, steam, or chemicals. Electrical burns, usually occurring from contact with faulty or uninsulated wiring, can be deceptive: Skin damage may be minimal, but internal injuries can be extensive.

How supplements can help

Self-care is most appropriate for first-degree and some small second-degree burns (more serious burns demand medical attention). To treat, immerse the burned area in cool water for about 15 minutes (be careful not to break any blisters) or apply cool compresses. Once the burn has cooled, apply **aloe vera gel,** a dressing soaked in **chamomile** tea, or

One of the most popular and effective natural remedies for a burn is the clear, soothing gel of the aloe plant.

Aloe vera gel	**Dosage:** Apply gel to affected areas of skin as needed. **Comments:** Use fresh aloe leaf or store-bought gel.
Calendula cream	**Dosage:** Apply cream to burns. **Comments:** Standardized to contain at least 2% calendula.
Gotu kola	**Dosage:** 200 mg extract or 400-500 mg crude herb twice a day. **Comments:** Extract standardized to contain 10% asiaticosides.
Vitamin A	**Dosage:** 50,000 IU a day for no more than 10 days. **Comments:** Women who are pregnant or considering pregnancy should not exceed 5,000 IU a day.
Vitamin C	**Dosage:** 1,000 mg 3 times a day until healed. **Comments:** Reduce dose if diarrhea develops.
Vitamin E	**Dosage:** 400 IU a day until healed. **Comments:** Creams containing vitamin E are available and may prevent scarring when applied topically.
Zinc	**Dosage:** 30 mg a day. **Comments:** Do not exceed 150 mg zinc a day from all sources.
Chamomile	**Dosage:** Use a strong tea: 2 or 3 tsp. dried herb for each cup of hot water. Cool quickly in freezer or with ice cubes. **Comments:** Apply tea-soaked cloth to burn for about 15 minutes.
Echinacea	**Dosage:** 200 mg 3 times a day. **Comments:** Standardized to contain at least 3.5% echinacosides.

Note: Consider using supplements in **blue** first; those in **black** may also be beneficial. Some dosages may be supplied by supplements you are already taking—see page 39.

Some dosages may be supplied by supplements you are already taking—see page 39.

FACTS & Tips

- If you don't have any aloe vera or chamomile on hand for your burn, try a potato instead. Put several slices of raw potato on the affected skin; replace them several times—every two or three minutes—before applying a dressing. The starch in the potato forms a protective layer that may help soothe the burn.
- Milk can also be a fairly effective first-aid remedy for minor burns. Soak a terry cloth towel or piece of cotton flannel in milk and use it as a compress for 15 minutes or so. Repeat this procedure every two to six hours. Be sure to rinse the skin between applications; soured milk can begin to smell.

LATEST FINDINGS

- Aloe vera gel significantly speeds healing, according to a study of 27 people with fairly bad burns. Those patients who were treated with aloe vera healed in 12 days on average, versus 18 days for those who used a regular gauze dressing.

lavender oil directly to the injured area to relieve pain and inflammation and soothe the skin. Then, use infection-fighting **calendula cream** or goldenseal cream on any raw areas and cover with a light dressing.

During the healing process, the body needs extra nutrients. These should be taken for a week or two, until the burn heals. In combination, the herbs **gotu kola** (which stimulates the growth of connective tissue in the skin) and **echinacea, vitamins A, C,** and **E,** and the mineral **zinc** all work together to boost the immune response, repair skin and tissues, and prevent scarring.

What else you can do

- ☑ Gently cleanse burns daily using mild soap, taking care not to break any blisters; rinse well. Use sterile gauze dressings to keep burns dry and protected from dirt and bacteria.
- ☑ Drink plenty of fluids while your skin is healing.
- ☑ Avoid exposing your burned skin to hot showers or the sun.

Did You Know?

Butter is an old folk remedy for burns—but don't use it. Just like other oils or greasy ointments, butter traps heat, slows healing, and increases the risk of later infection.

cancer

Conventional cancer treatments, including surgery, radiation, and chemotherapy, are often highly effective in battling this frightening illness. Gentle natural therapies may be used in conjunction with traditional methods to help curb their troublesome side effects and even boost their potency.

SYMPTOMS

- ■ *Unusual bleeding or discharge.*
- ■ *A change in either bowel or bladder habits.*
- ■ *Chronic indigestion or difficulty swallowing.*
- ■ *Unexplained increased appetite or weight loss.*
- ■ *A sore that doesn't heal.*
- ■ *Thickening or lump in the breast, testicles, or elsewhere.*
- ■ *Persistent cough, hoarseness, or sore throat.*
- ■ *A change in a wart or mole.*
- ■ *Unexplained fatigue.*

When to Call Your Doctor

- ■ If you have any symptom of cancer for two weeks or longer, and there is no other obvious cause.
- ■ Reminder: If you have a medical condition, talk to your doctor before taking supplements.

What it is

There are more than a hundred types of cancer, all marked by uncontrolled growth of abnormal cells. Most begin as solid tumors, from which cancer cells can spread (metastasize) to other parts of the body. Untreated, cancer cells can overpower normal cells and sap the body's vital nutrients, resulting in grave illness or even death.

What causes it

Why healthy cells turn cancerous is unknown. But such factors as smoking, excessive sun exposure, pollutants, stress, and a poor diet appear to play a role. Any of these may weaken the immune system, which is then unable to attack cancer cells effectively, or expose the body to free radicals, unstable oxygen molecules that can damage cells. Heredity also seems to be a key element in the development of many types of cancer.

How supplements can help

In cancer treatment, supplements stir especially intense debate. Studies conflict, and a parade of fraudulent "miracle cures" are offered—usually at a steep price. But a number of supplements, taken daily over the long term, do show special promise as valuable additions to conventional cancer therapies.

Vitamin A, along with the antioxidants **vitamin C, vitamin E, carotenoids** (especially beta-carotene and lycopene), **selenium,** and **coenzyme Q$_{10}$,** helps protect cells from free radicals and

Formulas that contain a mixture of various carotenoids provide a potent blend of cell-protecting antioxidants.

Supplement Recommendations

Vitamin A	**Dosage:** 50,000 IU a day for 1 month, then 25,000 IU a day. **Comments:** Take only 5,000 IU a day if you may become pregnant.
Vitamin C/ Vitamin E	**Dosage:** 2,000 mg vitamin C 3 times a day; 400 IU vitamin E twice a day. **Comments:** Vitamin C helps boost the effects of vitamin E.
Carotenoids	**Dosage:** 3 pills mixed carotenoids a day with food. **Comments:** Each pill should supply 25,000 IU vitamin A activity.
Selenium	**Dosage:** 200 mcg a day. **Comments:** Don't exceed 600 mcg daily; higher doses may be toxic.
Coenzyme Q$_{10}$	**Dosage:** 200 mg each morning. **Comments:** For best absorption, take with food.
Amino acids	**Dosage:** Mixed amino acids (see label for dosage), plus NAC (500 mg 3 times a day) and L-glutathione (250 mg twice a day). **Comments:** Take L-glutathione separately from other amino acids.
Echinacea	**Dosage:** 200 mg 3 times a day. **Comments:** Rotate in 3-week cycles with astragalus (400 mg twice a day), pau d'arco (500 mg twice a day), and mushrooms (below).
Mushrooms	**Dosage:** 500 mg reishi, 400 mg shiitake, 200 mg maitake 3 times a day; and/or 3,000 mg *Coriolus versicolor* divided into 2 daily doses. **Comments:** Avoid reishi mushrooms if you're on anticoagulants.

Some dosages may be supplied by supplements you are already taking—see page 39.

may inhibit the growth of cancerous cells. These supplements may be particularly beneficial for people who have undergone chemotherapy or radiation—procedures that damage healthy cells as they attack cancer cells. **Amino acids** may speed healing and slow tumor growth as well.

Rotating **echinacea** in three-week cycles with extracts of medicinal **mushrooms** and other immune-boosting herbs may help to strengthen overall immunity during cancer treatments. (Vitamin C also bolsters the immune system, aiding it in fighting off any cancer cells remaining in the body after treatment.) The *Coriolus versicolor* mushroom has shown particular promise against lung, stomach, and colon cancers. Taking a liver detoxification formula (sometimes called a lipotropic combination in health-food stores) to help prevent the buildup of dangerous cancer-promoting toxins in the body may also be a good idea.

What else you can do

- ☑ Eat a balanced diet, rich in vitamins and minerals.
- ☑ Join a support group: Studies show this step can prolong your survival.
- ☑ Try exercise, meditation, biofeedback, massage, or imaging techniques to help reduce stress, lessen anxiety, and ease symptoms.

cancer prevention

Lifestyle choices are thought to contribute to about 75% of all cancer cases. The strategies you can adopt to lower your risk of developing the disease range from getting regular screening exams to boosting your intake of cancer-fighting antioxidants.

What it is

Almost every cell in the body is replaced regularly, and within each cell is a code that tells it how and when to multiply and when to die. Cancer occurs when something goes wrong with this process, allowing cells to develop abnormally and grow uncontrollably. As these cells proliferate and spread, they damage healthy tissue, blood vessels, and nerves. Fortunately, in many cases the body is able to identify these changes and destroy the abnormal cells before they become a threat to health.

What causes it

Tobacco smoke, excessive exposure to radiation (from X rays or the ultraviolet light of the sun), some industrial chemicals, certain viruses, and some hormones all increase your risk of cancer. Heredity and dietary choices also play a major role in cancer risk: Excessive amounts of fat, alcohol, and pickled and smoked foods may contribute to cancer, just as fiber, certain nutrients, and fruits and vegetables help protect against it.

Not everyone exposed to cancer-causing agents, however, will be affected by the disease. A major factor in the development of cancer appears to be the immune system's ability to detect and destroy free radicals, unstable oxygen molecules that cause cell damage. Antioxidants, compounds produced by the body or derived from food and supplements, can inactivate free radicals and aid the immune system in eradicating early cancer cells.

How supplements can help

Though not a substitute for poor lifestyle choices, supplements may help protect against a variety of cancers. Taking several antioxidants daily is the first line of defense. **Vitamin C** with **flavonoids** play a role in preventing many cancers, such as those of the lung, esophagus, stomach, bladder, cervix, and colon. **Vitamin E** may reduce the risk of breast, colon, prostate, and possibly other cancers. The mineral **selenium** shows promise as a weapon against a number of cancers as well. Everyone who is concerned about cancer prevention should take these four supplements together.

Experts think green tea, in leaf or capsule form, may contain one of the most potent antioxidants ever discovered.

Supplement Recommendations

Vitamin C/ Flavonoids	**Dosage:** 1,000 mg vitamin C and 500 mg flavonoids 3 times a day. **Comments:** Reduce vitamin C dose if diarrhea develops.
Vitamin E	**Dosage:** 400 IU a day. **Comments:** Check with your doctor if taking anticoagulant drugs.
Selenium	**Dosage:** 400 mcg a day. **Comments:** Don't exceed 600 mcg daily; higher doses may be toxic.
Green tea extract	**Dosage:** 250 mg twice a day. **Comments:** Standardized to contain at least 50% polyphenols.
Grape seed extract	**Dosage:** 100 mg each morning. **Comments:** Standardized to contain 92%-95% proanthocyanidins.
Flaxseed oil	**Dosage:** 1 tbsp. (14 grams) a day. **Comments:** Can be mixed with food; take in the morning.
Coenzyme Q$_{10}$	**Dosage:** 50 mg each morning. **Comments:** For best absorption, take with food.
Glutathione	**Dosage:** 100 mg L-glutathione each morning. **Comments:** Take with food to minimize stomach irritation.
Carotenoids	**Dosage:** 1 pill mixed carotenoids a day with food. **Comments:** Each pill should supply 25,000 IU vitamin A activity.

Some dosages may be supplied by supplements you are already taking—see page 39.

For additional protection, the nutritional supplements **green tea extract** and **grape seed extract** may help prevent a host of cancers, including lung, breast, stomach, colon, prostate, and skin. Though it's not an antioxidant, **flaxseed oil** is important because it contains compounds called lignans, which may protect against breast, colon, and prostate cancers.

If you wish, you can add the nutrient **coenzyme Q$_{10}$** and the amino acid **glutathione,** both of which also support the immune system. Take **carotenoids** only if you don't eat many fruits and vegetables. These substances—which represent the yellow, orange, and red pigments in fruits and vegetables—help prevent a number of cancers. For example, the carotenoid lycopene (which gives tomatoes their red color) is particularly beneficial in warding off lung and prostate cancers.

What else you can do

☑ Don't smoke or chew tobacco. Drink alcohol only in moderation.

☑ Eat a diet low in saturated fat and high in fiber. Include plenty of fruits, vegetables, whole grains, and beans.

☑ Shield yourself from the sun and wear sunscreen when outdoors.

☑ Exercise for at least 30 minutes a day.

canker sores

Given their diminutive size, it's hard to fathom how canker sores can hurt as much as they do. Commonsense self-care measures can assist you in avoiding these painful mouth ulcers, and supplements may help you reduce their frequency and speed their healing.

SYMPTOMS

- *Small white or yellowish sores surrounded by a red area on the tongue, gums, or soft palate, or inside the lips or cheeks.*
- *Burning, itchiness, or a tingling feeling before a sore appears.*
- *Raw pain when eating and speaking; strongest during the first few days.*

When to Call Your Doctor

- If pain is too severe to consume adequate liquids.
- If more than four sores appear throughout your mouth.
- If sores persist longer than two weeks.
- If fever is 101°F or higher.
- If sores occur more than two or three times a year.
- Reminder: If you have a medical condition, talk to your doctor before taking supplements.

What it is

Though not serious, canker sores can be so bothersome that they can cause intense pain when talking, kissing, drinking, and eating. Affecting women more often than men, these shallow, ulcerated areas appear singly or in small clusters inside the mouth, and range in size from as tiny as a pinhead to as large as a quarter. Cankers emerge fairly suddenly and usually go away within one to three weeks. Fortunately, it is possible to ease the discomfort they cause.

What causes it

The prevailing view is that the sores are triggered by stress, which can cause the body's immune system to overreact to bacteria normally present in the mouth. Canker sores can also be precipitated by a number of actions, such as irritating the mouth cavity with a rough filling or a jagged or chipped tooth or wearing ill-fitting dentures. Maybe you've unconsciously gnawed the inside of your cheek, used a toothbrush with very hard bristles, or brushed too vigorously. Occasionally, even eating acidic, spicy, or salty foods—tomatoes, citrus fruits, hot peppers, cinnamon, nuts, or potato chips—can be the initiating factor.

Some experts believe recurring cankers are an allergic reaction to food preservatives (benzoic acid, methylparaben, or sorbic acid, to name a few) or to something in a food. They single out gluten, the protein found in wheat and some other grains, as the most likely offender.

A liquid form of goldenseal can promote healing when applied directly to a painful canker sore.

Supplement Recommendations

Lysine	**Dosage:** 500 mg L-lysine 3 times a day. **Comments:** Take on empty stomach; discontinue when sores heal.
Echinacea	**Dosage:** 200 mg 2 or 3 times a day at first sign of a sore. **Comments:** Begin with higher dose and reduce as sore heals. As a preventive, take 200 mg each morning for 3 weeks of each month.
Vitamin C/ Flavonoids	**Dosage:** 1,000 mg vitamin C and 500 mg flavonoids 3 times a day. **Comments:** Reduce vitamin C dose if diarrhea develops.
Licorice (DGL)	**Dosage:** Chew 1 or 2 deglycyrrhizinated licorice (DGL) wafers (380 mg) 3 or 4 times a day. **Comments:** Take between meals.
Goldenseal	**Dosage:** Apply liquid form to the sore 3 times a day. **Comments:** After application, wait at least an hour before eating.
Zinc lozenges	**Dosage:** 1 lozenge every 2 hours for 3 or 4 days. **Comments:** Do not exceed 150 mg zinc a day from all sources.
Vitamin B complex	**Dosage:** 1 pill each morning with food. **Comments:** Look for a B-50 complex with 50 mcg vitamin B_{12} and biotin; 400 mcg folic acid; and 50 mg of all other B vitamins.

Note: Consider using supplements in **blue** first; those in **black** may also be beneficial. Some dosages may be supplied by supplements you are already taking—see page 39.

How supplements can help

When canker sores erupt, turn to one or more of the following supplements. First try **lysine**—a deficiency in this amino acid has been associated with canker sores. **Echinacea** strengthens the immune system, and lower doses of this herb (200 mg each morning, three weeks a month) may also prevent cankers from forming. Another immune-booster, **vitamin C** helps heal the mouth's mucous membranes; **flavonoids** are natural compounds that enhance the effectiveness of this vitamin. **Licorice (DGL)** wafers coat and protect sores from irritants and help them heal. **Goldenseal** in liquid form applied directly to the sore also promotes healing. Instead of DGL or goldenseal, you may want to try **zinc lozenges** to speed healing and boost your resistance. People who get canker sores frequently may be deficient in B vitamins; a daily **vitamin B complex** is useful as a preventive.

What else you can do

☑ Keep your mouth clean and healthy by flossing and brushing your teeth at least twice a day. Be gentle and use a soft-bristled brush.

☑ See your dentist if a tooth problem is irritating your mouth.

☑ Be aware if you're constantly gnawing at the inside of your cheek.

☑ Don't eat spicy foods if you're prone to recurrent canker sores. Stay away from coffee and chewing gum, other known irritants.

FACTS & Tips

■ You might think that onions, with their strong flavor, would irritate the mouth and cause canker sores, but eating them regularly might actually prevent these sores. Onions contain sulfur compounds that have antiseptic properties, and they are also a leading source of quercetin, a flavonoid that stops the body from releasing inflammatory substances in response to allergens.

■ If supplements or other self-treatments don't help relieve the pain or frequency of canker sores, you might want to try a new prescription oral paste known by the generic name of amlexanox. A small amount applied as soon as sores appear seems to inhibit the formation and release of certain substances in the body that are known to cause allergic reactions and inflammation.

Did You Know?

Even the ancient Greeks were plagued by canker sores. It was Hippocrates, called the father of medicine, who in the fourth century B.C. coined the medical term for them: *aphthous stomatitis*.

carpal tunnel syndrome

If wrist pain wakes you at night or you feel pins and needles in your hands when you drive, you may have this disorder. Though considered a condition of modern times, carpal tunnel syndrome has actually been recognized since the 1880s.

SYMPTOMS

- *Numbness or tingling in the thumb and the first three fingers.*
- *Shooting pains in the wrist and forearm, which may radiate into the shoulder and neck.*
- *Weakness in the hand; difficulty picking up and holding objects.*
- *Feeling that the fingers are swollen when no swelling is visible.*

When to Call Your Doctor

- If your fingers feel stiff and painful—you may be suffering from arthritis.
- If wrist pain interferes with daily activities.
- If numbness and pain continue despite home care and supplements—your hands and wrists may need to be immobilized for a short period of time.
- Reminder: If you have a medical condition, talk to your doctor before taking supplements.

What it is

The bones and ligaments in the wrist (medically known as the carpus, from the Greek *karpos*) form a pathway called the carpal tunnel. Here the median nerve, which controls movement and feeling in most of the hand, and the tendons that connect the arm and hand muscles pass from the forearm into the hand. The tunnel can be narrowed by swelling of ligaments or tendons, bone dislocation, bone spurs, or fluid retention. This narrowing may compress the median nerve, causing the pain, numbness, and weakness characteristic of carpal tunnel syndrome.

Symptoms may develop gradually or suddenly, and they tend to be most painful at night (95% of patients with this condition report being awakened by pain). Symptoms may last for a few days and disappear without treatment or persist for months and require medical intervention.

What causes it

Carpal tunnel syndrome is usually a stress injury induced by prolonged, repeated movements of the hands or fingers. Overuse of the hands on the job (typing at a computer, working on an assembly line) or during leisure activities (knitting, playing musical instruments) can inflame the tendons or ligaments, causing them to swell and compress the median nerve.

Changes in hormonal balance during pregnancy, while taking birth control pills, or during menopause may also bring on or worsen carpal tunnel symptoms. Underlying disease (diabetes, hypothyroidism, Raynaud's disease, rheumatoid arthritis) or trauma to the wrist may result in carpal tunnel syndrome as well. About 5 million Americans suffer to some degree from this disorder. Carpal tunnel syndrome occurs three times more often in women than it does in men and is particularly common in overweight women ages 30 to 60 who have been pregnant.

Vitamin B₆ may reduce the nerve-related symptoms of carpal tunnel.

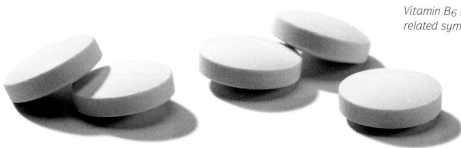

Supplement Recommendations

Vitamin B$_6$	**Dosage:** 50 mg 3 times a day until symptoms subside.
	Comments: 200 mg daily over long term can cause nerve damage.
Bromelain	**Dosage:** 1,000 mg twice a day during acute phase. Reduce to 500 mg twice a day when symptoms subside. Take between meals.
	Comments: Provides 8,000 GDU or 12,000 MCU in acute phase.
Turmeric	**Dosage:** 400 mg 3 times a day.
	Comments: Standardized to contain 95% curcumin. Should be used with bromelain.

Some dosages may be supplied by supplements you are already taking—see page 39.

Some dosages may be supplied by supplements you are already taking—see page 39.

How supplements can help

Several studies have suggested that a **vitamin B$_6$** deficiency can make you susceptible to the numbness and pain of carpal tunnel syndrome. This vitamin is important in maintaining healthy nerve tissue, relieving inflammation, and improving circulation. It also may increase the brain's production of the nerve chemical GABA (gamma-aminobutyric acid), which helps control pain sensations. If you don't notice any improvement after taking vitamin B$_6$ for three weeks, switch to pyridoxal-5-phosphate (P-5-P), a form of the vitamin that the body eventually produces as it breaks down vitamin B$_6$. Some people find this form works better for them.

In addition to B$_6$, **bromelain,** a powerful anti-inflammatory enzyme found in pineapple, is very effective in treating the inflammation and any resulting pain. The combination of bromelain and vitamin B$_6$ works better than either supplement alone. **Turmeric,** a member of the ginger family, is another useful herb. When turmeric is taken with bromelain, they enhance each other's anti-inflammatory properties and together may help relieve the pain of carpal tunnel syndrome. Though turmeric is safe to use over the long term, cut the dose in half once your symptoms subside. (This herb can be expensive.)

What else you can do

☑ Take frequent breaks when performing any repetitive hand activity, such as typing, knitting, or playing an instrument. Stop at least once an hour to flex your fingers and shake your hands.

☑ Apply ice to your wrists when pain strikes. Use a flexible ice pack—or even a bag of frozen peas—and put it on for 10 minutes every hour to ease the pain and reduce the inflammation.

☑ Elevate your wrists with a pillow when you lie down.

cataracts

Although half the people over age 50 and three-quarters of those over age 75 develop cataracts, the condition isn't an inevitable part of aging. Recent studies show that certain lifestyle strategies can lessen your chance of developing this serious but treatable vision disorder.

SYMPTOMS

- *Gradual and painless blurring or dimming of vision.*
- *Increased sensitivity to sun glare or car headlights at night.*
- *Seeing halos around lights.*
- *Changes in color perception.*

When to Call Your Doctor

- If you begin to develop cataract symptoms.
- Reminder: If you have a medical condition, talk to your doctor before taking supplements.

What it is

The eye's lens is normally transparent; it refracts and focuses light on the retina, which allows a clear image to form. When the proteins in the lens break down, they clump together and form opaque spots called cataracts. These spots hinder light from being transmitted properly to the retina, and vision becomes cloudy or blurry. The degree of impaired vision depends on the cataract's size, density, and location on the lens.

What causes it

Cataracts may develop as a result of age-related body changes; but some experts now think that the majority of cases can be attributed to smoking or to lifetime exposure to ultraviolet (UV) light from the sun. A low level of antioxidants (vitamins C and E, beta-carotene, and selenium) may also be a factor. These compounds can squelch free radicals—unstable oxygen molecules—that can damage the lens. (Normally, the lens has a high concentration of glutathione, an antioxidant produced by the body.) In addition, having diabetes or being overweight increases the risk of cataracts, probably because high levels of sugar (glucose) in the blood contribute to the destruction of lens proteins. Injury to the eye can cause cataracts too.

How supplements can help

Taking supplements before a cataract appears may postpone its development or prevent it altogether. In the early stages of a cataract, supplements may slow its growth. Only surgery will remove a cataract, however.

Both **vitamin C** and **vitamin E,** potent antioxidants, may protect the lens from damage from cigarette smoke and UV light. **Selenium,** another antioxidant, also helps neutralize free radicals. The herb **bilberry** is rich in flavonoids and helps eliminate toxins from the lens and retina. In one study, bilberry combined with vitamin E stopped the progression of cataracts in 48 of 50 participants.

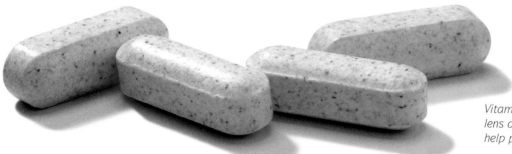

Vitamin C protects the lens of the eye and may help prevent cataracts.

Supplement Recommendations

Vitamin C

Dosage: 1,000 mg twice a day.
Comments: Reduce dose if diarrhea develops.

Vitamin E

Dosage: 400 IU a day.
Comments: Check with your doctor if taking anticoagulant drugs.

Selenium

Dosage: 400 mcg a day.
Comments: Don't exceed 600 mcg daily; higher doses may be toxic.

Bilberry

Dosage: 80 mg 3 times a day.
Comments: Standardized to contain 25% anthocyanosides. May be included in nutritional supplement eye formulas.

Ginkgo biloba

Dosage: 40 mg 3 times a day.
Comments: Standardized to have at least 24% flavone glycosides.

Alpha-lipoic acid

Dosage: 150 mg a day.
Comments: Take in the morning with or without food.

Grape seed extract

Dosage: 100 mg twice a day.
Comments: Standardized to contain 92%-95% proanthocyanidins.

Flaxseed oil

Dosage: 1 tbsp. (14 grams) a day.
Comments: Can be mixed with food; take in the morning.

Note: Consider using supplements in blue first; those in black may also be beneficial. Some dosages may be supplied by supplements you are already taking—see page 39.

This combination of supplements usually provides adequate cataract protection; however, the following nutrients may also be helpful: The herb **ginkgo biloba,** which improves circulation and has strong antioxidant properties, can be substituted for bilberry. Ginkgo may be a good choice for people who are already taking it for memory problems. **Alpha-lipoic acid** shows promise as a cataract preventive and also boosts the effectiveness of vitamins C and E. Because **grape seed extract** can have a therapeutic impact on even the tiniest blood vessels, it benefits circulation in the eye. Consider adding **flaxseed oil** to this regimen as well; its essential fatty acids nourish the eye. Riboflavin (vitamin B_2) is also important: Take 25 mg a day if you do not take a multivitamin or a B-complex supplement that supplies at least this amount.

What else you can do

☑ Quit smoking.
☑ Protect your eyes from UV rays by wearing sunglasses and a wide-brimmed hat when outdoors.
☑ Eat plenty of fresh fruits and vegetables; they're good sources of antioxidants.

chronic fatigue syndrome

Many people turn to supplements to combat the persistent tiredness and flulike symptoms that characterize this poorly understood and disabling disorder. Although no one knows its cause, a weakened immune system may be a factor.

SYMPTOMS

- *Continuing or recurring fatigue lasting at least six months and not relieved by sleep or rest.*
- *Memory loss, inability to concentrate, headaches.*
- *Low-grade fever, muscle or joint aches, sore throat, or swollen lymph nodes in neck or armpits.*

When to Call Your Doctor

- Fatigue that lasts longer than two weeks or is accompanied by sudden weight loss, muscle weakness, or other unusual symptoms may signal other, more serious ailments.
- Fatigue can be a side effect of certain medications. Your doctor can rule out other possible and often correctable causes.
- Have your doctor monitor your progress even if you are improving or if fatigue worsens despite home treatment.
- Reminder: If you have a medical condition, talk to your doctor before taking supplements.

What it is

Marked by profound and persistent exhaustion, chronic fatigue syndrome (CFS) affects more women than men, most younger than age 50. Patients feel weak and listless much of the time and often have difficulty sleeping, concentrating, and performing daily tasks; many also have underlying depression. Doctors disagree about whether CFS is a specific condition or a group of unrelated symptoms not attributable to a single cause.

What causes it

The specific cause of CFS is unknown, but an impaired immune response may play a role in its onset. People with CFS have other immune disturbances as well: About 65% are allergy sufferers (versus only 20% in the general population), and some have autoimmune disorders such as lupus, in which the immune system attacks the body's own healthy tissues.

Doctors aren't sure what triggers CFS. Many patients remember a flulike illness before their fatigue began, and CFS symptoms do suggest a lingering viral illness. Suspected infectious agents have included Epstein-Barr (the virus causing mononucleosis) and candida (the cause of yeast infections). Other theories suggest that CFS is caused by low blood pressure, brain inflammation, or abnormal levels of certain hormones. Nothing conclusive has been proved, however.

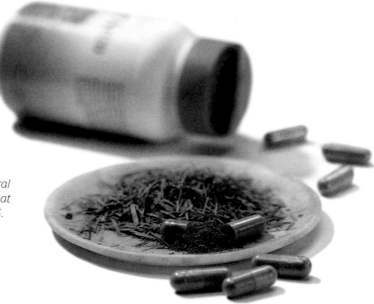

Pau d'arco is one of several immune-boosting herbs that may help people with CFS.

Supplement Recommendations

Vitamin C	**Dosage:** 2,000 mg 3 times a day. **Comments:** Reduce dose if diarrhea develops.
Carotenoids	**Dosage:** 2 pills mixed carotenoids a day with food. **Comments:** Each pill should supply 25,000 IU vitamin A activity.
Magnesium	**Dosage:** 400 mg once a day. **Comments:** Take with food; reduce dose if diarrhea develops.
Echinacea	**Dosage:** 200 mg twice a day. **Comments:** Standardized to contain at least 3.5% echinacosides. Limit consecutive use to 3 weeks or rotate with other herbs.
Siberian ginseng	**Dosage:** 100-300 mg twice a day. **Comments:** Standardized to contain at least 0.8% eleutherosides.
Licorice	**Dosage:** 200 mg 3 times a day. **Comments:** Standardized to contain 22% glycyrrhizin or glycyrrhizinic acid; can raise blood pressure.
Pantothenic acid	**Dosage:** 500 mg twice a day. **Comments:** Take with meals. Provides adrenal gland support.
Astragalus	**Dosage:** 200 mg standardized extract twice a day. **Comments:** Rotate in 3-week cycles with echinacea and pau d'arco.
Pau d'arco	**Dosage:** 250 mg twice a day. **Comments:** Standardized to contain 3% naphthoquinones.

Note: Consider using supplements in **blue** first; those in **black** may also be beneficial. Some dosages may be supplied by supplements you are already taking—see page 39.

How supplements can help

Supplement therapy aims to restore a healthy immune system, so begin with **vitamin C** and **carotenoids.** A powerful immune enhancer, **echinacea** can be added to the mix; it can be alternated with the herbs **astragalus,** which has antiviral and immunity-enhancing effects, **pau d'arco,** which fights many microbes (especially the yeast infections so common in those with low immunity), or goldenseal. For muscle pain, use **magnesium** too.

In addition, you can safely include the herbs **Siberian ginseng** and **licorice** and the B vitamin **pantothenic acid** to bolster the adrenal glands, which secrete hormones, such as cortisol, that counteract stress and boost energy. Allow a month for these supplements to take effect.

What else you can do

☑ Try behavioral counseling and relaxation techniques, such as hypnosis or meditation, to manage stress and treat any underlying depression.

☑ Get a good night's sleep. If needed, use supplements for insomnia, such as valerian, melatonin, or 5-HTP.

FACTS & Tips

■ Just one in every 10,000 adults who sees a doctor for fatigue actually has chronic fatigue syndrome. Many more have a condition called fibromyalgia, which can produce symptoms similar to those of CFS.

■ Chronic fatigue syndrome is not a new disease. In the 1800s, lingering fatigue was called neurasthenia; interestingly, it was often treated with licorice extract. From the 1930s through the 1950s, outbreaks of prolonged fatigue were reported in the U.S. and many other countries. But not until 1988 did the Centers for Disease Control and Prevention, the main federal public health agency, release comprehensive guidelines for diagnosing the syndrome, opening the way for further investigation of CFS in mainstream medicine.

LATEST FINDINGS

■ Mild aerobic exercise may be excellent for chronic fatigue syndrome, according to a recent study in the *British Medical Journal.* After a 12-week program of walking, swimming, or biking from 5 to 30 minutes a day, 55% of CFS patients felt "much" or "very much" better. Relaxation and stretching exercises may also work. But start and proceed slowly: If you do too much, you may suffer a setback. It may help to keep an energy diary—to record peaks and ebbs of energy—and plan your schedule around the times you routinely feel the best.

chronic pain

No matter where it hurts—in your head, toe, or anywhere in between—chronic pain can have a major impact on both physical and emotional well-being. Fortunately, natural therapies can be added to the wide range of treatments now available to help control pain.

What it is

The word "pain" evolved from the Latin *poena,* meaning punishment—a fitting derivation, as anyone who experiences chronic pain can attest. Whether it is in the form of aching, tingling, stabbing, shooting, or burning, prolonged and uncontrollable pain can adversely affect one's entire life. In addition to the physical discomfort, constant suffering can lead to anxiety, anger, and depression, which can all intensify the pain.

What causes it

Pain occurs when a nerve ending senses a source of distress and sends a signal to the brain. The pain can become chronic if this impulse continues. The causes of chronic pain are too numerous to list but include a poorly healing injury, arthritis, a pinched or irritated nerve, or an underlying disorder such as cancer. Unfortunately, in some cases, especially those involving the muscles and bones, the actual cause remains a mystery, making the condition especially difficult to treat.

How supplements can help

Under your doctor's supervision, you can use natural pain relievers, singly or together, for the long-term relief of all types of chronic pain. Most can also be taken with conventional painkillers: Generally, supplements are safer than those drugs and may reduce your need for them. The exception is **white willow bark,** which shouldn't be taken with aspirin; the two are so similar that combining them could increase the risk of aspirin-related side effects. (Both act to reduce levels of natural pain-causing compounds called prostaglandins.)

White willow bark can, however, be safely combined with other pain-relieving herbs. **Bromelain,** an anti-inflammatory protein derived from pineapple, may be particularly useful for inflammation-related pain and sports injuries. Other potentially helpful herbs include **ginger** (which, like white willow bark, acts on prostaglandins), meadowsweet, feverfew, cat's claw, devil's claw, pau d'arco, and turmeric.

Melatonin may be a good remedy if chronic pain keeps you from sleeping at night.

Supplement Recommendations

White willow bark	**Dosage:** 1 or 2 pills 3 times a day as needed for pain (follow package directions). **Comments:** Standardized to contain 15% salicin.
Bromelain	**Dosage:** 500 mg 3 times a day on an empty stomach. **Comments:** Should provide 6,000 GDU or 9,000 MCU daily.
Cayenne cream	**Dosage:** Apply cream thinly to painful areas several times a day. **Comments:** Standardized to contain 0.025%-0.075% capsaicin.
Ginger	**Dosage:** 100 mg 3 times a day. **Comments:** Look for supplements standardized to contain gingerols. Can use essential oil of ginger as part of a massage blend.
Peppermint oil	**Dosage:** Add a few drops oil to ½ ounce neutral oil. **Comments:** Apply to painful areas up to 4 times daily.
St. John's wort	**Dosage:** 300 mg 3 times a day. **Comments:** Standardized to contain 0.3% hypericin.
Kava	**Dosage:** 250 mg 3 times a day. **Comments:** Standardized to contain at least 30% kavalactones.
Melatonin	**Dosage:** 1-3 mg at bedtime. **Comments:** Start with lower dose and increase as needed.

Note: Consider using supplements in blue first; those in black may also be beneficial. Some dosages may be supplied by supplements you are already taking—see page 39.

Topical preparations can be beneficial too. **Cayenne cream** may be especially beneficial for arthritic joints, post-shingles pain, or nerve damage from diabetes or surgery (such as mastectomy or amputation); it may be less effective on large areas of the body because of the burning sensation it causes. Alternatively, try mixing a few drops of ginger, lavender, and birch oils with ½ ounce of a neutral oil (such as almond oil) and massaging the blend into the painful area. Other options include **peppermint oil,** wintergreen oil, or eucalyptus oil, which seem to work by quieting the nerve endings that transmit pain signals.

Supplements typically provide pain relief within three to four hours. If pain is accompanied by depression or anxiety, try **St. John's wort** first, and then **kava.** These herbs may have some direct pain-relieving properties as well. If pain is interfering with your ability to get a good night's sleep, consider **melatonin.**

What else you can do

☑ Consider acupuncture. Mind-body techniques—such as biofeedback, hypnosis, relaxation training, and behavioral counseling—may also help.

☑ Ask your doctor about pain clinics, which offer a range of treatments.

cold sores

Many people eventually become infected with the virus that causes the unsightly and painful lip blisters called cold sores. Using antioxidants, immune boosters, and especially the amino acid lysine, you'll have the tools to inhibit the virus and help heal the inflamed skin.

What it is

Cold sores are fluid-filled blisters that usually appear on the lips, though they can also develop on the gums, inner cheeks, roof of the mouth, or the area around the nostrils. In addition, the cold sore virus can spread by touch to the mucous membranes of the eyes, nose, and genitals—or to abrasions. Typically, cold sores (also called fever blisters) break and then form a scab, disappearing in a week to ten days.

What causes it

Cold sores are usually caused by herpes simplex type 1 virus (HSV-1). This virus is different from the one responsible for genital herpes—herpes simplex type 2—which is generally transmitted through sexual contact. Because the cold sore virus lies dormant in nerve cells after the first outbreak, new sores are likely to recur as frequently as every few weeks or as infrequently as every few years. Sores often reappear when the immune system is depressed by a fever or a viral infection such as a cold. Recurrences can also be triggered by fatigue, menstruation, stress, or exposure to sun and wind.

How supplements can help

The supplements listed can all help minimize outbreaks and speed healing. They should be used in combination at the first sign of a cold sore. Effects will be noticed in two or three days.

Most useful is the amino acid **lysine,** which, when taken orally, suppresses the growth of HSV-1; in cream form, lysine can be applied directly to the sores. It's fine to use long term and may help prevent cold sores from forming. Also effective is a **melissa cream** made from the potent antiviral herb *Melissa officinalis;* use at the first sign of tingling.

Vitamin C and **flavonoids** may help as well. As powerful antioxidants, they work to facilitate healing by eliminating naturally occurring, cell-damaging compounds known as free radicals; both also boost virus-fighting immune system cells. **Vitamin A** and **selenium** have antioxidant properties too. Along with **flaxseed oil,** they hasten the healing process

Lysine, the amino acid that helps prevent cold sores, is available in an easy-to-swallow tablet form.

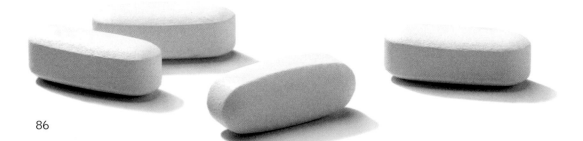

Supplement Recommendations

Lysine	**Dosage:** 1,000 mg 3 times a day for flare-ups, then 500 mg a day. **Comments:** Take on an empty stomach; don't take with milk.
Melissa cream	**Dosage:** Apply cream to sores 2-4 times a day. **Comments:** This herb is also called lemon balm.
Vitamin C/ Flavonoids	**Dosage:** 1,000 mg vitamin C and 500 mg flavonoids 3 times a day. **Comments:** Use for flare-ups; reduce dose if diarrhea develops.
Vitamin A	**Dosage:** 25,000 IU twice a day for 5 days. **Comments:** Women who are pregnant or considering pregnancy should not exceed 5,000 IU a day.
Echinacea/ Goldenseal	**Dosage:** 200 mg echinacea and 125 mg goldenseal 4 times a day. **Comments:** Sold singly or as combination supplement.
Selenium	**Dosage:** 600 mcg a day only during flare-ups. **Comments:** Don't exceed 600 mcg daily; higher doses may be toxic.
Flaxseed oil	**Dosage:** 1 tbsp. (14 grams) a day. **Comments:** Can be mixed with food; take in the morning.

Note: Consider using supplements in blue first; those in black may also be beneficial. Some dosages may be supplied by supplements you are already taking—see page 39.

by promoting cell renewal. (Vitamin A is also available in topical form; apply it directly to sores, alternately with vitamin E oil.) Flare-ups may be treated with the immune-enhancing herbs **echinacea** and **goldenseal,** which are natural antivirals and antibiotics.

To prevent cold sore recurrences, take a maintenance dose of 500 mg of lysine a day. (However, if you're using lysine long term, be sure to add an amino acid complex to provide a balanced mix of amino acids.) In addition, it's beneficial to alternate herbs: Try echinacea (200 mg a day); astragalus (200 mg a day); or a mixture of reishi (1,500 mg a day), shiitake (1,200 mg a day), and maitake mushrooms (600 mg a day). Take one herb for a week, then switch to another, and finally to the third.

What else you can do

☑ Apply sunscreen (SPF 15 or higher) to the lips to prevent recurrences. In a study involving people with recurrent cold sores, those who didn't use sunscreen developed a cold sore after 80 minutes in the sun.

☑ Don't touch the blisters. This can spread the virus, as can sharing personal items such as towels, razors, drinking glasses, or toothbrushes.

☑ Try meditation, yoga, or other forms of relaxation to reduce stress, which is thought to precipitate cold sores.

☑ Stay away from nuts, chocolate, whole-grain cereals, and gelatin. They contain a large amount of the amino acid arginine, which some doctors think triggers cold sores. Lysine may counteract its effect.

FACTS & Tips

■ As an alternative to using commercial melissa cream, try melissa tea, applied externally, to hasten the healing of cold sores. First, prepare a strong tea: Steep 2 or 3 teaspoons of the herb in a cup of very hot water for 15 minutes, then cool. Dab it on the sores with a cotton ball three times a day.

■ Supplements can be safely used with prescription antiviral creams, such as acyclovir or penciclovir, which also promote healing of cold sores.

LATEST FINDINGS

■ Vitamin C may be effective when applied topically, according to a recent study from Finland. Researchers soaked cotton pads in a vitamin C solution and applied them to cold sores. In those who were treated with vitamin C, blisters cleared up faster (3.4 days) than in those who received a placebo (5.9 days).

■ In studies at German hospitals, when a cream with a concentrated extract of melissa was used on patients during an initial outbreak of HSV-1, not one person had a recurrence. The cream also healed the cold sores more quickly than usual, often within five days. Patients with recurrent cold sores who applied melissa cream regularly either stopped developing sores or had less frequent recurrences.

Did You Know?

Holding an ice cube to the affected area for a few minutes several times a day can help reduce pain and dry out the cold sore.

colds and flu

Sooner or later, just about everyone comes down with a miserable cold or case of the flu—and some unfortunate people seem to get infected again and again. Vitamin C is probably the most familiar natural remedy for these viruses, but it's not the only one.

SYMPTOMS

- *Head and chest congestion.*
- *Sneezing and cough.*
- *Sore throat.*
- *Watery nasal discharge.*
- *Muscle aches.*
- *Fever and chills.*
- *Headache.*
- *Fatigue.*

When to Call Your Doctor

- If your temperature is above 100°F for three days or ever goes to 103°F or higher.
- If you have a sore throat combined with a fever that stays above 101°F for 24 hours—it may indicate strep throat, which requires antibiotics.
- If mucus is green, dark yellow, or brown—this may be a sign of a bacterial infection in the sinuses or lungs.
- If you have chest pain, shortness of breath, and difficulty breathing—this may mean you have pneumonia, especially if you also have a high fever.
- Reminder: If you have a medical condition, talk to your doctor before taking supplements.

What it is

Because the common cold and the flu are both respiratory infections, determining which you have may be difficult. Generally a cold comes on gradually, and the flu strikes suddenly—you can feel fine in the morning and lousy by afternoon. The classic cold symptoms—congestion, sore throat, and sneezing—are usually less severe than those of the flu, which often include fever, extreme fatigue, muscle aches, and headaches.

The amount of time needed to recover is different too. In general, a cold lasts about a week, but symptoms may trouble you for only three or four days if your immune system is in good shape. You can be sick with the flu for up to 10 days, and fatigue can persist for two to three weeks afterward. A cold rarely produces serious complications, but the flu can lead to bronchitis or pneumonia.

What causes it

Both colds and flu are caused by viruses that attach themselves to the lining of the nose or throat and then spread throughout the upper respiratory system and occasionally to the lungs as well. In response, the immune system floods the area with infection-fighting white blood cells. The symptoms of a cold or the flu aren't produced by the viruses but are actually the result of the body trying to stave off the infection. Colds and flu are more common in winter, when indoor heating reduces the humidity in the air; this lack of moist air dries out the nasal passages and creates the perfect breeding ground for the viruses.

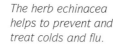

The herb echinacea helps to prevent and treat colds and flu.

Supplement Recommendations

Vitamin A	**Dosage:** 50,000 IU twice a day until symptoms improve; if needed beyond 7 days, reduce dose to 25,000 IU a day. **Comments:** Women who are pregnant or considering pregnancy should not exceed 5,000 IU a day.
Vitamin C	**Dosage:** 2,000 mg 3 times a day until symptoms improve; if needed beyond 5 days, reduce dose to 1,000 mg 3 times a day. **Comments:** Reduce dose if diarrhea develops.
Echinacea	**Dosage:** 200 mg 5 times a day. **Comments:** For prevention, take 200 mg a day in 3-week rotations with the herb astragalus (400 mg a day).
Zinc lozenges	**Dosage:** 1 lozenge every 3 or 4 hours as needed. **Comments:** Do not exceed 150 mg zinc a day from all sources.
Garlic	**Dosage:** 400-600 mg 4 times a day with food. **Comments:** Each pill should provide 4,000 mcg allicin potential.
Goldenseal	**Dosage:** 125 mg standardized extract 5 times a day for 5 days. **Comments:** Don't use during pregnancy or with high blood pressure.

Some dosages may be supplied by supplements you are already taking—see page 39.

How supplements can help

The supplements listed in the chart assist your body in combating cold and flu viruses, rather than suppressing symptoms. For this reason, you may not feel better immediately after taking them, but you'll probably recover faster. In some cases, prompt treatment may prevent a cold or the flu from fully developing. Start the supplements when symptoms first appear and, unless otherwise noted, continue until the illness passes.

At high doses, **vitamin A** has strong antiviral action, but take it for only seven days in these amounts. Contrary to popular belief, **vitamin C** won't prevent a cold, but it may shorten the duration or minimize the symptoms. The herb **echinacea** stimulates the immune system to mount an attack against the virus. **Zinc lozenges** may also help halt a cold, possibly by destroying the virus itself.

If you often develop a bacterial infection, such as sinusitis or bronchitis, from a cold or the flu, add **garlic** when you first notice symptoms. It contains compounds that may prevent bacteria from invading tissues. To give the immune system an extra boost, combine **goldenseal** with echinacea for the treatment (but not prevention) of colds and flu.

What else you can do

☑ Wash your hands often to reduce your chances of catching an infection.

☑ Use a humidifier or cool-mist vaporizer in winter to keep indoor air moist.

☑ Consider getting a flu shot. It takes six to eight weeks to build up a viral immunity, so get vaccinated in late fall before the flu season begins. Different flu strains emerge each year, so you'll need to have an annual shot.

FACTS
& Tips

■ Read the ingredient list of zinc lozenges carefully. Only zinc gluconate, ascorbate, and glycinate work against colds. And don't waste your money on products that contain sorbitol, mannitol, or citric acid. When combined with saliva, these chemicals make zinc ineffective.

LATEST FINDINGS

■ When it comes to cold prevention, researchers at Carnegie-Mellon University say you gotta have friends. In a study of 276 men and women, those with wide social networks developed fewer cold symptoms—even after researchers deposited a cold virus directly into the nose.

■ Smokers are twice as likely to catch colds as nonsmokers, according to a study from the Common Cold Unit of the Medical Research Council in Salisbury, England.

■ In one study, faster recovery from the flu was seen in men and women who took elderberry. Within two days, symptoms improved in 93% of those using the herb, whereas six days passed before improvement occurred in the group given a placebo.

congestive heart failure

It's the most frequent cause of hospitalization in people over age 65—and a serious condition that usually requires rigorous, lifelong treatment. Along with lifestyle changes and drugs, supplements can help ease symptoms of this ailment.

SYMPTOMS

- *Extreme fatigue and weakness.*
- *Shortness of breath after very little exertion or while reclining.*
- *Severe cough that produces reddish brown sputum.*
- *Unexplained extremely rapid or irregular heartbeat.*
- *Swelling (edema) of the extremities, especially ankles and feet.*

When to Call Your Doctor

- If you regularly feel extremely fatigued and short of breath after limited exertion.
- If you experience severe breathlessness or chest pain, which may indicate a heart attack—call an ambulance at once.
- If you have congestive heart failure and you develop fever or rapid or irregular heartbeat or symptoms worsen.
- Reminder: If you have a medical condition, talk to your doctor before taking supplements.

What it is

In congestive heart failure (CHF), a weakened, or "failing," heart doesn't pump as efficiently as it should. As a result, not enough oxygen-rich blood gets delivered to all parts of the body. Often simply called heart failure, CHF typically lingers and worsens over time. As blood flow from the heart slows, the blood returning to the heart backs up, leading to "congestion" in the tissues. Fluid can accumulate in the lungs, causing shortness of breath; can pool in the ankles, making them swell up; or can produce myriad other symptoms.

What causes it

A heart attack, which scars the heart and interferes with its pumping ability, frequently results in CHF. Other causes include persistent high blood pressure, chronic lung disease, long-term drug or alcohol abuse, and infections of the heart muscle or valves.

How supplements can help

Various medications can strengthen the heart's pumping action, expand blood vessels, increase blood flow, and eliminate excess fluid from the body. In consultation with your doctor, all these supplements can be taken long term along with conventional drugs to help slow the progression of CHF. Benefits may appear within three to four weeks.

A good starting strategy is to add antioxidants, including **vitamin C** and **vitamin E** and **coenzyme Q$_{10}$,** to your daily regimen. Taken regularly, they play a role in reducing damage from the highly reactive molecules known as free radicals, which can injure the heart and other organs. Coenzyme Q$_{10}$ also has energy-boosting properties.

Other supplements can be added to the mix as well. The herb **hawthorn** may be particularly effective in the early stages of CHF, helping

Often CHF patients benefit from thiamin supplements because diuretics prescribed for their condition deplete the body of this B vitamin.

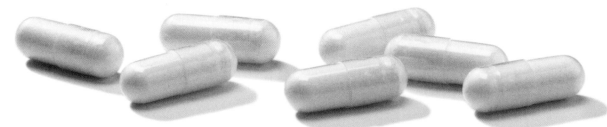

Supplement Recommendations

Vitamin C/ Vitamin E	**Dosage:** 1,000 mg vitamin C 3 times a day; 400 IU vitamin E daily. **Comments:** Check with your doctor if taking anticoagulant drugs.
Coenzyme Q$_{10}$	**Dosage:** 100 mg twice a day. **Comments:** For best absorption, take with food.
Hawthorn	**Dosage:** 100-150 mg 3 times a day. **Comments:** Standardized to contain at least 1.8% vitexin.
Carnitine	**Dosage:** 1,000 mg L-carnitine twice a day on an empty stomach. **Comments:** When using for longer than 1 month, add a mixed amino acid complex (follow package directions).
Taurine	**Dosage:** 500 mg L-taurine twice a day on an empty stomach. **Comments:** When using for longer than 1 month, add a mixed amino acid complex (follow package directions).
Magnesium	**Dosage:** 400 mg twice a day with food. **Comments:** Do not take if you have kidney disease.
Ginkgo biloba	**Dosage:** 40 mg 3 times a day. **Comments:** Standardized to have at least 24% flavone glycosides.
Thiamin	**Dosage:** 200 mg a day. **Comments:** Also called vitamin B$_1$.

Note: Consider using supplements in **blue** first; those in **black** may also be beneficial. Some dosages may be supplied by supplements you are already taking—see page 39.

FACTS & Tips

- Supplements may lessen the need for prescription heart medications, but never lower the dosage or stop taking any drug without consulting your doctor first.

- Regular walking and other types of mild aerobic exercise help many patients with CHF. However, always check with your doctor before beginning any exercise program.

LATEST FINDINGS

- A recent survey of more than 2,500 Italians with CHF found that adding coenzyme Q$_{10}$ to standard drug therapy significantly improved the quality of life of more than half of the patients after just three months.

- A report in the *International Journal of Cardiology* indicates that the antioxidant vitamin E may have a beneficial effect on patients with CHF. Tests showed that compared to healthy study participants, those with heart failure had higher levels of cell-damaging free radicals—and lower levels of antioxidants, which protect against free-radical damage. After four weeks of vitamin E therapy, levels of free radicals decreased in those patients with CHF.

- A recent study from Japan reported in the *Journal of the American College of Cardiology* suggests that vitamin C helps boost the effectiveness of nitroglycerin, a prescription drug commonly given to help open blood vessels and improve blood flow in patients with CHF.

widen blood vessels and improve blood flow throughout the body. **Carnitine** (an amino acid-like substance) plus the amino acid **taurine** help the heart beat more strongly and lower blood pressure. And taking the mineral **magnesium** can aid in reducing blood pressure and preventing dangerous arrhythmias, a common complication in those with CHF.

Finally, people with heart failure may benefit from two additional supplements. One is the herb **ginkgo biloba,** which improves blood circulation throughout the body, including the heart. The other is **thiamin.** Many people with CHF have low levels of this B vitamin because they take the diuretic Lasix (furosemide) in an effort to rid the body of excess fluids. But long-term use of Lasix depletes thiamin levels, so getting an extra amount may help boost the heart's pumping power.

What else you can do

- ☑ Get plenty of rest and don't undertake strenuous activity.
- ☑ Eat smaller, more frequent meals, which require less energy to digest.
- ☑ Reduce your salt intake and avoid caffeine, alcohol, and tobacco.

constipation

At the very least, constipation is uncomfortable, and sometimes it can be downright painful. Plenty of fiber, fluids, and exercise can help keep bowel movements regular. And for the times you need some gentle assistance, natural supplements might be the answer.

SYMPTOMS

- *Infrequent bowel movements.*
- *Hard, dry stools.*
- *Difficulty or pain when defecating.*
- *Swelling of the abdomen.*

When to Call Your Doctor

- If you notice an abrupt change in bowel habits.
- If symptoms of constipation persist for two weeks or longer, despite self-care measures.
- If fever or abdominal pain accompanies constipation.
- If cramping or pain is severe or disrupts your daily routine.
- If you notice blood in the stool.
- If you're on a new medication or supplement that may be causing constipation.
- Reminder: If you have a medical condition, talk to your doctor before taking supplements.

What it is

Bowel habits can vary widely from person to person, but most doctors would agree that anyone who passes hard stools less than three times a week is constipated. In addition, if you frequently have to strain to defecate, you also may benefit from therapies aimed at relieving constipation.

What causes it

In the majority of cases, constipation occurs because of a lack of fiber and fluids in the diet. Other contributing factors include insufficient exercise or prolonged inactivity; severe depression; and medical disorders, such as irritable bowel syndrome, diabetes, high blood calcium levels, a sluggish thyroid, or colon cancer. Overuse of laxatives or some antacids can impair bowel activity, and certain medications (including drugs for high blood pressure, antidepressants, and narcotic pain relievers) can also cause constipation.

How supplements can help

Any abrupt change in a person's usual frequency of bowel movements may be a sign of a more serious underlying disorder, such as cancer or a bowel obstruction, and requires medical evaluation. However, for occasional irregularity, various natural supplements may help. Benefits should be felt in a day or two. If needed, most of these supplements can be taken on a long-term basis.

Vitamin C is often useful for the treatment of constipation. Besides its role as an immune stimulant and antioxidant, this vitamin is a gentle

A tea made from the root of the dandelion plant may help relieve irregularity.

Supplement Recommendations

Vitamin C	**Dosage:** 1,000 mg 3 times a day.
	Comments: The dose can be increased by 1,000 mg a day (up to a total of 5,000 mg a day) until bowel movements become regular.
Magnesium	**Dosage:** 400 to 800 mg a day as needed.
	Comments: Take with food; reduce dose if diarrhea develops.
Psyllium	**Dosage:** 1-3 tbsp. powder dissolved in water or juice a day.
	Comments: Or take 1-3 tbsp. ground flaxseeds or 2 tsp. ground fenugreek seeds. Drink 8 glasses of water a day for these to work.
Prune	**Dosage:** Drink ½ cup juice or eat 3 or 4 prunes each morning.
	Comments: Can be used on a daily basis.
Dandelion root	**Dosage:** 1 cup tea 3 times a day.
	Comments: Use 1 tsp. dried root per cup of hot water.
Cascara sagrada	**Dosage:** 100 mg at bedtime.
	Comments: Look for a preparation that is standardized to contain 25% hydroxyanthracene derivatives.

Note: Consider using supplements in **blue** first; those in **black** may also be beneficial. Some dosages may be supplied by supplements you are already taking—see page 39.

laxative as well. A 3,000 mg daily dose loosens the stools in most people. If this amount doesn't work, gradually increase the dose or, alternatively, keep the daily dose at 3,000 mg and add the mineral **magnesium,** which, along with its many effects throughout the body, has gentle laxative properties too.

In addition to these nutrients, **psyllium,** ground flaxseed, or ground fenugreek seeds provide fiber and make the stools larger, softer, and easier to pass; they can be used on a daily basis. Be sure to have them with plenty of water to facilitate the passage of extra bulk through the digestive tract. You can also try **prune** juice or dried prunes for extra fiber; they're gentle enough to use with other supplements. Or, drink **dandelion root** tea, which has mild laxative properties.

If this combination of remedies does not provide relief within a day or two, consider the herb **cascara sagrada** as a last resort. Because this herb is a powerful laxative that stimulates the bowel muscles to contract, it should be used for no longer than one to two weeks at a time. Avoid it if you're pregnant or nursing.

What else you can do

☑ Eat foods high in fiber, including raw fruits and vegetables, whole grains, bran, and dried beans.

☑ Drink at least eight 8-ounce glasses of water or juice a day.

☑ Exercise regularly, and whenever possible, go to the bathroom as soon as the urge strikes.

■ If you're constipated, it's very important to drink plenty of fluids—but not all drinks are created equal. Alcohol and caffeinated beverages actually cause fluid loss, making constipation worse. On the other hand, water, vegetable and fruit juices, and clear soups are excellent fluid replenishers. A hot liquid in the morning may help trigger the reflex that gets the bowels moving.

LATEST FINDINGS

■ Taking psyllium significantly increased the frequency of bowel movements in patients with constipation, according to a recent study from the University of Nebraska. Those consuming psyllium also reported that their stools were softer and easier to pass, with far less pain during defecation.

■ A recent study from Seattle found that men and women with frequent constipation were much more likely to develop colon cancer. The researchers speculate that the stools of those with constipation remain in the intestine for a relatively long period, thus exposing the bowel to potentially cancer-causing chemicals for more time. These results provide yet one more reason to add psyllium or other natural supplements to your daily regimen.

cough

It's one of the most common medical complaints, and each year millions of people—up to 10% of the population by some estimates—seek their doctor's help for it. Often, however, using one or two natural treatments may be all that's necessary to get relief from a bothersome cough.

SYMPTOMS

■ *A cough is really a symptom— usually an indication of a respiratory infection or irritation of the throat, lungs, or air passages.*

■ *A cough can be dry (nonproductive) or wet (productive).*

When to Call Your Doctor

■ If cough persists day and night, is exhausting, or is accompanied by shortness of breath, chest pain, weight loss, wheezing, or severe headache.

■ If fever is 101°F or higher.

■ If breathing is painful.

■ If cough produces brown, pink, green, yellow, or bloody mucus.

■ If it lasts longer than a week.

■ Reminder: If you have a medical condition, talk to your doctor before taking supplements.

What it is

Despite its seemingly unhealthy sound, a cough is actually a vital bodily function. Even though you may not realize it, you probably cough once or twice every hour to clear your throat and air passages of debris. Coughing causes trouble only when an environmental substance or an illness makes you hack uncontrollably. Coughs can be dry and nonproductive, meaning they bring up no fluids or sputum; or they can be wet and productive, expelling mucus and the germs or irritants it contains.

What causes it

When an irritant enters your respiratory system, tiny cough receptors in the throat, lungs, and air passages begin producing extra mucus. This action stimulates nerve endings and sets in motion a sequence that culminates with the forceful expulsion of air and foreign material through the mouth—the cough. A variety of factors can trigger this reaction. Bacteria or viruses—such as those that cause the flu or the common cold—lead to an overproduction of mucus, which initiates a cough reflex (particularly at night, when sinuses drain and set off tickly coughs). Asthma, bronchitis, hay fever, and environmental pollutants—such as cigarette smoke, chemicals, or perfume—are other culprits. Heartburn can also provoke a cough (when stomach acid rises into the esophagus, burning and irritating the throat). Coughing is a side effect of certain prescription medications, especially those that treat high blood pressure. Less commonly, persistent coughing can result from a tumor in the lungs, throat, or voice box or from fluid in the lungs caused by congestive heart failure.

A tincture of licorice root helps make a cough more productive.

Supplement Recommendations

Slippery elm	**Dosage:** As a tea, 1 cup up to 3 times a day as needed. **Comments:** Use 1 tsp. dried herb per cup of hot water.
Marshmallow	**Dosage:** As a tea, 1 cup up to 3 times a day as needed. **Comments:** Use 2 tsp. dried herb per cup of hot water; can blend with slippery elm.
Licorice	**Dosage:** 45 drops tincture or 1 cup tea 3 times a day. **Comments:** Add tincture to water or to herbal cough teas. Or steep 1 tsp. dried herb in hot water with slippery elm or marshmallow.
Horehound	**Dosage:** As a tea, 1 cup up to 3 times a day as needed. **Comments:** Use 1 or 2 tsp. dried herb per cup of hot water. Can be taken alone or with other herbs listed.

Some dosages may be supplied by supplements you are already taking—see page 39.

How supplements can help

Natural cough remedies can be used in place of typical drugstore cough medicines. There are two primary goals in treating a cough: The first is to subdue the cough reflex, especially when a cough causes pain or interferes with sleep; the second is to thin the mucus, making it easier to bring up so the irritant can be flushed from the body.

A tea made from the herb **slippery elm** will soothe the throat and suppress dry coughs. You may want to include **marshmallow** in this mixture. When steeped in water, this herb releases mucilage, a gel-like plant substance that coats the throat and larynx and quiets the cough receptors. If you prefer, substitute mullein flowers instead; these also contain mucilage. Adding some **licorice**—one of the most effective expectorants—to the tea will loosen phlegm and relax bronchial spasms. (Using licorice for more than three weeks can raise blood pressure.) **Horehound** in tea form has the same benefit as licorice, but doesn't raise blood pressure. Combinations of these herbs are available as commercially prepared tea bags. If you don't like the tea, you can try tinctures of these herbs; follow package directions or add the tincture you're using to a small glass of warm water and drink three times a day.

Inhaling steam from hot water suffused with a few drops of eucalyptus or peppermint oil can open clogged sinuses, clear respiratory passages, and minimize bronchial spasms. Cough drops or hard candies containing eucalyptus, peppermint, anise, or fennel increase saliva, causing you to swallow more—which also suppresses the cough reflex.

What else you can do

☑ Drink lots of water, warm broth, tea, and room-temperature fruit or vegetable juice to help thin the mucus.

☑ Use a cool-mist vaporizer or humidifier to moisten the air.

☑ Don't smoke and avoid contact with irritating fumes or vapors.

FACTS
& Tips

■ The herb plantain (*Plantago lanceolata*) is an effective cough remedy. However, the FDA warns that many products claiming to be plantain actually contain digitalis, a substance that can cause heart abnormalities. Avoid products labeled "plantain" unless the botanical name is given. And don't confuse either type of plantain with the bananalike fruit *Musa paradisiaca*.

C·a·s·e H·i·s·t·o·r·y

VICKIE'S HERBAL COUGH TEA

It seemed to Vickie P. that just about every month she caught a cold from one of her young children. Her usual remedy: a prescription cough medicine. After reading that herbal practitioners often recommend herbal teas for colds, Vickie decided to compile her own list of curative herbs for a tea. She checked her choices with her doctor and was assured that they were safe.

She then began to experiment to find a tea that would ease her cold symptoms. After much trial and error, she came up with a recipe she now swears by. Each morning during a cold she prepares a pot of the tea, then drinks a cup of it three times a day.

Her recipe: 1 teaspoon slippery elm; 2 teaspoons marshmallow; 1 teaspoon hyssop; 45 drops echinacea tincture; and 45 drops licorice tincture for each pot of tea. She puts the dry herbs in a teapot, adds near-boiling water, steeps for 20 minutes, then strains. She adds the tinctures and honey to taste just before drinking it.

cuts and scrapes

Though often just an annoyance, these everyday injuries can become serious, especially if they are neglected. Basic hygiene, prompt first aid, and some of nature's own remedies can help prevent infections and speed healing.

SYMPTOMS

- *Narrow slices through the skin that usually bleed.*
- *Superficial skin abrasions that show redness or some bleeding.*
- *Punctures or holes that may penetrate deep into the skin.*

When to Call Your Doctor

- If a cut or scrape is dirty and can't be cleaned at home.
- If the cut will not close.
- If blood spurts out or bleeding can't be stopped.
- If signs of infection appear (pus in a cut or scrape, red streaks spreading from the injury, or an unusual discharge or fever).
- If you get a dirty cut or scrape or any puncture wound and haven't had (or can't recall) a tetanus shot for 10 years.
- Reminder: If you have a medical condition, talk to your doctor before taking supplements.

What it is

Cuts and scrapes are injuries that break the outer protective layer of skin. A cut occurs when the skin is pierced or sliced; a scrape, when the skin is visibly abraded or roughed up.

What causes it

A cut results from an encounter with a sharp implement, such as a knife, a razor blade, the edge of a piece of paper, or a jagged piece of glass or metal. When the skin is penetrated by an instrument with a sharp point such as a pin, nail, or pencil point, however, it causes a puncture wound. And a scrape occurs when the skin is literally rubbed away by a rough surface such as pebbles or a concrete pavement.

How supplements can help

Many topical supplements can ease or relieve pain, promote healing, prevent infection, and reduce the risk of scarring. They should be used only for minor cuts and scrapes. Gaping wounds that won't close or injuries that become infected require medical attention.

After stopping any bleeding and thoroughly cleaning the wound, apply **lavender oil** to the fresh cut or scrape to kill germs and to help it heal. **Tea tree oil** can be used instead as it helps halt infection and minimizes scarring as well. Or use **echinacea**, marigold, or myrrh tincture (dilute them in a little water first). Another option is comfrey ointment, which also may quicken the healing process.

Once you've completed these first-aid measures, bandage the wound. Change the

Diluted with a little water, echinacea tincture is a potent infection fighter when applied directly to skin wounds.

Supplement Recommendations	
Lavender oil	**Dosage:** Apply 1 or 2 drops of oil to wound after cleansing. **Comments:** Dab directly on any superficial wound.
Aloe vera gel	**Dosage:** Apply gel liberally to wound 3 or 4 times a day. **Comments:** Use fresh aloe leaf or store-bought gel.
Vitamin A	**Dosage:** 50,000 IU twice a day for 5 days. **Comments:** Women who are pregnant or considering pregnancy should not exceed 5,000 IU a day.
Vitamin C	**Dosage:** 1,000 mg 3 times a day for 5 days. **Comments:** Reduce dose if diarrhea develops.
Tea tree oil	**Dosage:** Apply 1 or 2 drops of oil to wound after cleansing. **Comments:** Can be used in place of lavender oil.
Echinacea	**Dosage:** Add 3 drops tincture to 1 tsp. water; apply to wound. **Comments:** A substitute for tea tree oil. In addition, drink 1 cup of echinacea-goldenseal tea 3 times a day until wound heals.
Calendula cream	**Dosage:** Apply cream to wound 3 times a day in place of aloe. **Comments:** Goldenseal cream or a combination of calendula and goldenseal is also effective; available at health-food stores.
Bromelain	**Dosage:** 500 mg 3 times a day on an empty stomach, for 5 days. **Comments:** Should provide 6,000 GDU or 9,000 MCU daily.

Note: Consider using supplements in **blue** first; those in **black** may also be beneficial. Some dosages may be supplied by supplements you are already taking—see page 39.

bandage three or four times a day, and spread either soothing **aloe vera gel** or **calendula cream** on the wound each time to relieve or limit inflammation, stop infection, and speed healing.

Take the remaining oral supplements together for five days after the injury. **Vitamin A** and **vitamin C** inhibit inflammation and accelerate healing. **Bromelain,** an enzyme derived from pineapples, has similar beneficial effects; and teas made with the herbs **echinacea** and goldenseal boost immunity and decrease the risk of infection.

What else you can do

☑ Stop any bleeding by applying steady pressure to the wound for a few minutes with a clean tissue or cloth. If the injury is a puncture wound, let it bleed for several minutes first to help flush out any embedded germs.

☑ Thoroughly clean the skin around the cut or scrape. Bandage the wound, especially if it's in an area likely to get dirty, such as a finger or knee. Antibiotics are not necessary unless signs of infection appear.

FACTS & Tips

■ To help clean and disinfect a wound, add a few drops of tea tree oil to a bowl of water. Soak a clean cloth in the mixture and use it to swab the injury. Or, hold the wound under running water for several minutes. Don't use hydrogen peroxide; it can damage the outer skin layer and slow healing.

■ An aloe vera plant is easily grown on a windowsill and makes an invaluable first-aid lotion for minor skin injuries. Break off one of the plumper leaves, slice it open lengthwise, and scrape or squeeze out the clear gel.

LATEST FINDINGS

■ In a study of people with scars, those who wore special silicon bandages containing vitamin E during the night showed greater improvement than patients not using vitamin E. Additional studies are needed to assess the role of this vitamin in halting or reversing scarring.

■ A small study of people who underwent surgery to remove tattoos found that those who took 3,000 mg of vitamin C and 900 mg of pantothenic acid (vitamin B_5) daily healed faster than those who consumed only 1,000 mg vitamin C and 200 mg of pantothenic acid a day.

Did You Know?

Tea tree oil was added to machine oils in Australian munitions factories during World War II to minimize infections when workers received cuts from the metal filings.

depression

A prevalent but little understood illness, depression afflicts nearly 18 million Americans each year. Along with innovative prescription medications has come additional research uncovering a new role for vitamin, mineral, and herbal supplements in dealing with this disease.

SYMPTOMS

- *Persistent sad or "empty" mood.*
- *Loss of pleasure in ordinary activities, including sex.*
- *Sleep disturbances, decreased energy, fatigue.*
- *Poor or increased appetite; weight loss or weight gain.*
- *Feelings of guilt, worthlessness, helplessness.*
- *Difficulty concentrating, irritability, excessive crying.*
- *Chronic aches and pains.*
- *Thoughts of death or suicide.*

When to Call Your Doctor

- If you or someone you know exhibits clear symptoms for at least two weeks.
- If you or someone you know has suicidal thoughts—get emergency help immediately.
- Reminder: If you have a medical or psychiatric condition, talk to your doctor before taking supplements.

What it is

More than just feeling blue, depression is a devastating illness that affects every aspect of a person's life—physical, mental, and emotional. It influences an individual's self-esteem and perception of others, and a person with depression has difficulty performing ordinary daily activities. There are various forms of depression, ranging from mild, long-term melancholy (dysthymia) to alternating moods of elation and despair (bipolar, or manic, depression) to the most serious form, despondency. The last leads to a total inability to function and even to thoughts of suicide.

What causes it

Depression doesn't seem to have a single underlying cause, although experts believe the illness is caused by an imbalance in the brain's production of neurotransmitters, chemical messengers that send signals from one nerve cell to another. A depressive episode can be triggered by the death of a loved one, the loss of a job, a divorce, a life-threatening illness, or another serious difficulty. Stress, reaction to medication (such as beta-blockers), shortage of daylight in winter, overconsumption of alcohol, smoking, food allergies, and nutritional deficiencies may also contribute to depression. Dysfunctional ways of coping with anger, guilt, and other emotions may be involved as well.

How supplements can help

Everyone afflicted with the disorder, even those on antidepressants, can benefit from all the vitamins and minerals listed. The herbs and 5-HTP can be added, but should not be combined with antidepressant drugs

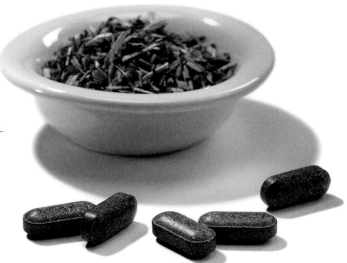

St. John's wort may be as effective as prescription anti-depressant medications.

Supplement Recommendations

Vitamin B complex	**Dosage:** 1 pill each morning with food. **Comments:** Look for a B-50 complex with 50 mcg vitamin B_{12} and biotin; 400 mcg folic acid; and 50 mg all other B vitamins.
Vitamin C	**Dosage:** 500 mg 3 times a day. **Comments:** Reduce dose if diarrhea develops.
Calcium/ Magnesium	**Dosage:** 250 mg of each twice a day. **Comments:** Extra dose can be taken before bedtime to aid sleep.
St. John's wort	**Dosage:** 300 mg 3 times a day. **Comments:** Standardized to contain 0.3% hypericin.
5-HTP	**Dosage:** 100 mg 3 times a day **Comments:** Don't use longer than 3 months without doctor's okay.
Ginkgo biloba	**Dosage:** 80 mg 3 times a day. **Comments:** Standardized to have at least 24% flavone glycosides.
Kava	**Dosage:** 250 mg 2 or 3 times a day as needed. **Comments:** Standardized to contain at least 30% kavalactones.

Note: Consider using supplements in **blue** first; those in **black** may also be beneficial. Some dosages may be supplied by supplements you are already taking—see page 39.

without your doctor's consent. And people using prescription drugs should never stop taking them without first talking it over with their doctor.

Low levels of the **B vitamins** and **vitamin C** have been associated with depression. All aid in the brain's production of neurotransmitters and may enhance the effectiveness of antidepressant medications. **Calcium** and **magnesium** have a soothing effect on the nerves and can be particularly helpful when depression interferes with sleep.

As for the herbs, **St. John's wort** may be a beneficial and safe alternative to prescription drugs, which often have side effects. For people over age 50, **ginkgo biloba** appears to combat depression better than—and may be used instead of—St. John's wort. A form of the amino acid tryptophan, **5-HTP** (5-hydroxytryptophan) seems to be effective at improving mood. For severe depression, it can be combined with St. John's wort or ginkgo. With your doctor's consent, **kava** can be used alone, or with St. John's wort, ginkgo, or 5-HTP if you're depressed and anxious.

What else you can do

☑ Exercise regularly. This may be the best natural antidepressant.

☑ Avoid tobacco, excessive caffeine, and alcohol.

☑ Seek counseling. Many current therapeutic techniques can help break the cycle of depressive behavior.

FACTS & Tips

■ Eating turkey, salmon, and milk products may help ease depression because they contain the amino acid tryptophan. Low tryptophan levels reduce the brain's production of the neurotransmitter serotonin, which helps regulate mood. Women may be particularly susceptible to low levels of tryptophan.

■ Women with depression may have porous bones, because imbalances in brain chemicals affect the production of the hormones that maintain bone density. This increased risk of osteoporosis may be offset by taking extra calcium.

LATEST FINDINGS

■ About 30% of the people who try antidepressants do not respond to them. A recent study suggests additional folic acid might help. After eight weeks of taking Prozac, about 35% of study participants with low folic acid levels did not improve. In contrast, 80% of those with adequate folic acid levels did respond to the drug.

■ According to preliminary studies, melatonin may aid people who suffer from seasonal affective disorder (SAD), also known as winter depression. In these people, the body's inner clock doesn't adjust to fewer hours of daylight. Taking small doses of melatonin several times in the afternoon seems to help the body shift its sleep and wake cycles and lift the depression.

diabetes

Approximately 16 million people in the United States suffer from diabetes. Many would do well to consider the use of herbs and nutritional supplements, which can complement conventional medical treatment and help prevent some complications of this chronic but manageable disease.

SYMPTOMS

- *Excessive thirst.*
- *Frequent and excessive urination.*
- *Extreme fatigue and weakness.*
- *Unintentional weight loss.*
- *Slow healing of cuts and wounds.*
- *Recurring infections, such as urinary tract infections or vaginal yeast infections.*
- *Blurred vision.*
- *Numbness or tingling in the hands and feet.*

When to Call Your Doctor

- If you experience any of the symptoms listed above.
- Reminder: If you have a medical condition, talk to your doctor before taking supplements.

What it is

A person with diabetes doesn't produce enough of the hormone insulin or is unable to use it effectively, which causes high blood sugar (glucose) levels. Over time, this imbalance can lead to heart disease, nerve damage, kidney disease, vision loss, and other complications. There are two types of diabetes. Less common is insulin-dependent diabetes (type 1), which usually develops before age 30. Non-insulin-dependent diabetes (type 2) accounts for 90% of cases; it usually appears after age 40.

What causes it

Type 1 diabetes occurs when the pancreas stops producing insulin. No one knows exactly why this happens, but some experts believe a virus or an autoimmune response, in which the body attacks its own pancreatic cells, is responsible. People with this type of diabetes must take insulin for life. Type 2 diabetes develops from insulin resistance. Here the pancreas secretes plenty of insulin, but the body's cells don't respond to it. Obesity plays a major role in most cases of type 2 diabetes. Genetic factors, however, can contribute to the onset of both types.

How supplements can help

All the supplements can be used along with prescription drugs and by people with both types of diabetes. Taking some supplements may require altering dosages for insulin or the hypoglycemic drugs used for type 2 diabetes. Dosage changes must be supervised by your doctor.

The **B vitamins** help produce enzymes that convert glucose to energy and may also aid in preventing diabetic nerve damage. The mineral **chromium** is effective in lowering blood glucose and reducing cholesterol levels in people with diabetes. **Gymnema sylvestre,** an herb from

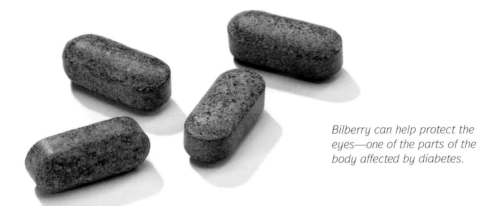

Bilberry can help protect the eyes—one of the parts of the body affected by diabetes.

Supplement Recommendations

Vitamin B complex	**Dosage:** 1 pill each morning with food. **Comments:** Look for a B-100 complex with 100 mcg vitamin B_{12} and biotin; 400 mcg folic acid; and 100 mg all other B vitamins.
Chromium	**Dosage:** 200 mcg 3 times a day with meals. **Comments:** May alter insulin requirements. Consult your doctor.
Gymnema sylvestre	**Dosage:** 200 mg twice a day. **Comments:** May alter insulin requirements. Talk to your doctor.
Essential fatty acids	**Dosage:** 1,000 mg evening primrose oil 3 times a day; 1,000 mg fish oils twice a day. **Comments:** Or use 1,000 mg borage oil once a day for primrose oil.
Antioxidants	**Dosage:** 1,000 mg vitamin C, 400 IU vitamin E, and 150 mg alpha-lipoic acid each morning. **Comments:** Alpha-lipoic acid may affect blood sugar; use with care.
Zinc/Copper	**Dosage:** 30 mg zinc and 2 mg copper a day. **Comments:** Add copper only when using zinc longer than 1 month.
Bilberry	**Dosage:** 160 mg twice a day. **Comments:** Standardized to contain 25% anthocyanosides.
Taurine	**Dosage:** 500 mg L-taurine twice a day on an empty stomach. **Comments:** If using longer than 1 month, add mixed amino acids.

Note: Consider using supplements in blue first; those in black may also be beneficial. Some dosages may be supplied by supplements you are already taking—see page 39.

India, improves blood sugar control, sometimes reducing the need for insulin or hypoglycemic medication.

Essential fatty acids protect against nerve damage and keep arteries supple. Fish oils, in particular, may raise "good" HDL cholesterol, reducing the risk of heart disease. **Antioxidants** prevent damage to the nerves, eyes, and heart as well. Vitamin E may block the buildup of plaque; alpha-lipoic acid improves glucose metabolism. Many people with diabetes have low levels of **zinc,** which helps the body use insulin and promotes wound healing (a function impaired by high glucose levels). Long-term zinc use may require extra **copper.** The herb **bilberry** helps prevent diabetic eye damage, and the amino acid **taurine** aids in the release of insulin and can prevent abnormal blood clotting, a factor in heart disease. New studies suggest magnesium may play a role in diabetes as well.

What else you can do

☑ Exercise regularly. Those who burn more than 3,500 calories a week through exercise are half as likely to develop type 2 diabetes as those burning less than 500. People with type 1 can benefit from exercise too.

☑ Lose weight. Being overweight is a major risk factor for type 2 diabetes.

☑ Eat whole grains, fruits, and vegetables to keep blood sugar in check.

FACTS & Tips

■ People with diabetes may find it beneficial to add soy foods to their diet. These products—including tofu, soy protein, soy milk, and soy flour—may improve glucose control, protect against heart disease, and lessen the stress on the kidneys.

■ The herb ginkgo biloba is useful for two common side effects of diabetes: nerve damage and poor circulation in the extremities. If you have signs of either complication or if you have trouble controlling your blood sugar levels, try taking ginkgo biloba at a dose of 40 mg three times a day.

LATEST FINDINGS

■ Poor control of glucose levels can deplete the body's stores of antioxidant nutrients, according to a study from Duke University Medical Center. Taking supplements such as vitamin C and vitamin E protects the body's cells against damage from free radicals (unstable oxygen molecules) and may reduce the risk of some serious complications of diabetes.

■ One in three people with diabetes may be deficient in magnesium, say researchers at Columbia University, and low magnesium levels may contribute to heart disease. Some experts recommend at least 250 mg of magnesium twice a day for people with diabetes. However, people with signs of kidney damage should not take magnesium supplements.

diarrhea

Unpleasant as it may be, diarrhea provides your body with a way to flush out harmful toxins. This common ailment usually subsides on its own in a day or so, but it can be uncomfortable and inconvenient. The goals of treatment are to prevent dehydration and restore bulk to the stool.

What it is

An increase in the frequency of stools or the passage of loose, watery stools is called diarrhea. It is not a disease itself, but a symptom of a variety of disorders—most benign, some serious. Diarrhea represents a disruption in the normal passage of food and waste through the large intestine. Ordinarily, water is absorbed through the intestinal walls as food passes through the large intestine, and fecal matter leaves the body as a solid mass. If something speeds up or otherwise interferes with this process, the fluid will be expelled from the body with fecal matter.

What causes it

Diarrhea is the inflammation or irritation of the intestine. It usually is the result of a bacterial or viral infection caused by eating or drinking contaminated food or water. Most people traveling to less developed areas of the world are aware of the risk of food or water contamination and take steps to avoid "traveler's diarrhea." At home, however, they may not be so careful. And often the diarrhea they chalk up to a 24-hour flu bug is more likely a consequence of food poisoning.

There are several other causes of diarrhea. Eating more fruits or vegetables than your digestive tract is accustomed to handling sometimes leads to diarrhea; citrus fruits and beans are typically the culprits. When consumed in large amounts, the low-calorie sweetener sorbitol may also trigger diarrhea. In addition, diarrhea may develop from taking therapeutic doses of vitamin C or magnesium (if this side effect occurs, reduce the dose). People with lactose intolerance—an

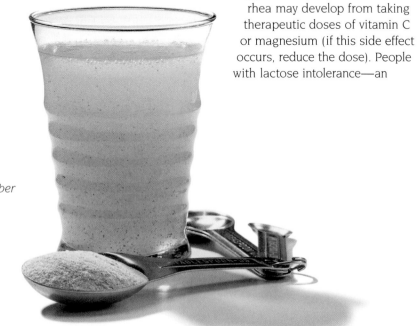

Psyllium relieves diarrhea by absorbing excess fluid in the intestine. To take it, mix the fiber with a glass of water or juice.

Supplement Recommendations

Agrimony	**Dosage:** As a tea, 1 cup up to 6 times a day.
	Comments: Use 1 tbsp. of leaves per cup of hot water; let it steep for 15 minutes and strain. Drink throughout the day as needed.
Blackberry/ Raspberry leaf	**Dosage:** As a tea, 1 cup up to 6 times a day.
	Comments: Use 1 tbsp. of leaves per cup of hot water; let it steep for 15 minutes and strain. Drink throughout the day as needed.
Psyllium	**Dosage:** 1-3 tbsp. powder dissolved in water or juice a day.
	Comments: Be sure to drink extra water throughout the day.
Acidophilus	**Dosage:** 2 pills 3 times a day on an empty stomach.
	Comments: Get 1-2 billion live (viable) organisms per pill.

Some dosages may be supplied by supplements you are already taking—see page 39.

see page 39.

inability to digest the sugar in dairy products (lactose)—often suffer from gas, bloating, and diarrhea after having milk, cheese, or ice cream. Antibiotics can bring on diarrhea because they destroy the intestine's "friendly bacteria." In some people, stress triggers diarrhea. It can also be a symptom of a gastrointestinal disorder, such as irritable bowel syndrome, colitis, Crohn's disease, pancreatic disease, or colon cancer.

How supplements can help

To combat diarrhea, try drinking **agrimony, blackberry leaf,** or **raspberry leaf** tea. These teas contain tannins, chemicals that have a binding effect on the mucous membranes in the intestine and help the body absorb fluids. The teas also replenish lost fluids, which is important in preventing the dehydration that may result from a prolonged bout with diarrhea.

If none of the teas provides relief, consider **psyllium.** Though this soluble fiber is more familiar as a constipation treatment, it absorbs excess fluid in the intestine and adds bulk to the stool. **Acidophilus** works to restore adequate levels of healthy bacteria to the intestine and is especially important if diarrhea is related to antibiotic use. All these remedies can be substituted for over-the-counter (OTC) diarrheal aids (except acidophilus, which can be used with OTC preparations, though not taken at the same time of day).

If food poisoning is to blame, wait a few hours before trying to treat the problem so that your body has enough time to get rid of the offending organism. Otherwise, start using the remedies immediately.

What else you can do

☑ Drink plenty of water and clear liquids to prevent dehydration.

☑ Avoid milk, citrus fruits, alcohol, and high-fiber foods for a day or two after having diarrhea; eat bland foods, such as bananas and white rice.

☑ When traveling to suspect areas, eat only cooked foods. Avoid ice cubes and use bottled water, even for brushing your teeth.

diverticular disorders

One in ten Americans over age 40 and half of those over age 60 have a diverticular disorder. But this isn't a disease of aging per se; it's a disease of lifestyle, particularly lack of fiber and exercise. A few simple measures can help.

What it is

There are two main types of diverticular disorders: diverticulosis and the more serious diverticulitis. In diverticulosis, the inner lining of the large bowel pushes through the muscular layer that usually confines it, forming pouches (diverticula) ranging from pea-size to more than an inch in diameter. Though diverticulosis often produces no symptoms, food can get trapped in these pouches, which then become inflamed and infected. The result is diverticulitis, whose symptoms are impossible to ignore.

What causes it

Most cases of diverticulosis probably stem from a low-fiber diet. A lack of fiber means the colon must work harder to pass the stool, and straining during bowel movements can aggravate the condition. A diet low in fiber also increases the likelihood of diverticulitis because waste moves slowly, allowing more time for food particles to become trapped and cause inflammation or infection. And lack of exercise makes the colon contents sluggish. The tendency toward such disorders may run in families.

How supplements can help

Although supplements cannot reverse diverticulosis once a pouch has developed, they (and changes in your diet) can help prevent or ease flare-ups. Providing fiber that forms bulk, **psyllium** acts to relieve or prevent constipation. Ground **flaxseeds** are also rich in fiber and ward off infection by keeping intestinal pouches clear. These two can be taken together long term first thing in the morning to assist with the initial bowel movement, along with probiotics such as **acidophilus.**

Acidophilus boosts levels of "friendly" bacteria in the gut, improving bowel health in those with diverticular disease.

Supplement Recommendations

Psyllium	**Dosage:** 1 tbsp. powder dissolved in water or juice twice a day. **Comments:** Be sure to drink extra water throughout the day.
Flaxseeds	**Dosage:** 2 tbsp. ground flaxseeds in glass of water twice a day. **Comments:** Be sure to drink extra water throughout the day.
Acidophilus	**Dosage:** 2 pills twice a day between meals. **Comments:** Get 1-2 billion live (viable) organisms per pill.
Aloe vera juice	**Dosage:** ½ cup juice twice a day. **Comments:** Containing 98% aloe vera and no aloin or aloe-emodin.
Glutamine	**Dosage:** 500 mg L-glutamine twice a day on an empty stomach. **Comments:** When using for longer than 1 month, add a mixed amino acid complex (follow package directions).
Slippery elm	**Dosage:** 1 cup bark powder, prepared like hot cereal each morning. **Comments:** Or use tea (1 tsp. per cup) 3 times a day.
Chamomile	**Dosage:** As a tea, 1 cup 3 times a day. **Comments:** Use 2 tsp. dried herb per cup of hot water; steep for 10 minutes, then strain. Alternatively, try melissa tea.
Wild yam/ Peppermint/ Valerian	**Dosage:** 1 cup tea 3 or 4 times a day. **Comments:** Use 2 parts wild yam, 1 part peppermint, 1 part valerian per cup of hot water; steep 10 minutes, strain. Sweeten to taste.

Note: Consider using supplements in **blue** first; those in **black** may also be beneficial. Some dosages may be supplied by supplements you are already taking—see page 39.

The fiber helps protect the acidophilus from stomach acids and carries it into the intestine, where it alters the bacterial balance in the digestive tract, enabling the body to fight off intestinal infections. Acidophilus is especially important if you're taking antibiotics during a flare-up.

Additional supplements, which may be particularly useful for treating flare-ups, are best taken at least two hours after taking psyllium, which can interfere with their absorption. **Aloe vera juice** promotes the healing of inflamed areas, as does the amino acid **glutamine,** which is essential for regenerating the cells that line the intestine. These two can be combined with one or more relieving herbs. **Slippery elm** is a mild natural laxative that soothes infected diverticula. **Chamomile** and **wild yam** are anti-inflammatories. **Peppermint** relaxes digestive spasms, and **valerian** and melissa likewise help soothe the digestive tract.

What else you can do

☑ Eat plenty of fruits, vegetables, and whole grains to boost your fiber intake to 20 to 30 grams a day.

☑ Drink at least eight 8-ounce glasses of water or other fluids every day.

LATEST FINDINGS

■ As part of the Health Professionals Follow-Up Study, Harvard University researchers monitored more than 43,000 men ages 40 to 75. Those who later developed diverticular disease ate significantly less fiber than those who didn't get the disease.

Did You Know?

Diverticulosis is almost unknown in rural areas of Africa and other "less developed" nations, where a high-fiber diet and regular exercise are the norm.

dizziness

Feeling light-headed? A bit woozy or off-balance? If you're traveling in a car, boat, or plane, it's probably motion sickness. But sometimes dizziness, also commonly called vertigo, becomes a lingering or recurrent problem. Regardless of the cause, natural remedies can bring relief.

SYMPTOMS

- *Unsteadiness or faintness.*
- *A feeling that the room is spinning or that you're whirling in space, sometimes accompanied by ringing in the ears.*
- *Nausea.*

When to Call Your Doctor

- If dizziness is accompanied by numbness, rapid heartbeat, fainting or a feeling of faintness, or blurred vision; if it affects your ability to speak.
- If dizziness comes on suddenly, especially if accompanied by nausea or vomiting.
- If dizzy spells increase in frequency or persist.
- Reminder: If you have a medical condition, talk to your doctor before taking supplements.

What it is

The terms "dizziness" and "vertigo" are often used interchangeably, but they are not synonymous. Dizziness simply refers to a feeling of unsteadiness or faintness, whereas vertigo usually involves a more serious disorientation, as if the world were spinning around you. (If you've ever been in a high place and felt as if you were falling, you've experienced vertigo.) Unfortunately, for some people, dizziness can persist and become disabling.

What causes it

Ordinary motion sickness—the queasy, light-headed feeling that comes while traveling—is by far the most common cause of dizziness. The problem arises when the eyes, which try to focus on constantly moving scenery, and the inner ear, which helps orient the body to movement, send conflicting signals to the brain. The result is a confusing, whirling sensation, often accompanied by nausea.

A number of medical conditions—including decreased blood flow to the brain or inner ear, ear infections, a head injury, high or low blood pressure, arrhythmias, nerve disorders, and allergies—can also bring on dizziness or vertigo. And certain medications, such as diuretics, tranquilizers, antidepressants, and antibiotics, can cause dizziness as well.

How supplements can help

A centuries-old remedy for delicate stomachs, **ginger** can act relatively quickly—even within minutes—to combat the dizziness and nausea associated with motion sickness or mild vertigo. In some tests, the herb

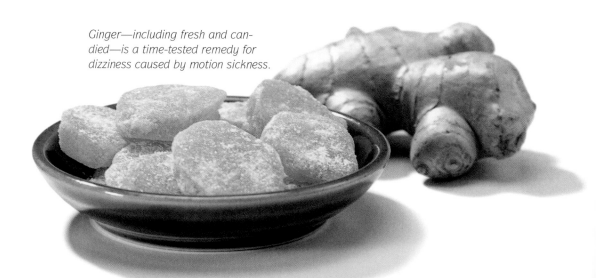

Ginger—including fresh and candied—is a time-tested remedy for dizziness caused by motion sickness.

has proved more effective—and longer lasting—than over-the-counter remedies. Moreover, ginger produces few of the side effects of conventional medications, such as drowsiness or blurred vision.

More persistent vertigo or dizziness requires medical attention to rule out serious underlying causes. Your doctor may prescribe drugs, though certain supplements, in addition to ginger, may also be beneficial. A French study showed that the herb **ginkgo biloba,** which boosts blood flow to the brain, helped almost half of the patients with chronic vertigo. It may, however, take eight to twelve weeks for ginkgo's effects to be noticed. In addition, **vitamin B$_6$,** essential to normal brain and nervous system function, may be useful in some cases of chronic dizziness.

What else you can do

For motion sickness

☑ Stop reading or staring at a computer screen if you begin to feel sick while in a moving car, train, or boat. Instead, face forward and focus on a fixed point, such as the distant scenery or the horizon, to keep your body and eyes simultaneously oriented to the movement.

☑ Opt for the front seat when riding in a car; at sea, stay amidship; and when flying, sit above the wing, where there is the least amount of motion.

For vertigo

☑ Steer clear of amusement park rides or virtual reality games that can wreak havoc with your sense of balance.

☑ Avoid sudden changes in body position (especially going from lying down to standing up) and extremes of head motion (particularly looking up, turning, or twisting).

☑ Try desensitization techniques: Move your head in a way that induces dizziness. Repeat several times a day for several weeks.

☑ Cut down on nicotine, caffeine, and salt, which can impair blood flow to the brain.

earache

Whether it's a middle ear infection, located deep in the ear, or swimmer's ear, affecting the outer ear canal, an earache hurts. It's most often a problem in children, but adults get earaches too. Though some conditions clear up on their own, supplements can speed up the healing process.

Symptoms

- *Throbbing or steady pain in ear; pain when pulling on lobe.*
- *Pressure or itching in the ear.*
- *A bloody, green, yellow, or clear discharge from the ear.*
- *Muffled hearing; popping in ear.*
- *Fever.*
- *Dizziness.*

When to Call Your Doctor

- If earache is accompanied by fever over 101°F, stiff neck, severe headache, or seepage of pus or other fluids; or if the ear or area behind it appears red or swollen—it is likely an infection requiring antibiotics.
- If pain or hearing loss is severe or worsens despite self-care.
- If an object is lodged in the ear or you have symptoms of a ruptured eardrum, such as sudden pain, partial hearing loss, bleeding, or ringing in the ears.
- Reminder: If you have a medical condition, talk to your doctor before taking supplements.

What it is

An earache results from inflammation, infection, or swelling in the outer canal of the ear or in the space adjoining the eardrum, which is the thin membrane that separates the outer and the middle ear. Normally, the eustachian tube, which extends from the middle ear to the throat, drains fluids from the ear, keeping it clear. But inflammation or infection can irritate the ear canal or block the eustachian tube, leading to the buildup of pus or other fluids and causing pain and other unpleasant symptoms.

What causes it

Earaches are typically caused by harmful bacteria, viruses, or fungi, usually preceded by an upper respiratory infection or seasonal allergies, or moisture trapped in the ear. Other causes include excessive ear wax, sudden changes in air pressure, a punctured eardrum, or exposure to irritating chemicals, such as hair dyes and chlorinated water.

How supplements can help

The supplements listed in the chart can play a supportive role in healing earaches. They can be used in conjunction with antibiotics, pain relievers, and other conventional remedies for short-term treatment of mild to moderate ear discomfort. All severe, lingering, or recurrent ear pain, however, requires medical evaluation.

Start with natural eardrops made from **garlic oil** or **mullein flower oil**—or a combination of

A few drops of garlic oil placed in a mildly aching ear may bring prompt relief.

Garlic oil	**Dosage:** A few drops in the ear twice a day.
	Comments: May be used alone or with mullein flower oil.
Mullein flower oil	**Dosage:** A few drops in the ear twice a day.
	Comments: May be used alone or with garlic oil.
Lavender oil	**Dosage:** Apply a few drops to the outer ear and rub in gently.
	Comments: Can be used as needed throughout the day.
Eucalyptus oil	**Dosage:** Add several drops essential eucalyptus oil to pan of water.
	Comments: Bring oil and water to boil and remove from heat; place towel over head and pan and inhale steam through the nose.
Vitamin A	**Dosage:** 50,000 IU twice a day until symptoms improve; if needed after 7 days, reduce to 25,000 IU a day until symptoms are gone.
	Comments: Women who are pregnant or considering pregnancy should not exceed 5,000 IU a day.
Vitamin C/ Flavonoids	**Dosage:** 1,000 mg vitamin C and 500 mg flavonoids 3 times a day until infection clears.
	Comments: Reduce vitamin C dose if diarrhea develops.
Echinacea	**Dosage:** 200 mg 3 times a day until infection clears.
	Comments: Standardized to contain at least 3.5% echinacosides.

Some dosages may be supplied by supplements you are already taking—see page 39.

see page 39.

FACTS & Tips

■ Herbal eardrops often bring rapid pain relief—within 10 minutes of administration. To make the application of drops more comfortable, warm the bottle under hot running tap water before placing the liquid in the ear.

LATEST FINDINGS

■ The latest study to look at the link between secondhand smoke and ear infections reported that exposure to smoke can affect the ears. Children who lived in households with at least two smokers were 85% more likely to suffer from middle ear infections than those who lived in nonsmoking homes. Although some studies have shown no link, it's always a good idea not to smoke, and to avoid smoke-filled rooms, especially if you're prone to earaches.

■ In a recent Finnish study, children who chewed gum sweetened with xylitol, a type of natural sugar (sometimes called birch sugar) that's found in a number of commercial chewing gums, had almost half the number of ear infections as those who chewed other types of gum. The researchers speculate that xylitol may help keep harmful microorganisms at the back of the mouth from reaching the ear, where they can cause infections.

the two. Eardrops should not be used, however, if ear pain is severe or if it's accompanied by partial hearing loss or puslike drainage from the ears; these symptoms suggest the eardrum may be ruptured. Garlic and mullein flower oils help fight disease-causing microbes and reduce inflammation and may relieve pain and itching. If the outer ear appears irritated, **lavender oil,** rubbed in gently, can be very soothing. In addition to applying topical herbal oils, prepare a **eucalyptus oil** steam bath, which will aid in opening the eustachian tube, easing pressure, and facilitating the drainage of infectious fluids from the ear. Repeat several times a day until pain subsides.

Supplements should also be taken internally. The immune-boosters **vitamin A** and **vitamin C** play an important role in fighting infections and preventing recurrences. Take vitamin C with the plant-based anti-inflammatories called **flavonoids,** which enhance its effectiveness. The immune-enhancing herb **echinacea** can be valuable as well, particularly when an earache is the result of an upper respiratory infection.

What else you can do

☑ Place a warm compress on the outside of your ear; use a heating pad or warm washcloth. Heat can bring quick pain relief and facilitate healing.

☑ Never insert a cotton swab, which can puncture the eardrum, into your ear. Don't use hydrogen peroxide as a cleaner; it can irritate the ear canal.

eczema

Applied to the skin, soothing creams can help relieve the red and often intensely itchy rashes of eczema. Various nutrients, taken internally, may also hasten healing. They may even be effective in preventing recurrences of this all-too-common—and bothersome—skin complaint.

Symptoms

- *Areas of itchy skin that are red, dry, scaly, rough, or cracked.*
- *Tiny pimplelike blisters.*
- *Thickened, dry patches of skin in persistent cases of eczema.*

When to Call Your Doctor

- If eczema is especially widespread or recurrent.
- If oozing or crusting sores appear—they may indicate a bacterial infection.
- If eczema doesn't respond to self-care measures within three or four days.
- Reminder: If you have a medical condition, talk to your doctor before taking supplements.

What it is

Known medically as dermatitis, eczema produces inflamed patches of red, scaly skin on the face, scalp, hands, and wrists; in front of the elbows and behind the knees; and in other areas of the body. Although eczema is frequently very itchy, scratching can aggravate it.

What causes it

Often triggered by an allergy to foods, pollen, animal fur, or other substances, eczema is likely to run in allergy-prone families. In fact, many people with eczema have (or later develop) hay fever. Those with eczema have higher than normal amounts of histamine in their bodies, a chemical that produces an allergic reaction when released in the skin. Some cases occur after contact with allergens, such as poison ivy or other poisonous plants, jewelry made of nickel or chrome, dyes, cosmetics, topical medications, and cleaning agents. People who have poor circulation in their legs may suffer from a type of eczema called stasis dermatitis, which causes scaly patches around the ankles. Eczema can also be triggered or aggravated by dry air, too much sun, and stress.

How supplements can help

Used individually, in combination with other supplements, or in conjunction with conventional drugs, various supplements can offer relief from flare-ups of eczema. Benefits should begin to appear within three or four days. The recommended supplements can also be continued long term to prevent recurrences.

A number of supplements, taken internally, are useful in countering inflammation and tempering the allergic response. Try a few and see which ones work for you. **Flaxseed oil** and **evening primrose oil** contain different types of skin-revitalizing essential fatty acids that can help relieve itching and inflammation. **Vitamins A** and **E** mitigate skin dryness and itchiness; the dosage of vitamin A can be reduced when

Zinc, taken with copper if used over the long term, helps relieve and prevent red, itchy flare-ups of eczema.

110

Supplement Recommendations

Flaxseed oil	**Dosage:** 1 tbsp. (14 grams) a day.
	Comments: Can be mixed with food; take in the morning.
Evening primrose oil	**Dosage:** 1,000 mg 3 times a day.
	Comments: Can substitute 1,000 mg borage oil once a day.
Vitamin A	**Dosage:** 25,000 IU daily for up to 10 days to treat flare-ups; reduce dose to 10,000 IU for maintenance therapy.
	Comments: Women who are pregnant or considering pregnancy should not exceed 5,000 IU a day.
Vitamin E	**Dosage:** 400 IU a day.
	Comments: Check with your doctor if taking anticoagulant drugs.
Zinc/Copper	**Dosage:** 30 mg zinc and 2 mg copper a day.
	Comments: Add copper only when using zinc longer than 1 month. Often sold in a single supplement.
Grape seed extract	**Dosage:** 100 mg twice a day.
	Comments: Standardized to contain 92%-95% proanthocyanidins.
Chamomile	**Dosage:** Apply cream or lotion to affected areas 3 or 4 times a day.
	Comments: Available ready-made in health-food stores.
Licorice	**Dosage:** Apply cream to affected areas 3 or 4 times a day.
	Comments: Also called glycyrrhetinic acid cream.

Note: Consider using supplements in blue first; those in **black** may also be beneficial. Some dosages may be supplied by supplements you are already taking—see page 39.

symptoms improve. The mineral **zinc** aids the healing process and boosts the functioning of the immune system; it's also necessary for the processing of essential fatty acids. When used long term, zinc should be taken with **copper,** because zinc depletes the body's copper reserve. In addition, **grape seed extract** is rich in antioxidant substances called flavonoids, which inhibit the body's allergic responses.

It's often a good idea to apply a topical cream containing **chamomile** or **licorice.** These herbs reduce skin inflammation and can be surprisingly soothing when applied directly to lesions.

What else you can do

☑ Eliminate any foods that may cause an allergic reaction. These often include milk, eggs, shellfish, wheat, chocolate, nuts, and strawberries.

☑ Wear loose-fitting cotton clothing, which is less likely than other fabrics to irritate the skin.

☑ Bathe or shower less frequently to keep skin from drying out. Use lukewarm water and avoid deodorant soaps, bubble baths, and perfumed products. After bathing, pat your skin dry instead of rubbing it.

FACTS
& Tips

■ As topical treatments for eczema, herbal liquids or lotions work best on oozing lesions. Creams and ointments are most effective on dry patches of eczema.

■ Licorice cream is especially good for those who also use prescription or over-the-counter cortisone creams to treat eczema. Licorice contains glycyrrhetinic acid, which both increases the effectiveness of cortisone and also reduces possible side effects, such as burning, itching, and irritation.

■ Another product worth considering is witch hazel cream. It's been shown to be as beneficial as 1% hydrocortisone cream for the treatment of eczema.

LATEST FINDINGS

■ Many conventional doctors question the effectiveness of evening primrose oil as a treatment for eczema, and studies conflict. One recent study, however, found that adults and children with eczema who took evening primrose oil for six months experienced less itching and decreased inflammation.

Did You Know?

Traditional Chinese herbalists often prescribe a tea for eczema that contains licorice and, depending on the symptoms, some nine other herbs. Although many complain that it tastes foul, this brew seems to be effective against the severe eczema that is resistant to other treatments.

endometriosis

Many women suffer from the pain and heavy bleeding of endometriosis. In the past, they often were told their complaints were "just cramps" or "all in your head." Today, doctors take this condition more seriously, but conventional medicine offers little to ease its symptoms.

SYMPTOMS

- *Intense menstrual cramps that begin before your period starts and reach their peak after it ends.*
- *Abnormally heavy menstrual bleeding, often with large clots.*
- *Nausea and vomiting just before a menstrual period.*
- *Sharp pain during sexual intercourse at any time of the month.*
- *Diarrhea, constipation, or pain during bowel movements.*
- *Blood in the stool or urine during menstrual period.*
- *Infertility.*

When to Call Your Doctor

- If you have any of the above symptoms.
- Reminder: If you have a medical condition, talk to your doctor before taking supplements.

Long used with other herbs as a uterine tonic in Asia, dong quai's medicinal properties are derived from its root. A tincture may ease endometriosis symptoms.

What it is

In endometriosis, bits of the uterine lining (endometrium) migrate out of the uterus and embed themselves in other abdominal tissues, often the ovaries, uterine ligaments, or intestines. Each month, as estrogen and other hormones cause the lining of the uterus to thicken with blood, the wayward cells also expand. The uterine tissues then slough off normally. But the stray cells have nowhere to release the blood they've amassed, leading to cysts, scarring, or adhesions (fibrous tissue that binds parts of the body that are normally not attached to each other). Although not all women with endometriosis have symptoms, the condition can cause severe pain. Endometriosis is a leading cause of female infertility.

What causes it

No one knows why endometriosis develops, but speculation abounds. According to the "reflux menstruation" theory, menstrual blood travels backward through the fallopian tubes, funneling endometrial cells into other abdominal areas where they seed and grow. Another hypothesis suggests that endometriosis is congenital—meaning that some endometrial cells have been outside the uterus since birth. Still another idea is that endometriosis is caused by a faulty immune system, which neglects to destroy the out-of-place cells.

How supplements can help

All of the supplements listed can be used together and with any medications prescribed by your doctor. Begin by taking the traditional combination of **chasteberry** and **dong quai**. These herbs aid in correcting the hormonal imbalances that can intensify the pain of

Supplement Recommendations

Chasteberry	**Dosage:** 225 mg standardized extract 3 times a day. **Comments:** Also called vitex. Should contain 0.5% agnuside.
Dong quai	**Dosage:** 200 mg, or 30 drops tincture, 3 times a day. **Comments:** Standardized to contain 0.8%-1.1% ligustilide.
Wild yam	**Dosage:** 500 mg twice a day. **Comments:** Take with food to minimize stomach upset.
Lipotropic combination	**Dosage:** 1 or 2 pills 3 times a day. **Comments:** Should contain milk thistle, choline, inositol, methionine, dandelion, and other ingredients.
Calcium/ Magnesium	**Dosage:** 500 mg calcium 4 times a day; 500 mg magnesium twice a day. **Comments:** Use this dose only during menstruation.
Vitamin C	**Dosage:** 1,000 mg 3 times a day. **Comments:** Reduce dose if diarrhea develops.
Vitamin E	**Dosage:** 400 IU twice a day. **Comments:** Check with your doctor if taking anticoagulant drugs.
Flaxseed oil	**Dosage:** 1 tbsp. (14 grams) a day. **Comments:** Can be mixed with food; take in the morning.
Evening primrose oil	**Dosage:** 1,000 mg 3 times a day. **Comments:** Can substitute 1,000 mg borage oil once a day.

Note: Consider using supplements in **blue** first; those in **black** may also be beneficial. Some dosages may be supplied by supplements you are already taking—see page 39.

Some dosages may be supplied by supplements you are already taking—see page 39.

endometriosis. They also relax the uterus, as does **wild yam.** In addition, take a **lipotropic combination,** which stimulates the liver to clear excess estrogen from the body. Use these supplements throughout your menstrual cycle for best results. If menstrual cramps are painful, take the high doses of **calcium** and **magnesium** listed, but only during your period. These minerals help to lower the body's production of prostaglandins, substances made by endometrial cells that cause menstrual cramps.

If a few months of taking these supplements doesn't help, try adding **vitamin C** to promote healing of the tissues damaged by cysts and scarring; **vitamin E** to balance hormone production further; and **flaxseed oil** and **evening primrose oil** to help control inflammation.

What else you can do

☑ Eat soy products, which contain phytoestrogens (plant estrogens) that may offset the effect of estrogen on symptoms of endometriosis.

☑ Exercise. In several studies, it has been shown to suppress symptoms and may actually prevent endometriosis.

C·a·s·e H·i·s·t·o·r·y

PAIN-FREE FOR GOOD

Each month Marie P. struggled with the pain of endometriosis and the fact that she'd never been able to conceive. The problem with conventional hormonal treatments for endometriosis, she had discovered, was the side effects. Though the pain improved, she wondered if the swelling, bloating, hot flashes, and nausea weren't worse than the condition itself.

Then she began reading about herbal and nutritional treatments. She decided to try supplements for three or four months and then go back to her old therapy if they didn't work. Marie began to watch her diet, adding soy and removing the highly processed foods she used to nibble on during the day. She also took the recommended vitamins and herbs.

The first thing she noticed was that she no longer dreaded the pain of intercourse. In fact, her libido perked up. Then menstrual cramps no longer confined her to bed. Finally, she took great delight in telling her husband the best news of all: She was pregnant.

LATEST FINDINGS

■ Women who do not get enough omega-3 fatty acids—found in fish oils and flaxseed oil—often have increased menstrual discomfort. In a Danish study that included 181 women, those who ate a lot of fish had milder menstrual cramps than the women who ate very little.

113

epilepsy

Throughout history, people prone to seizures were thought to be possessed by demons, to have special powers, or to be mentally ill. Today, we know none of this is true: Epilepsy is a condition that diminishes neither intellectual capacity, creativity, nor productivity.

SYMPTOMS

- *Short periods of blackouts, confusion, or altered memory.*
- *Repetitive blinking, chewing, or lip smacking, with or without a lack of awareness.*
- *Lack of attention: a blank stare, no response when spoken to.*
- *Loss of consciousness, sometimes with a loud cry, jerking muscles, or loss of bladder or bowel control; often followed by extreme fatigue.*

When to Call Your Doctor

- **If you experience any of the above symptoms.**
- **If you have a seizure for the first time. However, for later seizures, only falls causing an injury or one episode followed closely by another need a doctor's immediate attention.**
- **Reminder: If you have a medical condition, talk to your doctor before taking supplements.**

What it is

Technically not a disease, epilepsy is a disorder that results from excessive electrical activity in the brain and nervous system. Normally, brain cells transmit electrical impulses in a highly regulated manner. People with epilepsy, however, experience periods when many brain cells fire all at once. This uncontrolled discharge produces symptoms that can range from a blank stare to a loss of consciousness with convulsions. These episodes are called seizures (epilepsy is also known as seizure disorder). Having a single seizure is not necessarily a sign of epilepsy, which is actually defined as having recurrent seizures. In fact, only 27% of people who have a seizure will have another within three years.

What causes it

In more than half of epilepsy cases, the cause of the disorder is unknown. In the remaining cases, seizures can sometimes be traced to a previous head injury, stroke, brain tumor, or brain infection. Experts think that anyone is susceptible to seizures, but for some reason, certain individuals are particularly vulnerable. Heredity seems to play some role.

In people with epilepsy, low blood sugar levels (hypoglycemia) and low levels of certain nutrients (such as magnesium or B vitamins) can induce seizures. In addition, a lack of sleep, drinking too much alcohol, stress, or an illness may trigger a seizure even in people who do not have epilepsy.

How supplements can help

Under no circumstances should individuals using anticonvulsant drugs for epilepsy stop taking them or reduce the dosage on their own. The supplements in the chart are not a substitute for prescription drugs. Instead, they may help correct nutritional deficiencies that can contribute to seizures or aid in controlling seizures in people who continue to have

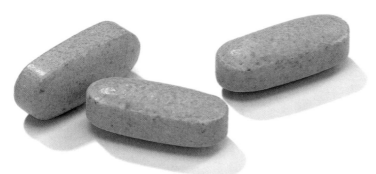

People with epilepsy may benefit from a balanced B-complex vitamin, which helps keep the brain and nerve tissues healthy.

Vitamin B complex	**Dosage:** 1 pill each morning with food. **Comments:** Look for a B-50 complex with 50 mcg vitamin B_{12} and biotin; 400 mcg folic acid; and 50 mg all other B vitamins.
Calcium/ Magnesium	**Dosage:** 250 mg each twice a day with food. **Comments:** Sometimes sold in a single supplement.
GABA	**Dosage:** 500 mg twice a day. **Comments:** Often combined with inositol; has tranquilizing effect.
Kava	**Dosage:** 250 mg twice a day. **Comments:** Standardized to contain at least 30% kavalactones.
Manganese	**Dosage:** 20 mg a day. **Comments:** Take with meals.
Taurine	**Dosage:** 500 mg L-taurine 3 times a day on an empty stomach. **Comments:** If using longer than 1 month, add mixed amino acids.

Note: Consider using supplements in **blue** first; those in **black** may also be beneficial. Some dosages may be supplied by supplements you are already taking—see page 39.

see page 39.

FACTS & Tips

- About 2.5 million Americans have epilepsy, and 125,000 people develop the disorder each year. Though it can develop at any age, 70% of new cases begin in people over age 18, and 12% occur in those over 55.

- Don't try to restrain a person having a seizure or insert a gag or anything else into his mouth to prevent him from biting his tongue. This could cause serious injury to the person or to you if he bites your fingers. Instead, cushion the person's fall and clear away any sharp or hard objects. When the seizure is over, turn him on his side to prevent possible choking.

LATEST FINDINGS

- Preliminary research suggests that vitamin E can help people with epilepsy. One theory on seizures suggests they're triggered by damage to the fatty membranes that surround nerve cells. With its antioxidant properties, vitamin E can inhibit the chemical changes in the body that lead to this damage. Although more study is needed, people with epilepsy can safely take 400 IU of vitamin E a day, either in a multivitamin or as a separate supplement.

them despite medication. Supplements may eventually allow a physician to reduce the dosage of anticonvulsant drugs, which often have unpleasant side effects.

Adequate amounts of B vitamins, especially B_6 and folic acid, are important because they are involved in the manufacture of brain chemicals (called neurotransmitters) that transmit messages throughout the nervous system. Because B vitamins work closely together, it's best to take a **vitamin B complex** supplement. Other nutrients that promote brain and nerve health are **calcium, magnesium,** and **manganese;** you may be getting the amounts you need from your daily multivitamin and mineral, or another supplement. To these, it is safe to add **GABA** (gamma-aminobutyric acid); low levels of this brain chemical appear to be linked to seizures. Though it does not directly control seizures, the herb **kava** may be useful in reducing stress and anxiety, which can trigger these episodes. The amino acid **taurine** may mimic the action of GABA in the body, so choose either it or GABA.

What else you can do

☑ Get plenty of sleep. Fatigue can predispose you to seizures.

☑ Avoid alcohol. It can interfere with anticonvulsant medications and possibly contribute to seizures.

eye infections

Reflexively reaching for over-the-counter eyedrops when your eyes become watery, itchy, red, or inflamed may actually make matters worse. Instead, give one of nature's gentle remedies a try—it may be just what the doctor ordered.

SYMPTOMS

- *Pinkness or redness in the whites of the eyes.*
- *Thick, oozing greenish yellow or white discharge from the eye.*
- *Excessive tearing.*
- *Dried crusts on the eyelid and eyelashes that form during sleep.*
- *Sensation of sand or grit in the eye when blinking.*
- *Swollen or flaking eyelids.*
- *A small, painful red bump at the base of an eyelash (sty).*

When to Call Your Doctor

- If the eye is red or swollen, with a thick discharge—you may need antibiotics for a bacterial infection. If you wear contact lenses, remove them.
- If the eye is painful or sensitive to sunlight, or you have blurring or loss of vision.
- If the pupils are different sizes or an object is lodged in an eye.
- If mild symptoms don't begin to wane in four days of self-care.
- Reminder: If you have a medical condition, talk to your doctor before taking supplements.

What it is

Eye infections are usually related to pinkeye (conjunctivitis), an inflammation of the sensitive mucous membranes that line the eyelids. Other causes of redness and irritation are a persistent scaliness on the eyelid edges (called blepharitis) and inflamed, painful bumps at the base of the eyelashes (known as styes). A doctor should evaluate eyes that are red and painful to determine the proper course of treatment and rule out more serious ailments, such as glaucoma.

What causes it

Viruses and bacteria cause eye infections. Inflammation and redness may also occur as a result of injuries to the eye, allergies, or irritants (such as smoke, makeup, or chlorine in a swimming pool).

How supplements can help

Any serious eye infection or injury requires immediate medical care. Mild eye infections can be treated at home with natural remedies, but see your doctor if the symptoms don't begin to clear up within three or four days.

First, use an herbal eyewash several times a day. **Eyebright** (as its name suggests) may reduce redness, swelling, or irritation from conjunctivitis, blepharitis, styes, or eye injuries. Eyewashes made from the herbs **chamomile** or **goldenseal** offer similar relief and are good alternatives to eyebright. Finely filter all eyewashes through a cheesecloth.

The eyes contain high levels of zinc. Taking this mineral can help boost immunity and combat eye infections.

Supplement Recommendations

Eyebright	**Dosage:** 1 tsp. dried herb per pint of hot water; cool and strain. **Comments:** Store in sealed container. Prepare fresh daily. Use an eyecup to wash affected eye 3 times a day.
Vitamin A	**Dosage:** 50,000 IU twice a day for 7 days, then 25,000 IU daily for 3 weeks. **Comments:** Women who are pregnant or considering pregnancy should not exceed 5,000 IU a day.
Vitamin C	**Dosage:** 1,000 mg 3 times a day for 1 month. **Comments:** Reduce dose if diarrhea develops.
Zinc	**Dosage:** 30 mg a day for 1 month. **Comments:** Do not exceed 150 mg zinc a day from all sources.
Chamomile	**Dosage:** 2 or 3 tsp. dried herb per cup hot water; cool and strain. **Comments:** Store in sealed container. Prepare fresh daily. Use an eyecup to wash affected eye 3 times a day.
Goldenseal	**Dosage:** 1 tsp. dried herb per pint of hot water; cool and strain. **Comments:** Store in sealed container. Prepare fresh daily. Use an eyecup to wash affected eye 3 times a day.

Note: Consider using supplements in **blue** first; those in **black** may also be beneficial. Some dosages may be supplied by supplements you are already taking—see page 39.

To promote healthy eyes, try taking vitamins A and C, as well as the mineral zinc, for a month. All these nutrients enhance immunity, helping to clear away an infection and prevent recurrences. Furthermore, **vitamin A,** well known for its role in maintaining vision, also is vital for the integrity of the mucous membranes, including those surrounding the eyes. **Vitamin C** may speed healing and protect the eye from further inflammation. And **zinc,** which is found in one of its highest concentrations in the eye, may boost the effectiveness of vitamin A.

What else you can do

☑ Wash your hands often with an antiseptic soap, and don't touch or rub your eyes. Change pillowcases and towels frequently; don't share them with others. Most eye infections are highly contagious.

☑ Avoid wearing eye makeup or contact lenses during an eye infection.

☑ Wipe the discharge from the infected eye with a tissue and dispose of it immediately to prevent the infection from spreading.

☑ For styes, apply a warm, moist compress for 10 minutes three or four times a day until the sty comes to a head and drains.

☑ For blepharitis, try a warm, moist compress; apply for 15 minutes to loosen the infected scaliness on the eyelids. Then scrub the eyelid gently with water and baking soda, or with diluted baby shampoo.

☑ Use a separate compress or eyecup for each eye to prevent inadvertently spreading any infection.

fatigue

Hippocrates wrote about it; so did Shakespeare: Throughout the ages, fatigue has doggedly plagued humankind. Today, this complaint accounts for more than 7 million doctor visits a year, and Americans consistently rank it as one of their top 10 health concerns.

SYMPTOMS

■ Persistent, lingering weariness, either intermittent or continuous, that lasts longer than two weeks.

■ Personality changes, particularly a tendency to become angry, impatient, or depressed because of feeling tired all the time.

■ Diminished concentration; difficulty accomplishing familiar tasks; less interest in activities that were once appealing.

When to Call Your Doctor

■ If fatigue lasts longer than two weeks or is accompanied by other symptoms, such as fever, weight loss, nausea, hoarseness, or muscle aches.

■ If fatigue causes daytime drowsiness that interferes with normal everyday activities.

■ Reminder: If you have a medical condition, talk to your doctor before taking supplements.

What it is

Not a true ailment in itself, fatigue is usually a classic symptom of some other problem: poor nutrition; overwork; lack of (or too much) exercise; insomnia or poor sleeping habits; or a specific medical disorder, such as premenstrual syndrome. Though everyone has an occasional energy slump, fatigue is a generalized, persistent feeling of exhaustion.

What causes it

In many sufferers, fatigue can be traced to stress, anxiety, depression, or lowered immunity and chronic infections. It's been linked to diabetes; thyroid or adrenal gland imbalance; and heart, liver, or kidney disease. Vitamin and mineral deficiencies decrease red blood cell production and can lead to fatigue because these cells transport oxygen used for energy. In women, fatigue can result from fluctuating hormone levels in pregnancy and menopause, or from anemia caused by heavy periods. Sleeping disorders and medications, including blood pressure drugs, can also bring it on.

How supplements can help

The supplements listed here should be used only when an underlying fatigue-causing medical condition has been ruled out. A two-month course should bring relief. Start with the vitamins and the two ginsengs. Then add magnesium, amino acids, and flaxseed oil if fatigue persists.

The **B-complex vitamins** support the nervous and immune systems. They enhance the effectiveness of white blood cells, which fight bacteria and viruses, and they are also needed for proper replication of red blood cells. Also important is **vitamin C;** it promotes immune function,

In Asia, Panax ginseng has been prescribed as an energy tonic for literally thousands of years.

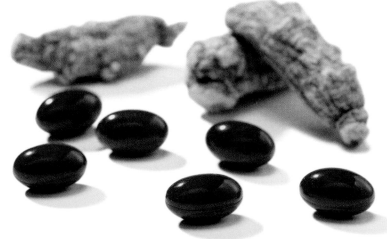

Supplement Recommendations

Vitamin B complex	**Dosage:** 1 pill twice a day with food. **Comments:** Look for a B-50 complex with 50 mcg vitamin B_{12} and biotin; 400 mcg folic acid; and 50 mg all other B vitamins.
Vitamin C	**Dosage:** 1,000 mg 3 times a day. **Comments:** Reduce dose if diarrhea develops.
Panax ginseng	**Dosage:** 100-250 mg twice a day. **Comments:** Standardized to contain at least 7% ginsenosides.
Siberian ginseng	**Dosage:** 100-300 mg twice a day. **Comments:** Standardized to contain at least 0.8% eleutherosides.
Magnesium	**Dosage:** 400 mg a day for 2 months. **Comments:** Take with food; reduce dose if diarrhea develops.
Amino acid complex	**Dosage:** 1 pill twice a day. **Comments:** Take on an empty stomach.
Flaxseed oil	**Dosage:** 1 tbsp. (14 grams) a day. **Comments:** Can be mixed with food; take in the morning.

Note: Consider using supplements in **blue** first; those in **black** may also be beneficial. Some dosages may be supplied by supplements you are already taking—see page 39.

see page 39

FACTS & Tips

- Fatigue is often a symptom of an unrecognized vitamin B_{12} deficiency. But B_{12} injections, which were once routinely given to boost energy, are beneficial only when a deficiency has been confirmed by blood tests. Even then, the problem can usually be resolved with very high oral doses, which must be monitored by your doctor.

LATEST FINDINGS

- Measures to prevent and treat fatigue may help increase longevity, especially among the elderly. Researchers studied more than 1,000 people born in 1914. They found that long-term fatigue is a more accurate predictor of death than traditional yardsticks, such as smoking or eating habits.

Did You Know?

Caffeinated beverages can wreak havoc with your ability to fall and remain fast asleep for up to 10 hours after you drink them.

helps repair tissues, and supports the adrenal gland, which controls production of stress hormones in the body.

One of the most popular uses of ginseng is to boost the body's own energy levels. **Panax ginseng** has long been used for this purpose in Asia. **Siberian ginseng** contains compounds that have been shown to fight fatigue. A mild **magnesium** deficiency may be the cause of fatigue in some people. A two-month course of the mineral should address any shortage. Every cell in the body needs a mixture of **amino acids** to make protein, and in some cases low levels may contribute to fatigue. **Flaxseed oil** helps by supplying essential fatty acids, which protect the integrity of cell membranes and enhance the immune system.

What else you can do

☑ Take a 20-minute nap in the afternoon or after work. But set the alarm: A longer nap can interfere with nighttime sleep.

☑ Don't skip breakfast. Near bedtime, avoid large meals, fatty foods, alcohol, and caffeinated beverages.

☑ Go to sleep and get up at the same time every day; get at least eight hours of sleep a night.

☑ Keep active. Moderate exercise is a prescription for feeling less tired.

☑ Don't expect an energy boost from sugary foods. Instead eat complex carbohydrates (pasta, whole grains, beans) and lots of fruits and vegetables.

☑ Have blood tests for thyroid problems or anemia if fatigue persists.

fibrocystic breasts

Most doctors no longer call the pain and lumpiness of fibrocystic breasts a disease because this condition affects virtually half of all women under age 50. Selected supplements and a shift in diet may help diminish the symptoms of this disorder.

SYMPTOMS

- *Breast lumps or nodules that may be tender or not painful at all.*
- *An increase in the size of lumps or in breast discomfort a week or so before a menstrual period.*

When to Call Your Doctor

- If a new lump develops, especially if you have not always had lumpy breasts.
- If a lump grows larger, hardens, or does not diminish after your menstrual period ends.
- If you have any discharge from either nipple.
- If your breast pain is severe.
- Reminder: If you have a medical condition, talk to your doctor before taking supplements.

What it is

Normal breasts vary in density and texture. Before menopause, women tend to have more tissue (which can make the breasts feel firm or lumpy) and less fat in their breasts than they do in their later years. Occasionally, women develop fluid-filled cysts or fibrous areas, which can be tender just before menstruation. Though most women experience some mild breast discomfort in their life, some have monthly pain so severe that it interferes with daily activities.

Such premenstrual changes have long been labeled "fibrocystic breast disease." But this condition is not a disease, and it doesn't increase your risk of breast cancer (though having lumpy breasts may make identifying a cancerous growth more difficult if one develops). Normal lumps can usually be distinguished from cancerous ones because they move freely in the breast, changing with the menstrual cycle.

What causes it

Fibrocystic changes in the breast are linked to the rise and fall of hormones associated with the menstrual cycle. Women who produce a particularly high level of estrogen in conjunction with a low level of progesterone after ovulation may suffer more. This combination can cause the body to produce too much prolactin, a hormone that triggers milk production in new mothers but increases breast tenderness in women who are not breast-feeding.

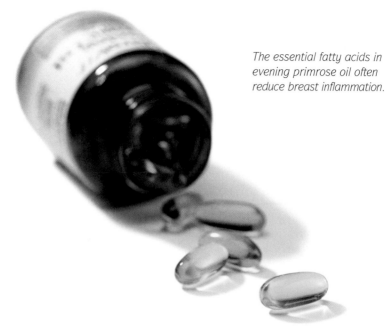

The essential fatty acids in evening primrose oil often reduce breast inflammation.

Supplement Recommendations

Vitamin E	**Dosage:** 400 IU twice a day. **Comments:** Check with your doctor if taking anticoagulant drugs.
Chasteberry	**Dosage:** 225 mg standardized extract each morning. **Comments:** Also called vitex. Should contain 0.5% agnuside.
Essential fatty acids	**Dosage:** 1,000 mg evening primrose oil 3 times a day; 1 tbsp. (14 grams) flaxseed oil a day. **Comments:** Or use 1,000 mg borage oil once a day for primrose oil.
Magnesium	**Dosage:** 600 mg a day. **Comments:** Take with food; reduce dose if diarrhea develops.
Vitamin B₆	**Dosage:** 100 mg twice a day for 1 week. **Comments:** Take this amount only the week before menstruation; this dose can cause nerve damage if taken daily over the long term.

Note: Consider using supplements in **blue** first; those in **black** may also be beneficial. Some dosages may be supplied by supplements you are already taking—see page 39.

Many experts think caffeine stimulates the growth of lumps or fluid-filled breast cysts (and some women showed improvement when they eliminate caffeine), but other researchers maintain there's no firm evidence of any connection between caffeine and breast tenderness.

How supplements can help

All the supplements listed can be used together and as needed; you should see improvement in a month or two. Many women report relief from breast pain after taking **vitamin E.** Just how it works is unknown, but some experts believe this vitamin blocks the changes in breast tissue possibly caused by caffeine.

Because it works to restore the hormonal balance between estrogen and progesterone, the herb **chasteberry** may be useful in reducing menstrual-related breast changes. **Essential fatty acids** often act as anti-inflammatory compounds; they also help the body absorb iodine (low iodine levels have been linked to fibrocystic breasts). **Magnesium** may also reduce inflammation and pain. **Vitamin B₆** may be beneficial for women who experience PMS symptoms with breast pain; it may also help the liver process excess estrogen.

What else you can do

☑ Eliminate caffeine and see if that helps. Besides coffee and tea, caffeine is found in chocolate, colas, and some over-the-counter medications. Be patient: Six months may pass before you notice any improvement.

☑ Wear a bra with good support when your breasts are tender.

fibromyalgia

If you can't explain why every muscle in your body seems to hurt lately, you may have fibromyalgia, an elusive disorder that affects millions of Americans. This condition is most common among women between the ages of 20 and 50, although it can strike anyone at any age.

SYMPTOMS

- *Chronic muscle pain and stiffness (at its worst in the morning) for three consecutive months.*
- *Sensitivity in 11 of 18 specific body sites, called tender points.*
- *Poor quality of sleep.*
- *Fatigue (chronic or occasional), even after adequate sleep.*
- *Depression, often with anxiety.*
- *Headaches.*
- *Impaired memory, concentration, and muscle coordination.*

When to Call Your Doctor

- If symptoms last for three months; sooner if you can't carry out your daily routine.
- If other causes, such as flu or arthritis, have been eliminated.
- If sleep disturbances are severe.
- If you are depressed.
- Reminder: If you have a medical or psychiatric condition, talk to your doctor before taking supplements.

What it is

Defined as a rheumatic disorder, fibromyalgia is characterized by wide-spread muscle pain and fatigue. In the morning, a person with this condition frequently feels unrefreshed and experiences aching or stabbing muscle pain (which often improves as the day progresses). Symptoms may be constant or disappear for months at a time and then recur.

Because blood tests and X rays show no abnormalities, fibromyalgia can be hard to diagnose. To distinguish this disorder from others that cause similar symptoms, such as chronic fatigue syndrome or depression, doctors often apply pressure to specific areas of the body (called tender points); the pressure causes enough pain to make the person flinch or cry out. The diagnosis of fibromyalgia is made when fatigue and muscle pain persist for three months and can't be linked to another cause, and when extreme sensitivity is found at 11 of 18 tender points, at the base of the skull and in the neck, shoulders, ribs, upper chest (near the collarbone), elbows, knees, lower back, and buttocks.

What causes it

The cause of fibromyalgia is not known. Once thought to be a psychological disorder, the condition is now ascribed by some to low levels of serotonin, one of the chemicals that transmit messages throughout the brain and nervous system. Lack of serotonin may produce the muscle pain directly or, more likely, interfere with sleep, thus aggravating the pain.

Others suggest that individuals with fibromyalgia have extremely high levels of substance P, which is believed to transmit pain messages from the body to the brain. Therefore, those with the condition may simply be abnormally sensitive to pain-producing stimuli. In addition, a particularly severe case of the flu, a physical injury such as whiplash, a weak immune system, or some long-standing psychological stress have all been associated with the disease. Fibromyalgia also seems to be closely linked to chronic fatigue syndrome, and the two may occur together.

Magnesium and malic acid may relieve the pain of fibromyalgia by helping the muscles to relax.

Supplement Recommendations

Magnesium/ Malic acid	**Dosage:** 150 mg magnesium and 600 mg malic acid twice a day. **Comments:** Sometimes sold in combination as magnesium malate.
St. John's wort	**Dosage:** 300 mg 3 times a day. **Comments:** Standardized to contain 0.3% hypericin.
5-HTP	**Dosage:** 100 mg 3 times a day. **Comments:** If drowsiness occurs, reduce to 50 mg 3 times a day.
Vitamin C	**Dosage:** 1,000 mg 3 times a day. **Comments:** Reduce dose if diarrhea develops.
Grape seed extract	**Dosage:** 100 mg twice a day. **Comments:** Standardized to contain 92%-95% proanthocyanidins.
Coenzyme Q$_{10}$	**Dosage:** 100 mg twice a day. **Comments:** For best absorption, take with food.
Melatonin	**Dosage:** 3 mg before bedtime. **Comments:** Helpful if sleep disorders accompany pain.

Note: Consider using supplements in **blue** first; those in **black** may also be beneficial. Some dosages may be supplied by supplements you are already taking—see page 39.

How supplements can help

Everyone with fibromyalgia should take **magnesium** and **malic acid.** These are important for energy and muscle relaxation. Many people with this condition are deficient in magnesium; the malic acid enhances its absorption as well as its fatigue-fighting effect. Consider adding either the herb **St. John's wort** or **5-HTP** (5-hydroxytryptophan, a form of the amino acid tryptophan); both raise serotonin levels, ease depression, and improve pain tolerance. Unless directed to do so by a doctor, don't use either of these with prescription antidepressants. To help protect muscle cells from damage, take **vitamin C** with or without **grape seed extract;** both are powerful antioxidants. If you feel you need more support, add **coenzyme Q$_{10}$.** It helps relieve the symptoms of chronic fatigue syndrome, which may accompany fibromyalgia. And if you're having difficulty sleeping, try **melatonin** or the herb valerian.

What else you can do

☑ Eat several small meals during the day to keep a steady supply of protein and carbohydrate available for proper muscle function.

☑ Take hot baths or showers—especially in the morning—to soothe soreness, increase circulation, and relieve stiffness.

☑ Find a massage therapist familiar with fibromyalgia. A technique called trigger point therapy can be extremely helpful in reducing pain.

☑ Cut back on caffeine, alcohol, and sugar, which often cause fatigue.

☑ Get at least eight hours of sleep a night.

LATEST FINDINGS

■ In a study of 24 people with fibromyalgia, high doses of magnesium and malic acid were effective in reducing pain and tenderness. At least two months of treatment were necessary before results appeared.

■ Rather than further taxing chronically sore muscles, aerobic exercise may actually help them and relieve symptoms of fibromyalgia, according to a recent study. When combined with stress management techniques, 45 minutes of exercise three to five times a week eased pain and fatigue. If you don't currently exercise much, gradually work your way up to 45-minute sessions. Doing too much too fast can backfire.

■ Meditation, movement therapy, and knowledge of the connections between mind and body helped 20 fibromyalgia patients in one study. After eight weeks, standardized tests showed improvements in the sleep, fatigue, pain level, and mood of the study's participants.

flatulence

Passing gas may not be life-threatening, but it can be uncomfortable—and embarrassing—especially if it happens too often. Commonsense changes in your diet and some helpful supplements can provide welcome relief for you—and for those around you.

What it is

Passing intestinal gas is normal. A typical adult does it as often as 15 times a day, generating one to three pints of gas. But normal doesn't necessarily mean worry-free. Even the average amount of gas can cause discomfort for some people, and in others the frequency of flatulent episodes and the amount of gas emitted are much greater than average. The only good thing about flatulence is that by itself it is not a symptom of cancer or any other serious intestinal disease.

What causes it

Flatulence results when excess gases build up in the digestive tract and are then expelled through the rectum. Chemical reactions that occur after eating certain foods are the most common cause. The most likely culprits are broccoli, brussels sprouts, cabbage, cauliflower, onions, and beans. Because they contain complex carbohydrates, these foods are often incompletely digested in the stomach and small intestine. After they arrive in the large intestine, they are broken down by the harmless bacteria that live there, and certain gases—carbon dioxide, hydrogen, and methane—are by-products of this bacterial action. In some people, milk and milk products induce gas and bloating; this milk-related flatulence is often the result of lactose intolerance.

Hydrogen sulfide and other compounds containing sulfur are responsible for the unpleasant odor of some intestinal gas—though not all gas has an odor. Passing excessive gas can be a symptom of disorders that hinder normal digestion, such as celiac disease. It can also result from stressful situations, because people under stress often swallow a lot of air.

How supplements can help

If flatulence is more than an occasional problem, try a combination of the first four supplements in the chart. **Ginger,** in tablet form or as freshly

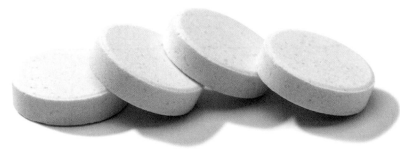

Acidophilus supplements help control intestinal tract bacteria that can produce excess gas.

Ginger	**Dosage:** 100 mg 2 or 3 times a day as needed. **Comments:** Standardized to contain gingerols.
Acidophilus	**Dosage:** 1 pill twice a day between meals. **Comments:** Get 1-2 billion live (viable) organisms per pill.
Bifidus	**Dosage:** 1 pill twice a day with meals. **Comments:** Get 1-2 billion live (viable) organisms per pill.
FOS	**Dosage:** 2,000 mg twice a day. **Comments:** Use in combination with acidophilus and bifidus.
Activated charcoal	**Dosage:** 500 mg after each meal and every 2 hours as needed. **Comments:** Do not exceed 4,000 mg a day.

Note: Consider using supplements in **blue** first; those in **black** may also be beneficial. Some dosages may be supplied by supplements you are already taking—see page 39.

grated root (mixed with a little lime juice), is a good all-purpose digestive aid. It soothes the digestive tract and is useful for relieving flatulence.

Acidophilus and **bifidus,** two of the friendly bacteria that inhabit the large intestine, help keep the growth of gas-producing bacteria in check. **FOS** (fructo-oligosaccharides), indigestible carbohydrates that are present in certain foods, promote the growth of friendly bacteria. Replenishing these bacterial good guys will often relieve gas, bloating, and other digestive complaints. If this course of action is unsuccessful, use **activated charcoal** to absorb gas in the intestine and help reduce the accompanying odor. It is also available as pills or a tasteless powder, which can be mixed in a glass of cold water and sipped through a straw to prevent staining the teeth.

What else you can do

☑ Avoid carbonated beverages.

☑ Chew food thoroughly. Large particles cause gas when they pass into the large intestine without being completely digested.

☑ Eat slowly. If you eat too quickly, you tend to swallow more air.

☑ Soak beans before cooking, which removes some indigestible sugars. Discard the soaking water and cook the beans in fresh water.

FACTS & Tips

- Before you even consider supplements for flatulence, try giving up all dairy products for a few days and see if you feel better. If you do, you may be lactose intolerant. You can minimize the effects of lactose intolerance by eating dairy products in small portions with other foods or by choosing lactose-reduced products.

- Be cautious about using the sweeteners sorbitol and xylitol, which are found in many commercial products. They often promote gas.

- Some people swear by an old folk remedy for flatulence: a teaspoon of apple cider vinegar with every meal.

LATEST FINDINGS

- A recent Veterans Administration study of young and middle-aged men dispelled the myth that flatulence increases with age. It also confirmed that indigestible carbohydrates are at the root of the problem. Both groups of men passed gas an average of 10 times a day while on their normal diets. This frequency nearly doubled when they were also given 10 grams of such carbohydrates each day.

Did You Know?

Even the Founding Fathers were concerned with flatulence. Benjamin Franklin once noted: "It is universally well known, that in digesting our common food, there is created or produced in the bowels of human creatures, a great quantity of wind."

gallstones

Some 20 million Americans have gallstones, crystallized pellets in the gallbladder that can suddenly cause painful spasms a few hours after eating a rich meal. A high-fiber diet, along with certain supplements, can help prevent, relieve, or even dissolve these troublesome stones.

SYMPTOMS

- *Intermittent pain on the right side of the upper abdomen. The pain typically develops after a meal, lasts from 30 minutes to 4 hours, and may move to the back, chest, or right shoulder.*

- *Nausea and vomiting may accompany pain. Heartburn, gas, or bloating may also be present.*

When to Call Your Doctor

- If you develop severe abdominal pain, or pain with nausea, vomiting, or fever. Either symptom may signal gallbladder inflammation or a blockage of the bile duct. Both are medical emergencies.

- If you have upper right abdominal pain and nausea with shortness of breath and sweating—this may be a heart attack. Call an ambulance right away.

- Reminder: If you have a medical condition, talk to your doctor before taking supplements.

What it is

Gallstones are rocklike clumps of cholesterol or other digestive substances that form in the gallbladder, the pear-shaped organ that sits in the upper right section of the abdomen, just under the liver. The gallbladder stores and concentrates bile—a thick greenish yellow fluid that's produced by the liver—and eventually releases it through the bile duct into the small intestine to aid in the digestion of fats. Gallstones can develop if the bile contains very high levels of cholesterol, bile acids, pigments, or other substances. Whether they're really tiny or as big as a golf ball, gallstones often produce no symptoms and need no special care. Sometimes, though, they can block the bile duct or inflame the gallbladder, causing intense abdominal pain and requiring prompt treatment.

What causes it

Though the exact cause of gallstones is not known, several factors may contribute to their formation, including a low-fiber, high-fat diet; intestinal surgery; inflammatory bowel disease; or other disorders of the digestive tract. Gallstones tend to occur in people over age 40 and are three times more common in women than in men. Obesity is also strongly linked to gallstones, as is rapid weight loss. There may be a genetic component as well: Among Arizona's Pima Indians, nearly 70% of women over age 30 have gallstones.

How supplements can help

The supplements recommended in the chart may all aid in preventing or dissolving gallstones. Three months of treatment may be effective in dissolving small existing stones, though those supplements in blue (except taurine) can also be used long term to help prevent gallstone attacks.

Extra **vitamin C** is important because it lowers bile cholesterol levels, decreasing the chance that cholesterol-laden bile will clump to form stones. Vitamin C should be combined with various other supplements.

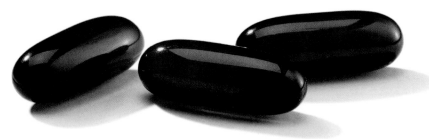

Gallstone-fighting flaxseed oil comes in capsule form for those who dislike the taste of the oil.

Supplement Recommendations

Vitamin C	**Dosage:** 1,000 mg 3 times a day.
	Comments: Reduce dose if diarrhea develops.
Lipotropic combination	**Dosage:** 1 or 2 pills twice a day.
	Comments: Need 250 mg milk thistle (take extra if needed); may also include choline, inositol, methionine, and dandelion.
Taurine	**Dosage:** 1,000 mg L-taurine twice a day for up to 3 months.
	Comments: After 6 weeks, add a mixed amino acid complex.
Lecithin	**Dosage:** 2 capsules of 19 grains (1,200 mg) each twice a day.
	Comments: Or 2 tsp. granular form twice a day before meals.
Flaxseed oil	**Dosage:** 1 tbsp. (14 grams) a day in liquid or pill form.
	Comments: Can be mixed with food; take in the morning.
Peppermint oil	**Dosage:** 2 capsules (containing 0.2 ml of oil each) twice a day.
	Comments: Buy enteric-coated capsules. Take between meals.
Psyllium	**Dosage:** 1 tbsp. powder dissolved in water or juice twice a day.
	Comments: Be sure to drink extra water throughout the day.

Note: Consider using supplements in **blue** first; those in **black** may also be beneficial. Some dosages may be supplied by supplements you are already taking—see page 39.

A good general choice is a **lipotropic** ("fat-metabolizing") **combination,** containing milk thistle, choline, inositol, and methionine, which bolsters liver function and promotes a healthy flow of fats and bile from the liver and gallbladder. The herb milk thistle, for example, alters bile composition, helping to dissolve gallstones and eliminate stones that may have formed. Choline and inositol (related to the B vitamins) and the amino acid methionine aid in fat and cholesterol metabolism as well. They also strengthen liver and gallbladder function. Methionine may increase levels of another amino acid, **taurine,** which improves bile flow and helps dissolve existing stones. Choline and inositol are also vital to the fatty bile component **lecithin** (inadequate levels may precipitate gallstones).

Other supplements may be worth adding to the mix, either singly or together. **Flaxseed oil** contains essential fatty acids that may be useful in preventing or even dissolving gallstones. **Peppermint oil,** taken in enteric-coated capsules, also has gallstone-dissolving effects. And daily doses of **psyllium** can promote bowel movements, which may be of value in blocking the formation of gallstones.

What else you can do

☑ Eat a diet high in fiber and low in refined carbohydrates, sugar, and fat. Fruits and vegetables, oat bran, and pectin (found in apples, bananas, cabbage, carrots, oranges, peas, and okra) may be especially important in preventing and dissolving gallstones.

☑ Keep your weight down and drink plenty of water daily.

gout

At least one male in a hundred over age 40 suffers from gout. Women can develop it too, mainly after menopause. Though people with gout feel fine much of the time, an attack can occur without warning, bringing on breath-catching joint pain that demands fast-acting, effective relief.

SYMPTOMS

- *Sudden and severe joint pain, usually involving the big toe, heel, ankle, or instep first. Subsequent attacks may affect the knee, wrist, elbow, fingers, or other areas.*
- *Redness and swelling in affected joint or joints.*
- *Kidney stones develop occasionally, causing fever, severe low back pain, nausea, vomiting, or a swollen abdomen.*

When to Call Your Doctor

- If you experience symptoms of an acute gout attack—your doctor can prescribe medications to ease the initial pain.
- If you suffer the severe pain of passing a kidney stone.
- Reminder: If you have a medical condition, talk to your doctor before taking supplements.

What it is

Gout is a metabolic disorder linked to high levels of uric acid in the blood. Uric acid, a by-product of various body processes, is also formed after eating certain foods. The body rids itself of uric acid through the urine. But some people produce too much uric acid—or can't dispose of it fast enough—and levels build up. Often, the excess uric acid is converted into needle-shaped crystals that settle in and around joints and other tissues, triggering inflammation and the excruciating pain associated with gout.

What causes it

It's uncertain what precipitates a gout attack, though some factors may put you at risk. A quarter of those who suffer from gout have a family history of the illness, and three-quarters have high triglyceride levels. Men who gain a lot of weight between ages 20 and 40 are particularly vulnerable. Excessive alcohol intake (including "binge" drinking), high blood pressure, kidney disease, exposure to lead, crash diets, and certain medications (including antibiotics, diuretics, and cancer chemotherapy drugs) may also play a role. For a few people, eating foods high in chemicals called purines (such as liver or anchovies) can cause flare-ups.

How supplements can help

Uric acid can accumulate in the blood for years with no symptoms. An acute attack often happens suddenly and is best treated with conventional drugs. The main supplement that seems to help during an acute attack is bromelain. The others, taken together, may prevent future attacks. All can be safely used for long periods, though cherry extract, vitamin C, and nettle may be the simplest regimen to follow for long-term maintenance.

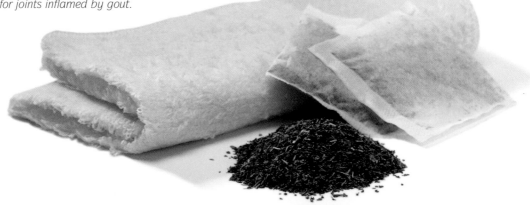

A compress soaked in tea brewed from the green leaves of the nettle plant may supply soothing relief for joints inflamed by gout.

Supplement Recommendations

Bromelain	**Dosage:** 500 mg every 3 hours during an attack; reduce to twice a day to help prevent further attacks. **Comments:** Each dose should provide 2,000 GDU or 3,000 MCU.
Quercetin	**Dosage:** 500 mg twice a day between meals. **Comments:** Take with bromelain to help prevent gout attacks.
Cherry fruit extract	**Dosage:** 1,000 mg 3 times a day following an acute attack. **Comments:** Reduce dosage to 1,000 mg a day for maintenance.
Vitamin C	**Dosage:** 500 mg a day. **Comments:** Add 500 mg every 5 days until you reach 1,000 mg twice a day. Reduce dose if diarrhea develops.
Nettle	**Dosage:** 250 mg standardized extract 3 times a day. **Comments:** Also effective as a nettle tea compress applied to sore joints. (Use 1 or 2 tsp. dried herb per cup of hot water.)
Flaxseed oil	**Dosage:** 1 tbsp. (14 grams) a day. **Comments:** Can be mixed with food; take in the morning.

Note: Consider using supplements in **blue** first; those in **black** may also be beneficial. Some dosages may be supplied by supplements you are already taking—see page 39.

An enzyme derived from pineapples, **bromelain** is a popular natural anti-inflammatory that may relieve gout pain. When not using it for acute flare-ups, decrease the dosage and add **quercetin**. This flavonoid reduces uric acid levels and is better absorbed if taken with bromelain.

Cherries, an old folk remedy for gout, are rich in flavonoids and often effective at lowering uric acid levels. **Cherry fruit extract** is available at many health-food stores; cherry or blueberry juice (a half cup a day) also works well. In incremental doses, **vitamin C** helps uric acid to free itself from the tissues and be excreted in the urine. (High initial doses may release so much uric acid that a kidney stone develops.) **Nettle** can be helpful internally and externally: Capsules clear out excess uric acid, and topical nettle tea compresses may relieve inflamed joints.

Finally, **flaxseed oil** may deter the production of leukotrienes, substances involved in the inflammatory reaction of gout. Other natural therapies to reduce uric acid levels include eating celery or avocados, or drinking teas made from the herbs cat's claw, devil's claw, or olive leaf.

What else you can do

☑ Drink at least eight glasses of water a day to dilute the urine and help lower uric acid levels. Stay away from alcohol, which can trigger attacks.

☑ Keep weight down. Obesity may play an important role in gout attacks.

☑ Avoid fats, refined carbohydrates, excess protein, and, if you're sensitive to purines, foods containing them (including organ meats, anchovies, legumes, oatmeal, spinach, asparagus, cauliflower, and mushrooms).

FACTS & Tips

■ One of the oldest known remedies for gout—a drug called colchicine—is derived from the autumn crocus, also known as meadow saffron. Unfortunately, colchicine in pill form causes severe cramping and diarrhea in up to 80% of those who take it in the high doses needed to combat gout attacks. An injectable form of colchicine administered by your doctor, however, appears to work quickly and without side effects.

■ Eating fresh or canned cherries (a half pound a day) may help keep gout at bay by reducing levels of uric acid. Some people swear by them; and a small study conducted many years ago found that eating cherries may indeed lower uric acid levels. An easier way to get the benefits of cherries is to take 1,000 mg daily of cherry fruit extract pills (available at health-food stores). Strawberries, blueberries, celery, or celery seed extracts may have a similar beneficial effect.

Did You Know?

Although between 10% and 20% of Americans have high uric acid levels, only a small percentage of them ever actually develop gout.

gum disease

If you haven't had gum problems yet, chances are you will: Three out of four adults over age 35 experience tender, swollen, or bleeding gums at some point in their lives. But there are plenty of things you can do to relieve pain, heal the gums, and preserve your teeth.

SYMPTOMS

- *Gums that bleed after brushing.*
- *Red, swollen, and tender gums.*
- *A toothache made worse by hot, cold, or sweet foods or liquids.*
- *Chronic bad breath or a bad taste in the mouth.*
- *Loose or missing teeth.*

When to Call Your Doctor

- See your dentist if you experience red, swollen gums or loose teeth. It may save your teeth.
- Have your teeth professionally cleaned if you haven't done so in the previous year.
- Reminder: If you have a medical condition, talk to your doctor before taking supplements.

What it is

There are two main types of gum disease: gingivitis and periodontitis. Gingivitis—marked by tender, inflamed gums—occurs when bacteria in the mouth form a thin, sticky film called plaque that coats the teeth and gums. If ignored, plaque will turn into tartar, a hard mineral shell that erodes gum tissue. Over time this will lead to the more serious—and harder to treat—condition known as periodontitis. In advanced periodontal disease, the gums recede in places and pockets form around the teeth, allowing bacteria to eat away at the bone anchoring the teeth.

What causes it

Poor oral hygiene—including improper brushing, flossing, or rinsing—is the leading cause of gum disease. Other precipitating factors include a high-sugar diet, lack of vitamin C or other nutrients, and smoking (the chemicals in tobacco smoke harm gums and teeth). In addition, certain medications can make gum disease worse because they inhibit saliva production, which helps wash away bacteria and sugars. Genetic factors likely make some people particularly susceptible to gum disease. Women seem to be more prone to gum problems during pregnancy and menopause because of hormonal changes. Diabetes and other chronic diseases that can lower resistance to infection also increase the risk.

How supplements can help

Various supplements—used together—can help heal sore and bleeding gums. Benefits should be noticed within two weeks. People at high risk for gum disease can also take them on a long-term preventive basis.

When consumed orally on a daily basis, **vitamin C, flavonoids,** and **coenzyme Q$_{10}$,** all powerful antioxidants, protect gum tissue against cell damage and speed healing. They also boost immunity, helping to keep

Chewable vitamin C tablets are a convenient way to get this superstar antioxidant, but rinse your mouth after chewing one to prevent damage to tooth enamel.

Supplement Recommendations

Vitamin C/ Flavonoids	**Dosage:** 1,000 mg vitamin C and 500 mg flavonoids twice a day. **Comments:** Reduce vitamin C dose if diarrhea develops.
Coenzyme Q₁₀	**Dosage:** 50 mg twice a day. **Comments:** For best absorption, take with food.
Vitamin E	**Dosage:** Break open a 400 IU capsule; rub contents on gums. **Comments:** Alternate with folic acid/vitamin C treatments.
Folic acid liquid	**Dosage:** Dip swab in liquid; apply along gum line every other day. **Comments:** Follow up with vitamin C powder. Alternate with vitamin E gum treatment every other day.
Vitamin C powder	**Dosage:** Using ½ tsp. powder, brush along gum line every other day. **Comments:** Alternate with vitamin E treatment every other day.

Some dosages may be supplied by supplements you are already taking—see page 39.

gum-attacking bacteria in check. Studies of coenzyme Q₁₀, for example, show that it reduces the depth of pockets formed around the teeth by bacteria; this stabilizes the teeth and aids in shortening the recovery period after dental surgery. Other studies suggest that vitamin C and flavonoids may strengthen connective tissue in the gums and decrease inflammation, and that they are most effective when used together.

In addition, various topical therapies may reduce gum inflammation and bleeding. Every other day, break open a **vitamin E** capsule and rub the oil on the inflamed tissue to soothe the area and promote quicker healing. On alternate days, apply **folic acid liquid** to your gums with a cotton swab. Follow up by gently brushing along the gum line with **vitamin C powder,** using a very soft toothbrush. These topical treatments should be carried out twice a day, after regular tooth brushing.

What else you can do

☑ Floss at least once a day and brush at least twice with a soft-bristle brush. It is important to use the proper technique, including brushing the tongue, which collects the same bacteria that stick to your teeth. If you're not sure you're flossing or brushing correctly, ask your dentist or dental hygienist to show you how. Plan to spend five minutes or so each session.

☑ Limit your intake of sweets and sticky carbohydrates—or at least brush as soon as possible after eating them. These foods can accumulate in gum spaces and pockets, particularly in older people, who tend to have more exposed roots in their teeth.

☑ See a dentist at least once a year for a professional cleaning—or more often if you have a problem that needs special attention.

FACTS & Tips

- Try natural toothpastes and mouthwashes containing the herb bloodroot. These supply an antibacterial substance called sanguinarine that helps reduce and prevent the accumulation of dental plaque—the first step in gum disease.

- Commission E, a noted panel of health experts in Germany that reviews herbal supplements, officially recognizes chamomile as an effective gargle or mouthwash for the treatment of gingivitis. Make a chamomile tea using 2 or 3 teaspoons of herb per cup of hot water. Steep for 10 minutes, strain, and cool. Use as a daily mouthwash or gargle.

LATEST FINDINGS

- Maintaining healthy gums with natural supplements and good dental care may produce more than just a pretty smile. Now researchers at several medical centers report a possible link between the most common type of bacteria causing dental plaque and the development of heart disease. This link is still under investigation, but one theory is that the gum bacteria can enter the bloodstream and promote blood clots or damage the heart muscle.

Did You Know?

Fluoridation of drinking water dramatically cuts the risk of tooth loss. The trace mineral fluoride interacts with tooth enamel and hardens it, making it 50% to 70% less susceptible to decay.

hair problems

Americans face a variety of hair problems: dandruff, balding, brittle and graying hair, to name just a few. Though most are signs of the natural progression of aging, or basic genetic predispositions, various simple measures can contribute to a healthier head of hair.

SYMPTOMS

- *Flaking or crusting of the scalp.*
- *Increased loss of hair, such as when washing or combing.*
- *Changes in hair color, texture, or growth patterns.*
- *Irritated skin patches on the scalp.*

When to Call Your Doctor

- If hair loss occurs suddenly, especially when accompanied by symptoms such as the cessation of the menstrual cycle.
- If the scalp develops dry, crusty patches or itches intensely.
- Reminder: If you have a medical condition, talk to your doctor before taking supplements.

What it is

Hair is a nonliving tissue, made up mainly of a fibrous protein called keratin—the same material found in your fingernails and toenails. The health of your hair requires a plentiful supply of nutrient-rich blood to nourish the hair follicles in the scalp, from which new hair sprouts. On average, hair grows about half an inch a month. It's not unusual for people to shed up to a hundred hairs a day—fortunately, when one falls out, another usually grows in. Problems can arise when hair becomes dry or brittle, stops growing back, or becomes flecked with dandruff caused by excess flaking and shedding of skin on the scalp.

What causes it

Stress, a poor diet, and hormonal changes (such as those accompanying pregnancy) can all contribute to hair loss. Some hair conditions may also be the result of nutritional deficiencies, environmental circumstances, an underactive thyroid gland, immune disorders, or genetic factors.

How supplements can help

The recommended supplements, which can be taken together, may help your hair grow stronger and healthier by nourishing it at the roots. Though there's no miracle remedy that can guarantee a luxurious head of hair, you may notice improvement within six months, when new hair has had time to grow in.

Supplements containing essential fatty acids, such as flaxseed oil and evening primrose oil, provide various benefits. **Flaxseed oil** is rich in omega-3 fatty acids—without them, hair is often dry and lifeless; flaxseed oil may also cut down on itching and flaking dandruff and be useful for treating eczema and psoriasis of the scalp. **Evening primrose oil** moisturizes the hair and the scalp as well.

Vitamins and minerals, such as zinc, promote healthy hair growth and may slow hair loss. Because it can boost thyroid function, **zinc** may be especially beneficial for people who have brittle or thinning hair as a result of an

Taking biotin and other B vitamins is good for your hair.

Supplement Recommendations

Flaxseed oil	**Dosage:** 1 tbsp. (14 grams) a day.
	Comments: Can be mixed with food; take in the morning.
Evening primrose oil	**Dosage:** 1,000 mg 3 times a day.
	Comments: Can substitute 1,000 mg borage oil once a day.
Zinc/Copper	**Dosage:** 30 mg zinc and 2 mg copper a day.
	Comments: Add copper only when using zinc longer than 1 month.
Biotin	**Dosage:** 1,000 mcg a day.
	Comments: Can combat excessive oiliness and flaking; take with vitamin B complex.
Vitamin B complex	**Dosage:** 1 pill twice a day with food.
	Comments: Look for a B-50 complex with 50 mcg vitamin B_{12} and biotin; 400 mcg folic acid; and 50 mg all other B vitamins.
PABA	**Dosage:** 100 mg a day.
	Comments: Promotes the health of the skin and scalp.
Selenium	**Dosage:** 200 mcg twice a day.
	Comments: Don't exceed 600 mcg daily; higher doses may be toxic.

Note: Consider using supplements in **blue** first; those in **black** may also be beneficial. Some dosages may be supplied by supplements you are already taking—see page 39.

Some dosages may be supplied by supplements you are already taking—see page 39.

FACTS & Tips

■ The hair is very sensitive to vitamin or mineral imbalances in the body. A lack of vitamin A, for example, can result in a flaky scalp, but too much vitamin A (more than 100,000 IU a day) over a long period can cause hair loss. Call your doctor if you notice excessive hair loss after taking any supplements.

■ Supplements can be safely used along with prescription drugs, such as minoxidil, which helps restore hair in some people.

■ Thinning hair may be a sign that your gastrointestinal (GI) tract is not absorbing zinc and other nutrients properly. Taking acidophilus (one or two pills twice a day) may improve GI function and boost your body's ability to absorb important hair-nourishing substances from the foods you eat.

LATEST FINDINGS

■ Need another reason to quit smoking? Scientists in England recently reported that, age notwithstanding, smokers were four times more likely to have gray hair than nonsmokers. The researchers also reported a link between smoking and hair loss.

Did You Know?

The average youthful head contains about 100,000 hairs. But nearly two-thirds of all adults develop some balding or thinning by age 50.

---

underactive thyroid. Zinc needs to be taken with **copper** to maintain a proper mineral balance in the body. Copper also serves another useful purpose: It is an essential ingredient in melanin, the pigment that colors hair and skin, and may reverse the graying of hair caused by a copper deficiency. Both **biotin** and **vitamin B complex** may strengthen hair, condition the hair and scalp, and prevent excessive hair loss. Biotin may also restore lost hair, but only if the loss is due to a biotin deficiency.

As for **PABA** (para-aminobenzoic acid), it may protect hair follicles and prevent hair loss. It's sometimes recommended for restoring gray hair to its natural color, but may work only if you're deficient in PABA or other B vitamins. Finally, **selenium** may also foster healthy hair growth.

What else you can do

☑ Eat sensibly. Avoid fad diets that may deprive you of essential nutrients.

☑ Wash your hair with a mild shampoo. Afterward, gently towel it dry and apply a conditioner. Avoid harsh chemicals, such as the chlorine in pools, and high heat from blow dryers or curling irons.

☑ Protect your hair and scalp from the sun by wearing a hat.

☑ Perform a weekly scalp massage. Not only does it stimulate blood flow, but it also helps relieve stress, which can contribute to hair loss.

heart disease prevention

Lifestyle and dietary strategies can help you avoid a host of diseases, but they are probably most effective in preventing heart disease. Recent research confirms that certain nutrients can provide many heart-healthy benefits.

What it is

What most people consider heart disease is really atherosclerosis—a buildup of fatty deposits (called plaque) within the walls of the arteries. As plaque grows, it hinders the flow of blood that carries oxygen and nutrients throughout the body. The tiny arteries that thread through the heart and nourish it with blood are particularly susceptible to plaque accumulation. If any of them become blocked, a heart attack can occur.

What causes it

The primary cause of atherosclerosis is high blood cholesterol levels. LDL ("bad") cholesterol sticks to artery walls, and this accumulation eventually leads to plaque growth. High blood pressure, smoking, a sedentary lifestyle, obesity, and stress can also contribute to plaque buildup, as well as reduce the ability of the arteries to widen and constrict as necessary. In their younger years, men are at higher risk for heart disease than women, because estrogen may have a heart-protective effect. After menopause, however, women are as susceptible to heart disease as men.

How supplements can help

Supplements can never be substitutes for a healthy lifestyle, nor are they meant to target any one risk factor, such as high cholesterol. People who already have heart disease may benefit from the supplements listed here. Except for vitamin E and fish oils, which may interact with anticoagulants, these are safe to use with prescription drugs for heart disease.

The first four are antioxidants, substances that inactivate free radicals (unstable oxygen molecules that damage cells). Each one has a different function, so take them all. **Vitamin E** prevents the first step in the development of plaque—the oxidation of LDL cholesterol. **Vitamin C** helps recycle vitamin E and also keeps arteries flexible. Beta-carotene and lycopene are **carotenoids** thought to protect against heart disease;

Vitamin E (shown in dry powder capsules) is one of the most important supplements for combating the development of heart disease.

Supplement Recommendations

Vitamin E	**Dosage:** 400 IU a day.
	Comments: Check with your doctor if taking anticoagulant drugs.
Vitamin C	**Dosage:** 1,000 mg 3 times a day.
	Comments: Reduce dose if diarrhea develops.
Carotenoids	**Dosage:** 1 pill mixed carotenoids twice a day with food.
	Comments: Each pill should supply 25,000 IU vitamin A activity.
Grape seed extract	**Dosage:** 100 mg twice a day.
	Comments: Standardized to contain 92%-95% proanthocyanidins.
Vitamin B_{12}/ Folic acid	**Dosage:** 1,000 mcg vitamin B_{12} and 400 mcg folic acid a day.
	Comments: Sometimes sold in a single supplement.
Vitamin B_6	**Dosage:** 50 mg a day.
	Comments: 200 mg daily over long term can cause nerve damage.
Flaxseed oil	**Dosage:** 1 tbsp. (14 grams) a day.
	Comments: Can be mixed with food; take in the morning.
Fish oils	**Dosage:** 1,000 mg 3 times a day.
	Comments: Take only if you don't eat fish at least twice a week.
Magnesium	**Dosage:** 400 mg a day.
	Comments: Do not take if you have kidney disease.

Some dosages may be supplied by supplements you are already taking—see page 39.

but use a mixed carotenoid supplement for a proper balance. **Grape seed extract** contains procyanidolic oligomers (PCOs), flavonoids thought to have many times the antioxidant power of vitamins C and E.

In addition to antioxidants, **folic acid** is a key supplement for reducing homocysteine, an amino acid by-product linked to an increased risk of heart disease. **Vitamins B_{12}** and **B_6** help lower homocysteine levels as well, and vitamin B_6 may also be of value in ensuring that the arteries stay pliable. The omega-3 fatty acids in **flaxseed oil** and **fish oils** help keep triglyceride levels (a blood fat related to cholesterol) in check. The mineral **magnesium** aids in stabilizing heart rhythm.

What else you can do

☑ Maintain a diet low in fat, especially saturated fat.

☑ Include at least five servings of fruits and vegetables in your daily diet.

☑ Eat lots of soluble fiber (oats, beans, citrus fruits) to control cholesterol.

☑ Have salmon, tuna, sardines, or other fatty fish twice a week.

☑ Exercise for at least 30 minutes every day. Activity strengthens the heart, raises the level of protective HDL cholesterol, and eases weight loss.

☑ Don't smoke. Nothing makes up for damage smoking does to the heart.

heartburn

In many cases, this digestive problem can be prevented with some simple lifestyle changes. But when heartburn hits—as it does daily for more than 25 million Americans—natural remedies can provide quick relief from the disorder's fiery sensations.

SYMPTOMS

- *A burning sensation behind the breastbone lasting from a few minutes to several hours.*
- *Burning in the throat or regurgitation of a hot, sour fluid into the back of the throat.*
- *Belching.*
- *Discomfort that worsens when lying down.*

When to Call Your Doctor

- If you have heartburn twice a week or more.
- If you have difficulty swallowing or if food gets stuck in your esophagus.
- If you are vomiting or passing black stools.
- If your chest pain is crushing rather than burning or is accompanied by dizziness, shortness of breath, sweating, or pain that radiates to your arm or jaw—these are signs of a possible heart attack. Get medical help immediately.
- Reminder: If you have a medical condition, talk to your doctor before taking supplements.

What it is

To help digest food, the stomach produces about a quart of hydrochloric acid a day. Usually, the acid isn't a problem, because the gastrointestinal tract is coated with a protective mucous lining. But when acid moves up the esophagus (the tube running from the throat to the stomach), look out. Lacking a protective coating, the delicate tissue of the esophagus is vulnerable to the acid's corrosive action, which produces a burning sensation doctors label gastroesophageal reflux—and the rest of us call heartburn.

What causes it

Stomach acid generally stays where it belongs, thanks to the lower esophageal sphincter (LES). This muscle relaxes only to admit food into the stomach and then shuts tightly. But sometimes the LES doesn't close properly, allowing the stomach's contents to wash up into the esophagus.

Several factors can cause heartburn. Being overweight, pregnant, or a smoker weakens the LES. Smoking also dries up saliva, which neutralizes acid in the esophagus and washes it down into the stomach. Some foods—chocolate, alcohol, fatty foods, garlic, and onions—and certain medications make the LES relax. Acidic foods—tomatoes, citrus fruits, and coffee—may produce extra stomach acid. Waist-pinching clothing puts additional pressure on the abdomen, forcing the stomach contents upward. Overeating also increases pressure and stimulates prolonged acid production to digest the extra food. Avoid lying down too soon after a meal, it tilts digestive juices toward the esophagus.

How supplements can help

All the suggested supplements are effective for relieving heartburn—the ones in blue immediately, those in black within a month or so. Try each

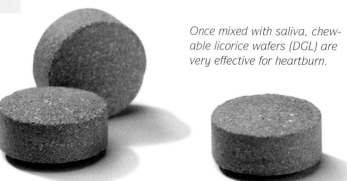

Once mixed with saliva, chewable licorice wafers (DGL) are very effective for heartburn.

Supplement Recommendations

Calcium carbonate	**Dosage:** 250-500 mg 3 times a day **Comments:** Chewable tablets provide the quickest relief.
Licorice (DGL)	**Dosage:** 2 deglycyrrhizinated licorice (DGL) wafers (380 mg). **Comments:** Take 3 or 4 times a day between meals as needed.
Aloe vera juice	**Dosage:** ½ cup juice 3 times a day between meals. **Comments:** Containing 98% aloe vera and no aloin or aloe-emodin.
Gamma-oryzanol	**Dosage:** 150 mg 3 times a day on an empty stomach. **Comments:** Also known as rice bran oil.
Choline	**Dosage:** 500 mg 3 times a day. **Comments:** For chronic heartburn, use in combination with pantothenic acid and thiamin for 1 month to see if symptoms abate.
Pantothenic acid	**Dosage:** 1,000 mg twice a day. **Comments:** For chronic heartburn, use in combination with choline and thiamin for 1 month to see if symptoms abate.
Thiamin	**Dosage:** 500 mg a day, taken first thing in the morning. **Comments:** Also called vitamin B_1. For chronic heartburn, combine with pantothenic acid and choline for 1 month.

Note: Consider using supplements in **blue** first; those in **black** may also be beneficial. Some dosages may be supplied by supplements you are already taking—see page 39.

see page 39

FACTS & Tips

- Strange as it may seem, heartburn can be the result of insufficient stomach acid. You may have this problem if you don't feel the typical burning sensations of heartburn but still suffer from routine stomachaches, bloating, belching, and flatulence after meals. Consider taking a supplement supplying 10 grains of betaine hydrochloride and 2 grains of pepsin with each meal for one month. (Before using this combination, make sure you don't have an ulcer; betaine can make it worse.) If your symptoms don't improve, see your doctor.

- Instead of coffee after meals, try one or a combination of these herbal teas: slippery elm, marshmallow, ginger, meadowsweet, or chamomile. They provide a warm, soothing end to a meal and have the added benefit of alleviating the irritation of heartburn.

LATEST FINDINGS

- Chewing gum can give quick heartburn relief. A recent study found that a stick of sugarless gum reduced heartburn in 70% of the participants. The gum stimulates saliva production and washes away stomach acid. Drinking a glass of lukewarm water after a meal may produce a similar effect.

methodically to see which one or combination works best for you. All can be used in addition to prescription or over-the-counter heartburn drugs.

Probably the most familiar heartburn-related supplement, **calcium carbonate** is used in antacid tablets such as Tums and is a good choice for occasional reflux. Deglycyrrhizinated **licorice (DGL)** helps repair the mucous lining of the stomach and can bring relief. You can also try **aloe vera juice** to soothe an irritated esophagus.

The remedies above can halt an attack of heartburn. To enhance the whole digestive process—which will most benefit people with chronic heartburn—take **gamma-oryzanol,** a rice bran oil extract. The supplement appears to work on the central nervous system's control of digestion. Alternatively, use the B vitamins **choline, pantothenic acid,** and **thiamin** in combination for a month and see if your symptoms diminish. If they do not, consult your doctor.

What else you can do

☑ Eat smaller, more frequent meals to minimize stomach acid production.

☑ Avoid fatty foods, limit alcohol, and shun coffee (even decaf).

☑ Eat your last meal or snack at least three hours before going to bed.

☑ Sleep with the head of your bed elevated six inches or so to allow gravity to help prevent reflux.

hemorrhoids

Nearly three-quarters of all Americans will develop hemorrhoids during their lives. Yet many people aren't aware they have them, because hemorrhoids often have few symptoms. When they flare up, natural remedies may have more to offer than conventional treatments.

SYMPTOMS

- *Streaks of blood on toilet tissue.*
- *Bloody, painful bowel movements.*
- *Itching in the anal area.*
- *Painful bump on or near the anus.*
- *Mucus discharge from the anus.*

When to Call Your Doctor

- If you note blood-streaked toilet tissue for the first time—it's probably hemorrhoids, but anal bleeding can have other causes.
- If bleeding isn't related to a bowel movement, even when you have hemorrhoids.
- If blood is dark, not bright red.
- If there's a throbbing pain in the anal area—this may be a blood clot in the hemorrhoid.
- If you've been diagnosed with hemorrhoids and daily bleeding is severe—you could be developing iron deficiency anemia.
- Reminder: If you have a medical condition, talk to your doctor before taking supplements.

What it is

Hemorrhoids (also known as piles) are essentially enlarged (varicose) veins in the anus or rectum. Veins are vessels that return deoxygenated blood to the heart, but sometimes the laws of gravity slow down this process in the lower half of the body. Blood can pool in the veins, stretching and weakening them. The veins in the rectum and anus are particularly susceptible. Not only are they in the lower body, but unlike other veins, these do not have valves to prevent the backward flow of blood. (Weak or faulty valves contribute to varicose veins in the legs.)

There are two types of hemorrhoids. The internal ones develop inside the rectum; they sometimes cause bleeding after a bowel movement, but otherwise have no symptoms because there are no pain sensors in the rectum. External hemorrhoids occur around the anal opening. They may be painful and can be fragile, bleeding easily after a bowel movement or when wiped with toilet tissue.

What causes it

Straining during a bowel movement is a primary cause of hemorrhoids, because it puts excess pressure on the veins in the anus and rectum. Being overweight or pregnant also weakens these veins. Experts disagree as to whether constipation directly causes hemorrhoids, but people who are constipated often strain to defecate, so at the very least this problem makes hemorrhoids worse. Studies show frequent diarrhea also increases the likelihood of hemorrhoids.

In addition, long periods of standing or sitting can lead to the development of hemorrhoids. The muscles that help propel blood through

St. John's wort ointment can relieve hemorrhoidal pain.

Supplement Recommendations	
Vitamin C/ Flavonoids	**Dosage:** 1,000 mg vitamin C and 500 mg flavonoids 3 times a day. **Comments:** Reduce vitamin C dose if diarrhea develops.
Butcher's broom	**Dosage:** 150 mg 3 times a day. **Comments:** Standardized to contain 9%-11% ruscogenin.
Zinc/Copper	**Dosage:** 30 mg zinc and 2 mg copper a day. **Comments:** Add copper only when using zinc longer than 1 month.
Psyllium	**Dosage:** 1 tbsp. powder dissolved in water or juice a day. **Comments:** Be sure to drink extra water throughout the day.
Flaxseeds	**Dosage:** 1 tbsp. ground flaxseeds in large glass of water each day. **Comments:** Drink at least 8 glasses of water a day.
St. John's wort ointment	**Dosage:** Apply ointment 3 or 4 times a day, as needed. **Comments:** Very beneficial when used after a bowel movement.

Note: Consider using supplements in **blue** first; those in **black** may also be beneficial. Some dosages may be supplied by supplements you are already taking—see page 39.

see page 39

the veins lose tone with age, so it is not surprising that hemorrhoids are more common in older people. The tendency to develop hemorrhoids also seems to run in families.

How supplements can help

Supplements are meant to be used in conjunction with a high-fiber diet and regular exercise. Fiber is of value in bulking up and softening the stool, which makes it easier to pass. Exercise is important in toning the muscles that surround the veins and promotes regular bowel movements.

Unlike over-the-counter ointments, the recommended vitamins and herbs will aid in strengthening the veins and minimizing irritation as they heal. In combination, try **vitamin C, flavonoids,** and the herb **butcher's broom** to help tone and shrink the veins. **Zinc** plays a role in wound healing; **copper** is needed with long-term use of zinc, however, because zinc interferes with copper absorption. If you don't get enough fiber in your diet or need an extra fiber boost, take **psyllium** or **flaxseeds.** Both are effective in easing the passage of stool. When hemorrhoids are painful, apply an ointment containing the herb **St. John's wort** several times a day, especially after bowel movements. This ointment is also useful in shrinking swollen tissues.

What else you can do

☑ Increase fiber by eating lots of fruits, vegetables, grains, and legumes.

☑ Drink at least eight glasses of water a day. Fluid is important in preventing the constipation associated with hemorrhoids.

☑ Breathe normally when lifting weights or heavy objects, or during a bowel movement. Holding your breath increases pressure in the abdomen.

hepatitis

Knowing the ABCs of this liver disorder can save your life. Though some hepatitis viruses cause an acute but temporary flulike illness, others can produce a chronic, festering liver infection. Natural therapies are designed to protect the liver and boost your immune system.

SYMPTOMS

- *Fatigue.*
- *Fever.*
- *Loss of appetite.*
- *Nausea and vomiting.*
- *Aching muscles or joints.*
- *Abdominal discomfort, pain, or swelling.*
- *Jaundice (yellowish tinge of skin and whites of eyes).*
- *Dark urine and pale stools.*

When to Call Your Doctor

- If you think you have been exposed to hepatitis, either through contaminated food or water or by sexual contact with an infected person.
- If you develop lingering flulike symptoms. During its acute phase, viral hepatitis so closely resembles the flu that it is frequently misdiagnosed.
- If you develop jaundice or other symptoms of hepatitis.
- Reminder: If you have a medical condition, talk to your doctor before taking supplements.

What it is

Hepatitis is an inflammation of the liver. Of the two forms—acute and chronic—the first is the easier to treat. Hepatitis can be caused by any of six viruses, called A, B, C, D, E, and G. Hepatitis A, the most common, is highly contagious; it produces acute flulike symptoms but usually no long-lasting damage. Hepatitis B and C, on the other hand, can linger for years, often causing few or no symptoms but in some cases leading to irreversible liver scarring (cirrhosis) or liver cancer. Types D, E, and G are rare. All forms of hepatitis attack the liver, impairing its ability to process sugars and carbohydrates, to secrete fat-digesting bile, and to rid the body of toxins and waste. But the chronic forms are the most dangerous because they may ultimately lead to liver failure.

What causes it

Whether contracted through contaminated food or water (type A), or through blood transfusions, infected hypodermic needles, or sexual intercourse (types B and C), hepatitis is most often caused by a viral infection. Certain medications, toxic chemicals, or years of alcohol abuse can also result in hepatitis. Rarely, an autoimmune dysfunction—in which the immune system attacks the body's own tissues—is to blame. And sometimes, no cause can be determined.

How supplements can help

Conventional medicines have achieved only limited success in treating hepatitis, particularly the more dangerous chronic form. The natural therapies listed in the chart are designed to protect and strengthen the liver

Capsules of the liver-protecting herb milk thistle may benefit hepatitis sufferers.

140

Vitamin C	**Dosage:** 1,000 mg 3 times a day.
	Comments: Reduce dose if diarrhea develops.
Vitamin E	**Dosage:** 400 IU a day.
	Comments: Check with your doctor if taking anticoagulant drugs.
Milk thistle	**Dosage:** 150 mg 3 times a day.
	Comments: Standardized to contain at least 70% silymarin.
Licorice	**Dosage:** 200 mg 3 times a day for a maximum of 10 days.
	Comments: Standardized to contain 22% glycyrrhizin or glycyrrhizinic acid; can raise blood pressure. Don't use DGL form.
Lipotropic combination	**Dosage:** 2 pills twice a day.
	Comments: Should contain milk thistle, choline, inositol, and other ingredients.
Alpha-lipoic acid	**Dosage:** 200 mg 3 times a day.
	Comments: Can be taken with or without food.
Dandelion root	**Dosage:** 500 mg standardized extract twice a day.
	Comments: May be contained in lipotropic combination formulas.

Note: Consider using supplements in blue first; those in black may also be beneficial. Some dosages may be supplied by supplements you are already taking—see page 39.

and boost general immunity. They should be used together, along with conventional drugs, until symptoms of acute hepatitis subside. Benefits may be noticed within a week. For chronic disease, take them long term.

Vitamin C and **vitamin E** are powerful antioxidants that act together to help protect liver cells against damage from free radicals; the nutritional supplement **alpha-lipoic acid** affords antioxidant protection as well and may enhance the potency of these vitamins. Not only does the herb **milk thistle** protect the liver, it also promotes growth of new liver cells and improves liver function.

Other liver-protecting herbs are **licorice,** which contains antiviral and antioxidant compounds, and **dandelion root.** A better way to get dandelion may be as part of a liver-detoxifying combination product called a **lipotropic combination** (which also includes the B vitamins choline and inositol, as well as milk thistle); this blend is thought to speed the flow of bile and cell-damaging toxins away from the liver.

What else you can do

☑ Watch what you eat and drink when traveling in areas where sanitation is poor and disease rates high. Have only bottled water and cooked foods.

☑ Refrain from alcohol, especially during and for a month after an acute illness, or until your doctor says your liver function tests are normal.

☑ Make sure disposable or sterilized needles are used during acupuncture, body piercing, tattooing, and similar procedures.

FACTS & Tips

■ About 4 million Americans have hepatitis C, and nearly 150,000 new cases are diagnosed each year. Because so few recognized treatments are available, natural supplements may well be worth trying. Traditional options include taking the antiviral drug interferon, which has serious side effects and only limited benefits, and having a liver transplant (hepatitis is the leading reason this major surgical procedure is performed).

■ Natural therapies have few of the side effects of common over-the-counter and prescription drugs. Acetaminophen, aspirin, and some antibiotics can all damage the liver, which is especially dangerous for those with hepatitis.

LATEST FINDINGS

■ Recent research indicates that patients with liver disease have depleted levels of antioxidants, and that in severe cases of viral hepatitis, patients may primarily be deficient in vitamin E. When administered to a pilot test group of several patients who had not responded to chemical treatment with antiviral drugs, vitamin E was found to inhibit scarring and destruction of liver cells. Further study is needed. In the meantime, be sure you get extra vitamin E (400 IU a day) either as a separate supplement or as part of your daily multivitamin.

Did You Know?

Vaccines against both hepatitis A and hepatitis B are available. Ask your doctor if you should have one or both.

high blood pressure

Called the silent killer, this condition has no symptoms but can lead to serious health problems. New studies show lifestyle changes and natural supplements may be viable alternatives to prescription drugs for some cases of high blood pressure.

What it is

Defined as the force the blood exerts on arteries and veins as it circulates through the body, blood pressure is controlled by a complex regulatory system involving the heart, blood vessels, brain, kidneys, and adrenal glands. It's normal for blood pressure to fluctuate often—even minute to minute. In some people, however, blood pressure remains chronically high, a condition known medically as hypertension.

Blood pressure is recorded as two numbers. Systolic pressure (the top number in a reading) denotes when the heart contracts and forces blood through the arteries; diastolic pressure (the bottom number) reflects when the heart relaxes. Normal blood pressure is 120 (systolic) over 80 (diastolic) or lower. Hypertension is defined as blood pressure averaging 140/90 or higher in at least two separate measurements.

What causes it

In 90% of people with hypertension, the cause isn't known; this type is called essential hypertension. However, risk factors include smoking, obesity, gender (men are twice as likely to suffer hypertension as women), a high-sodium diet, and a family history. In addition, blacks are more prone to hypertension—and suffer greater consequences from it—than whites.

How supplements can help

If you have mild hypertension (140 to 159 systolic and 90 to 99 diastolic), start making lifestyle changes and take calcium and magnesium. If your blood pressure is higher, see your doctor before using supplements.

In some studies, **calcium** has been shown to lower blood pressure; it is also involved in muscle contraction, so it's good for the heart and blood vessels. **Magnesium** relaxes the muscles that control blood vessels, permitting blood to flow more freely. It also helps to maintain a

The mineral calcium is an important nutrient in helping to lower blood pressure.

142

Supplement Recommendations

Calcium/ Magnesium	**Dosage:** 1,000 mg calcium and 500 mg magnesium a day. **Comments:** Do not use magnesium if you have kidney disease.
Vitamin C	**Dosage:** 1,000 mg 3 times a day. **Comments:** Reduce dose if diarrhea develops.
Coenzyme Q$_{10}$	**Dosage:** 50 mg twice a day. **Comments:** For best absorption, take with food.
Essential fatty acids	**Dosage:** 1 tbsp. (14 grams) flaxseed oil a day; 1,000 mg fish oils 3 times a day. **Comments:** Take fish oils if you don't eat fish at least twice a week.
Hawthorn	**Dosage:** 100-150 mg 3 times a day. **Comments:** Standardized to contain at least 1.8% vitexin.
Taurine	**Dosage:** 500 mg L-taurine twice a day on an empty stomach. **Comments:** If using longer than 1 month, add mixed amino acids.
Arginine	**Dosage:** 1,000 mg L-arginine twice a day on an empty stomach. **Comments:** Don't take if you have kidney disease or genital herpes, or are prone to cold sores. Take with a mixed amino acid complex.

Note: Consider using supplements in **blue** first; those in **black** may also be beneficial. Some dosages may be supplied by supplements you are already taking—see page 39.

balance between potassium and sodium in the blood, which has a positive effect on blood pressure. The mineral potassium is also effective in reducing blood pressure. But potassium supplements are almost never necessary; eating more fruits and vegetables is sufficient for most people.

If your blood pressure does not decline after a month, stop taking calcium and magnesium (stick with lifestyle changes) and begin **vitamin C** and **hawthorn.** Both widen blood vessels; hawthorn helps moderate the heart rate as well. Alternatively, try **coenzyme Q$_{10}$;** more than a third of people with high blood pressure are thought to have an inadequate supply of this substance. To these, add **essential fatty acids** in the form of flaxseed oil and fish oils to foster good circulation. Amino acids may also help: **Taurine** is believed to normalize the increased nervous system activity associated with high blood pressure, and **arginine** appears to widen blood vessels. Use them together along with a mixed amino acid complex to be sure you are getting the proper balance.

What else you can do

☑ Lose weight. Even a few extra pounds can raise blood pressure.

☑ Walk or do some other form of aerobic exercise regularly.

☑ Eat plenty of fruits, vegetables, and low-fat dairy products; reduce fat and salt intake. A new study found such a diet may be an alternative to prescription drugs for mild hypertension.

■ If you have mild hypertension, you may want to try lifestyle changes and supplements before turning to prescription drugs, which often have unpleasant side effects. Begin a two or three-month trial with supplements. If your blood pressure drops, you can use the supplements indefinitely. If your blood pressure doesn't respond, you may need prescription antihypertensive drugs. If you already take such medication, don't stop or reduce your dose without your doctor's approval.

LATEST FINDINGS

■ Vitamin C can help lower blood pressure by widening blood vessels. In a preliminary study, 3,000 mg of intravenous vitamin C relaxed blood vessels in 17 people with hypertension. Scientists speculate that constricted arteries may be partly caused by the type of cell damage that vitamin C corrects. More research is needed to see if vitamin C supplements produce the same results.

■ Some experts theorize that a deficiency of vitamin D might contribute to high blood pressure. One scientist from the University of Alabama has noticed that hypertension is less common in areas where there is more daylight (the sun triggers vitamin D production in the body) and thinks vitamin D may affect hormones that are involved in blood pressure. If this theory is proved, vitamin D supplements may begin to be recommended for some people with hypertension.

high cholesterol

A high level of cholesterol in your blood can increase your risk of heart attack and possibly stroke. Along with dietary changes, vitamins C and E and some potent herbal compounds can help control your cholesterol level and reduce your risk.

SYMPTOMS

- *High cholesterol usually has no obvious symptoms, but it is a risk factor for other disorders with evident symptoms, such as angina.*
- *When levels are very high, cholesterol may appear as yellow nodules beneath the skin of the elbows or knees, or under the eyes.*

When to Call Your Doctor

- Have cholesterol levels measured at least once every five years, more often if total cholesterol is 200 mg/dl (milligrams per deciliter) or higher.
- Ask about conventional prescription drugs if home remedies don't lower your total cholesterol sufficiently in two or three months. These drugs are effective, reducing heart attack risk by up to 25%.
- Reminder: If you have a medical condition, talk to your doctor before taking supplements.

What it is

In itself, cholesterol—a fatlike substance circulating in the blood—isn't harmful; in fact, your body needs some of it to help maintain cell membranes and perform other vital functions. But too much cholesterol can be unhealthy. Doctors focus on total blood cholesterol and on two types of cholesterol that your body manufactures: the "bad" cholesterol (called LDL), which in excess amounts can lead to blocked arteries and possibly a heart attack, and the "good" type (HDL), which helps clear away cholesterol before it builds up in the arteries. High total blood cholesterol and LDL levels increase the risk of a heart attack, as does a low level of HDL (below 35 mg/dl). Experts recommend keeping total cholesterol below 200 mg/dl and your HDL level as high as possible.

What causes it

Although genetic factors affect cholesterol levels, in many people high levels are linked to a diet rich in saturated fat and cholesterol. Both are present chiefly in animal foods, such as beef, butter, and whole-milk dairy products. (Coconut, palm, and hydrogenated oils in processed foods are high in saturated fat but not cholesterol.) Excess weight, smoking, and lack of exercise can have an undesirable effect on cholesterol levels as well.

How supplements can help

Several nutritional and herbal remedies can help control cholesterol levels. Begin by taking vitamins E and C, and garlic, either together or separately. These are beneficial and safe to use for long periods—even if

Taken in enteric-coated softgels or as fresh cloves, garlic can help fight high cholesterol.

Supplement Recommendations

Vitamin E	**Dosage:** 400 IU twice a day.
	Comments: Check with your doctor if taking anticoagulant drugs.
Vitamin C	**Dosage:** 1,000 mg twice a day.
	Comments: Reduce dose if diarrhea develops.
Garlic	**Dosage:** 400-600 mg a day.
	Comments: Each pill should provide 4,000 mcg allicin potential.
Inositol hexaniacinate	**Dosage:** 500 mg 3 times a day.
	Comments: Safest form of niacin to use; does not cause flushing and may be less harmful to the liver than other forms.
Red yeast rice	**Dosage:** 2 capsules (600 mg each) twice a day with meals.
	Comments: Sold as Cholestin. Discontinue if muscle pain, tenderness, or weakness occurs.
Gugulipid	**Dosage:** 25 mg guggulsterones 3 times a day.
	Comments: Guggulsterones are the active ingredient in gugulipid.
Psyllium	**Dosage:** 1 tbsp. powder dissolved in water or juice twice a day.
	Comments: May have a laxative effect. Drink lots of extra water.

Note: Consider using supplements in blue first; those in black may also be beneficial. Some dosages may be supplied by supplements you are already taking—see page 39.

FACTS & Tips

- Garlic pills are best absorbed if they are enteric-coated. This covering allows them to pass intact to the small intestine, where chemical reactions release garlic's cholesterol-lowering components most effectively. This coating also helps minimize the herb's pungent taste and odor.

- Home cholesterol tests are convenient and can give you results in a matter of minutes. But such test kits are not always reliable, and they don't measure your HDL level. Therefore, it's usually best to have your cholesterol tested (and results confirmed) by a physician.

you're on a cholesterol-lowering prescription drug. Although it does not lower your cholesterol directly, **vitamin E** seems to prevent free radicals (unstable oxygen molecules) from damaging LDL cholesterol—the first step in the buildup of coronary plaque. **Vitamin C** helps boost the effectiveness of vitamin E and may even increase the level of protective HDL cholesterol. Studies have been conflicting on the power of **garlic** to lower cholesterol levels, but many nutritionally oriented physicians believe it has a positive effect and is worth trying. And anyone whose diet lacks soluble fiber, which can lower total cholesterol, should add the herb **psyllium.**

Inositol hexaniacinate, red yeast rice, and gugulipid may all provide alternatives to cholesterol-lowering medications; these supplements should never be taken in conjunction with such drugs. Used for three or four months, **inositol hexaniacinate,** a form of the B vitamin niacin, may reduce LDL and raise HDL. Either of the herbal remedies **red yeast rice** or **gugulipid** can be tried in place of—or as an adjunct to—inositol hexaniacinate. Red yeast rice inhibits cholesterol formation; gugulipid increases your body's ability to metabolize LDL.

What else you can do

☑ Improve your diet by reducing saturated fats and dietary cholesterol. Substitute fish for meat, eat high-fiber foods (grains, vegetables, and fruits), and use monounsaturated oils (olive or canola) in place of butter.

☑ Follow a program of regular exercise to help raise your HDL level.

LATEST FINDINGS

- In studies examining gugulipid, subjects' cholesterol levels fell between 14% and 27% over a 12-week period—an effect comparable to that of prescription drugs for lowering cholesterol.

- Taking psyllium is one of the least expensive ways to lower cholesterol. A new study indicates most people with high cholesterol can achieve a 10% drop in cholesterol levels when they combine a low-fat diet with 5 grams of psyllium taken twice daily. The effect of psyllium is more pronounced in people with higher cholesterol levels.

Did You Know?

Dietary cholesterol can raise blood cholesterol levels. But it's the saturated fat in foods that affects cholesterol levels even more. Even if a food label boasts "No Cholesterol," don't just assume the product is healthy. Check carefully for its saturated fat content.

HIV/AIDS

New drugs have brought renewed hope to the battle against HIV infection and AIDS. Yet opinions about the role of alternative therapies for HIV and AIDS remain heated. Research suggests that a number of supplements can serve as vital additions to conventional treatments.

SYMPTOMS

- *Persistent fatigue; recurring or prolonged fever, possibly with chills or night sweats; joint or muscle pain.*
- *Frequent sore throats, swollen glands, coughs, colds, cold sores, yeast infections, or other types of infections.*
- *Loss of appetite and weight; frequent diarrhea.*
- *Unusual rashes or skin discoloration, especially purplish markings (Kaposi's sarcoma).*
- *Many people infected with HIV have no symptoms.*

When to Call Your Doctor

- If you experience any of the above symptoms.
- If you suspect you've been exposed to HIV, the virus that causes AIDS.
- If you've been diagnosed with HIV, and symptoms suddenly become worse.
- Reminder: If you have a medical condition, talk to your doctor before taking supplements.

What it is

The human immunodeficiency virus, or HIV, is the underlying cause of acquired immune deficiency syndrome, or AIDS. Following the initial infection with the virus, it may take years before the immune system is damaged to the extent that AIDS-related illnesses arise. AIDS develops when the body can no longer fight off such diseases as pneumonia, fungal or parasitic infestations, and certain cancers. So far, there is no cure and no vaccine against HIV or AIDS.

What causes it

HIV is carried in the body fluids (such as blood, semen, vaginal secretions, and breast milk) of those who are infected. It is spread when others come into contact with these fluids, particularly during sex or through exposure to contaminated blood (which can happen among drug users who share needles). Nonetheless, the virus is hard to transmit because it dies very quickly outside the host's body. Thus HIV does not spread through air or water, nor does it travel easily from person to person (through coughing or sharing drinking cups, for example), as many other viruses do.

How supplements can help

The recommended supplements, all aimed at boosting immunity, should be taken together. They can be used along with conventional AIDS drugs, and should be continued long term. Benefits may be felt within a month.

Antioxidant therapy—especially megadoses of **vitamin C**—shows promise in slowing the disease and strengthening the immune system. Vitamin C appears to fight viruses and fungal infections, and it has anti-inflammatory properties. The nutrient **coenzyme Q_{10}** plays a vital role in energy production and may improve stamina in people with AIDS. It also has an antioxidant effect. Other useful antioxidants include **vitamin E** and alpha-lipoic acid.

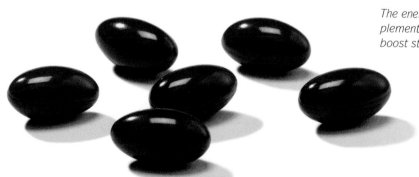

The energizing effects of the supplement coenzyme Q_{10} may help boost stamina in those with AIDS.

Supplement Recommendations

Vitamin C/ Vitamin E	**Dosage:** 2,000 mg vitamin C 3 times a day; 400 IU vitamin E daily. **Comments:** Vitamin C helps boost the effects of vitamin E.
Coenzyme Q$_{10}$	**Dosage:** 100 mg twice a day. **Comments:** For best absorption, take with food.
Zinc/Copper	**Dosage:** 30 mg zinc and 2 mg copper a day. **Comments:** Add copper only when using zinc longer than 1 month.
NAC/Amino acid complex	**Dosage:** 500 mg NAC 3 times a day; follow label for amino acids. **Comments:** Take both on an empty stomach but at different times.
Turmeric/ Bromelain	**Dosage:** 400 mg turmeric and 500 mg bromelain 3 times a day. **Comments:** Bromelain to provide 6,000 GDU or 9,000 MCU daily.
Essential fatty acids	**Dosage:** 1,000 mg evening primrose oil 3 times a day; 1 tbsp. (14 grams) flaxseed oil a day. **Comments:** Or use 1,000 mg borage oil once a day for primrose oil.
DHEA	**Dosage:** 100 mg each morning. **Comments:** Take only under medical supervision. Don't use if you're at risk for hormone-related (breast, prostate, etc.) cancers.
Reishi/Maitake mushrooms	**Dosage:** 500 mg reishi and 200 mg maitake 3 times a day. **Comments:** Avoid reishi mushrooms if you're on anticoagulants.

Some dosages may be supplied by supplements you are already taking—see page **39**.

Zinc is crucial to the healthy functioning of the immune system and may help maintain body weight. Don't exceed the recommended dose because excessive intake may impair immunity. Zinc may be most beneficial in the later stages of AIDS, to combat pneumonia and fungal infections. Zinc depletes **copper** stores, so take both minerals.

The amino acid **NAC** (N-acetylcysteine), balanced with a mixed **amino acid complex,** acts as an antioxidant, stimulates the immune system, assists in repairing body tissues, and fights weight loss. Most notably, NAC seems to interfere with the replication of all viruses, including HIV. The herb **turmeric** (take it with **bromelain** for better absorption) may also block HIV reproduction. **Essential fatty acids** improve immune function, and **DHEA,** a hormone, works to reduce the muscle wasting that is associated with AIDS. Some studies suggest that extracts of **reishi** and **maitake mushrooms,** as well as other Japanese varieties, can stimulate immunity and improve survival rates in those with certain AIDS-related cancers.

What else you can do

☑ Exercise regularly and stop smoking.

☑ Reduce stress. Meditation, yoga, or a support group may help.

impotence

For one man in four over the age of 50—and some much younger men too—a durable erection is an elusive thing. In most cases, the cause of what doctors call "erectile dysfunction" is physical and correctable, often by making some surprisingly simple changes.

What it is

An erection occurs when blood vessels in the penis fill with blood, stiffening the organ. The process is sparked by sexual stimulation, which causes nerves in the brain and spine to signal arteries in the penis to expand. The inability to get or maintain an erection is called impotence.

What causes it

The main cause of impotence is poor circulation and impaired blood flow through the penis, which is often the result of atherosclerosis ("hardening of the arteries"). Other possible reasons include hormonal imbalances, prostate disease, diabetes, nerve disorders, or medication side effects. Only one in ten cases is purely psychological. Because erections occur involuntarily during sleep, a man may be able to determine if the problem is physical or psychological by using the "postage stamp test." Encircle the penis with stamps from a roll, gluing them end to end. If nighttime erections occur, the stamps will be torn in the morning, and the cause is probably psychological. This type of impotence is usually stress-related and often temporary.

How supplements can help

A number of supplements, when taken together, may improve blood flow to the penis. **Vitamin C** plays a role in keeping blood vessels supple, allowing them to expand and let more blood pass through. **Flaxseed oil** and **evening primrose oil** contain different types of essential fatty acids that also improve blood flow; taken long term, they can help by lowering cholesterol and preventing blood vessel narrowing. And **ginkgo biloba**, which increases blood flow in the brain, may have a similar effect on the penis. Ultrasound examinations of 60 impotent men who took ginkgo biloba showed improved penile blood circulation after six weeks. After six months, 50% of the patients had regained potency. All these supplements should be used long term

The herb Panax ginseng may help restore sexual function in men suffering from impotence.

Supplement Recommendations

Vitamin C	**Dosage:** 1,000 mg 3 times a day. **Comments:** Reduce dose if diarrhea develops.
Flaxseed oil	**Dosage:** 1 tbsp. (14 grams) a day. **Comments:** Can be mixed with food; take in the morning.
Evening primrose oil	**Dosage:** 1,000 mg 3 times a day. **Comments:** Can substitute 1,000 mg borage oil once a day.
Ginkgo biloba	**Dosage:** 80 mg 3 times a day. **Comments:** Standardized to have at least 24% flavone glycosides.
Pygeum africanum	**Dosage:** 100 mg twice a day between meals. **Comments:** Standardized to contain 13% sterols. Side effects may include nausea and upset stomach.
Panax ginseng	**Dosage:** 100-250 mg twice a day; rotate with Siberian ginseng. **Comments:** Standardized to contain at least 7% ginsenosides.
Siberian ginseng	**Dosage:** 100-300 mg standardized extract twice a day. **Comments:** Alternate with Panax ginseng every two weeks.
Muira puama	**Dosage:** As tea, 1 tsp. dried herb per cup hot water each morning. **Comments:** May be hard to find. Also available as a tincture.

Note: Consider using supplements in **blue** first; those in **black** may also be beneficial. Some dosages may be supplied by supplements you are already taking—see page 39.

(at least six months) for best results, though benefits may be noticed in a month. Because they have largely positive effects on the body, they can also be part of your general nutritional maintenance program.

Other supplements may help when impotence is related to different causes. The African herb **pygeum africanum** may be useful when impotence is a result of prostate disease. Studies in animals have shown that both **Panax** and **Siberian ginseng** boost testosterone levels and increase mating behavior; they may produce similar effects in humans. And if those are ineffective, make a tea with the herb **Muira puama** (also known as potency wood), long used in Brazil as an aphrodisiac.

What else you can do

☑ Ask your doctor about the prescription drug Viagra (sildenafil). Like supplements, the little blue pill is easy to use. The manufacturer did not test Viagra to see if it was compatible with herbal treatments, but there have been no reports of drug-supplement interactions so far.

☑ Exercise regularly to improve blood flow throughout the body, boost energy, and reduce stress.

☑ Limit alcohol intake and don't smoke; both can aggravate impotence.

☑ Consider counseling if stress or anxiety is contributing to the problem.

FACTS & Tips

■ "Men's Mixtures," sold in health-food stores, sometimes tout the herb yohimbe, which shows some promise against impotence. But most mixtures contain tiny—and useless—amounts of the herb. The pure herb is very difficult to obtain. Even if you can find it, yohimbe has many side effects, including anxiety, high blood pressure, and a racing pulse. Ask your doctor about the prescription drug yohimbine, which contains the purified active ingredient in yohimbe. It's the safest and most effective way to get this herb—but even the drug has serious side effects.

LATEST FINDINGS

■ According to the results of a recent study, ginseng may be a valuable treatment for impotence. Men who took Panax ginseng experienced a 60% improvement in their ability to achieve an erection, compared with a 30% improvement in men using a placebo.

■ Only one study to date has been done on the little-known Brazilian herb Muira puama: a 1990 study from the Institute of Sexology in Paris. Of 262 men who had trouble getting or keeping erections, more than half responded positively to the herb within two weeks.

Did You Know?

Supplements that improve blood flow to the penis may also help prevent heart disease because both disorders often involve blocked blood vessels.

infertility, female

Not being able to conceive can be frustrating and stressful. Conventional infertility treatments often have side effects and pose financial and ethical dilemmas. For some women, herbal and nutritional supplements may be an effective alternative.

SYMPTOMS

- *You have been trying to conceive for six months to a year and have not been successful.*
- *You have been diagnosed with endometriosis, chlamydia, or pelvic inflammatory disease.*
- *You do not menstruate, or menstruate infrequently or irregularly.*

When to Call Your Doctor

- **Every woman who suspects she is infertile should see a doctor for an evaluation.**
- **Reminder: If you have a medical condition, talk to your doctor before taking supplements.**

What it is

A woman may be infertile if she has not become pregnant within a year despite having regular unprotected intercourse during her most fertile times of the month (before and during ovulation). Because fertility does decline with age, experts recommend that a woman over age 35 wait only six months before seeking help. Infertility affects 10 million Americans, or 15% of couples. In one-fifth of those cases, both the man and woman have problems that make it difficult for them to conceive. In the remaining cases, the problem is equally likely to affect either partner.

What causes it

Normally, an egg is released from a woman's ovary midway through her menstrual cycle (ovulation). The egg then travels from the ovary through the fallopian tubes, where it can be fertilized by sperm if the woman has sex. Infertility occurs in some women because they ovulate irregularly or don't ovulate at all; in others, the fallopian tubes may be scarred and/or obstructed. Though a medical evaluation is necessary to pinpoint the cause of infertility, women whose periods are irregular or absent probably are not ovulating normally. In some cases, despite extensive testing, no cause can be found.

Irregular ovulation becomes more frequent as a woman enters her late 30s. Hormonal imbalances caused by a variety of factors—weight problems or excess exercise—can also inhibit or halt ovulation. And certain medical conditions, such as endometriosis, chlamydia, and pelvic inflammatory disease, can result in scarring and physical obstructions.

How supplements can help

Most of the supplements in the chart can be used regardless of the cause of infertility; they can also be combined with conventional treatments. It may take three to six months to notice any effect; don't hesitate to consult a fertility specialist if these treatments don't work for you.

The essential fatty acids in evening primrose oil softgels are important for the healthy functioning of the uterus.

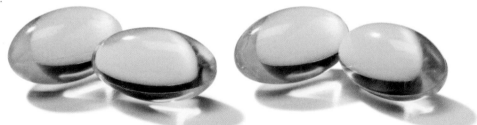

Supplement Recommendations

Vitamin B complex	**Dosage:** 1 pill each morning with food. **Comments:** Look for a B-50 complex with 50 mcg vitamin B_{12} and biotin; 400 mcg folic acid; and 50 mg all other B vitamins.
Vitamin B_6	**Dosage:** 50 mg a day. **Comments:** 200 mg daily over long term may cause nerve damage.
Zinc/Copper	**Dosage:** 30 mg zinc and 2 mg copper a day. **Comments:** Add copper only when using zinc longer than 1 month.
Essential fatty acids	**Dosage:** 1,000 mg evening primrose oil 3 times a day; 1 tbsp. (14 grams) flaxseed oil a day. **Comments:** Or use 1,000 mg borage oil once a day for primrose oil.
Siberian ginseng	**Dosage:** 100-300 mg standardized extract twice a day. **Comments:** Do not use while menstruating. Stop using as soon as you find out you are pregnant.
Chasteberry/ False unicorn root	**Dosage:** ½ tsp. tincture of each twice a day. **Comments:** Do not take while menstruating. Stop using as soon as you find out you are pregnant.

Some dosages may be supplied by supplements you are already taking—see page 39.

The **B complex** family of vitamins, along with extra **vitamin B_6,** are important for a healthy reproductive system. In addition, should you become pregnant, they will play an essential role in early fetal development; folic acid, in particular, helps prevent birth defects. **Zinc** is necessary for proper cell division; **copper** is needed to prevent copper deficiency when taking zinc long term. **Essential fatty acids** and **Siberian ginseng** support healthy uterine function.

If infertility results from irregular ovulation, try a blend of **chasteberry** (also called vitex) and **false unicorn root** to stimulate ovulation in place of medications designed for this purpose (such as clomiphene citrate), which often have adverse side effects. Chasteberry has been shown to enhance a woman's production of the hormone progesterone and to suppress the production of the hormone prolactin. Either low progesterone or high prolactin levels may inhibit the ovulation process.

What else you can do

☑ Don't smoke. Cigarette smoke can reduce fertility. And it can seriously affect your baby's health and development if you do get pregnant.

☑ Lose weight if overweight; gain weight if underweight.

☑ Exercise moderately. Strenuous exercise can interfere with ovulation.

FACTS & Tips

■ Many women use home tests to determine exactly when they are ovulating. However, once ovulation does occur, the window of opportunity for conception may already have passed. A study of 221 healthy women ages 25 to 35 found the peak time for conception is five days before and the day of ovulation. Intercourse at other times is unlikely to result in pregnancy.

LATEST FINDINGS

■ Women who drink more than a half cup of black or green tea a day may double their chances of getting pregnant, according to a recent study. Researchers investigated the effect of caffeine consumption on the fertility of 187 women. Although coffee and caffeine did not seem to affect fertility, researchers could not conclusively rule out a negative impact. They noted that the benefits of tea may be related to some compound in the brew, or it may be that tea drinkers simply have better health habits than coffee drinkers do.

infertility, male

An unfortunate fact of life is that when the time comes to father a child, some men have great difficulty doing so. Though in certain cases surgery or other medical treatments may be necessary, in others safe and gentle natural therapies may be the answer.

SYMPTOMS

- *Unsuccessful attempts to conceive for a year.*
- *A diagnosis of chlamydia or other reproductive-tract infection, which may have left scar tissue blocking the exit of sperm.*

When to Call Your Doctor

- If you suspect you are infertile, your doctor can assess the problem and help uncover any underlying causes. Your partner may also need to be examined, because one or both of you may have fertility problems.
- Reminder: If you have a medical condition, talk to your doctor before taking supplements.

What it is

Doctors recognize infertility as a problem if a man does not impregnate his partner after a year of having unprotected sex with her, particularly during her most fertile days of the month. In every case, there is a 50/50 chance that the source of the infertility is in the male partner; in one-fifth of cases, both partners have a problem. Researchers can't say exactly how many sperm a man needs to be fertile, but they know that the higher the sperm count, the greater the chances of conception.

What causes it

Some cases of infertility in men are linked to anatomical defects or scar tissue from a long-healed infection in the reproductive tract. But most of the time, the precise cause can't be identified. Many infertile men have a low sperm count caused by low levels of testosterone, a hormone that signals the testes to manufacture sperm. But the amount of sperm a man produces is not the only determinant of fertility. A high percentage of the sperm must be healthy and motile (active). Because they are fragile, sperm are easily damaged by naturally occurring molecules called free radicals. Numerous factors can affect levels of both free radicals and testosterone: Drinking, smoking, poor nutrition, even stress. Some prescription drugs can also alter sperm motility and make conception difficult.

How supplements can help

Surgery may be the best way to correct anatomical defects. But for many infertile men, supplements are worth a try. They provide benefits at any age: Unlike female fertility, which declines after age 35, fertility in men is not age-dependent. A study of 240 couples undergoing in vitro fertilization found that sperm collected from men in their 60s was just as lively as sperm collected from men in their 30s. Supplements should usually be taken for at least several months—and often longer. Those listed here are generally safe for prolonged use.

Taken together, **vitamin C, vitamin E,** and mixed **carotenoids** provide a powerful medley of antioxidants that sweep up cell-damaging

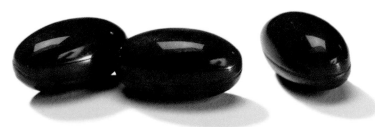

Carotenoid supplements contain a rich blend of sperm-protecting antioxidants.

Supplement Recommendations

Vitamin C	**Dosage:** 1,000 mg 3 times a day. **Comments:** Reduce dose if diarrhea develops.
Vitamin E	**Dosage:** 400 IU twice a day. **Comments:** Check with your doctor if taking anticoagulant drugs.
Carotenoids	**Dosage:** 1 pill mixed carotenoids twice a day with food. **Comments:** Each pill should provide 25,000 IU vitamin A activity.
Zinc/Copper	**Dosage:** 30 mg zinc and 2 mg copper a day. **Comments:** Add copper only when using zinc longer than 1 month.
Flaxseed oil	**Dosage:** 1 tbsp. (14 grams) a day. **Comments:** Can be mixed with food; take in the morning.
Arginine	**Dosage:** 500 mg L-arginine 4 times a day for 3 months. **Comments:** Don't use if you have kidney disease or genital herpes, or are prone to cold sores. Take with a mixed amino acid complex.
Panax ginseng	**Dosage:** 100-250 mg twice a day; rotate with Siberian ginseng. **Comments:** Standardized to contain at least 7% ginsenosides.
Siberian ginseng	**Dosage:** 100-300 mg twice daily; rotate with Panax ginseng. **Comments:** Standardized to contain at least 0.8% eleutherosides.

Some dosages may be supplied by supplements you are already taking—see page 39.

free radicals and protect the sperm. Vitamin C also increases sperm motility, partly by preventing sperm from clumping together; this vitamin may be especially important for smokers, who tend to be deficient in it.

Men may benefit from zinc and flaxseed oil as well. **Zinc** plays a crucial role in male reproduction, increasing testosterone production and raising sperm count. (Take it with **copper,** because zinc inhibits the body's absorption of this mineral.) **Flaxseed oil** provides essential fatty acids that among other functions help keep sperm healthy. In addition, try the amino acid **arginine,** which can enhance sperm motility and increase the sperm count; three months of arginine treatment is sufficient to correct any deficiency that may be contributing to infertility.

The supplements above can also be combined with one or more herbal therapies. **Panax ginseng** stimulates testosterone production and sperm formation. Rotate it every three weeks with **Siberian ginseng,** which may also raise sperm count. Another herb worth trying is pygeum africanum (take 100 mg standardized extract twice a day). It may be particularly effective in men who have prostate problems.

What else you can do

☑ Avoid alcohol. If you smoke, quit.

☑ Try yoga, meditation, and other stress-reducing relaxation techniques.

inflammatory bowel disease

This chronic condition, which actually encompasses several related disorders, is marked by an often painful inflammation of the intestines. Symptoms may be eased with dietary changes, vitamin supplements, and soothing herbs.

Symptoms

- *Early symptoms may include constipation and the frequent urge to defecate, with passage of only small amounts of blood or mucus.*

- *Later symptoms include chronic diarrhea with rectal bleeding, abdominal pain, low-grade fever, general malaise, arthritis, mouth sores, blurred vision, painful joints, poor appetite, low energy, and weight loss. After a decade, there's increased risk for colorectal cancer.*

- *Symptoms may come and go. A severe attack can cause nausea, vomiting, dehydration, heavy sweating, loss of appetite, high fever, and heart palpitations.*

When to Call Your Doctor

- If you have black or bloody stools, or painful, mucus-filled diarrhea.
- If symptoms suddenly worsen.
- If you have a swollen abdomen or severe pain (especially on the lower-right side)—it may be a sign of appendicitis.
- If severe abdominal pain accompanies fever over 101°F.
- Reminder: If you have a medical condition, talk to your doctor before taking supplements.

What it is

Inflammatory bowel disease (IBD) is a general term for several related disorders (including Crohn's disease and ulcerative colitis) that often first strike people in their 20s or 30s. Typically, all or part of the digestive tract becomes chronically inflamed and develops small erosions, or ulcers. Bouts of inflammation are followed by periods of remission lasting weeks or years.

What causes it

Experts are not entirely sure why people develop IBD, although heredity plays a part. More than a third of IBD sufferers know of a family member afflicted with the disease, and it's four times more common in Caucasian and Jewish families. The disease may be triggered by a bacterium or a virus, or by a malfunctioning immune system. Factors such as stress and anxiety, or sensitivity to certain foods, can all contribute to flare-ups.

How supplements can help

IBD usually causes a decreased ability to absorb nutrients from food, so a daily high-potency multivitamin is essential. Additional supplements, taken together, may also be beneficial, especially during flare-ups.

Many people with IBD are deficient in B_{12}, folic acid, and other B vitamins. Taking **vitamin B complex** helps replace lost vitamins and restores proper digestion. Another B vitamin worth taking is **PABA** (para-aminobenzoic acid), which has an anti-inflammatory effect similar to the prescription drug sulfasalazine. **Licorice (DGL)** has healing properties as well, as do **vitamins E** and **A**. Once symptoms improve, the latter two can be continued long term, along with a high-potency antioxidant,

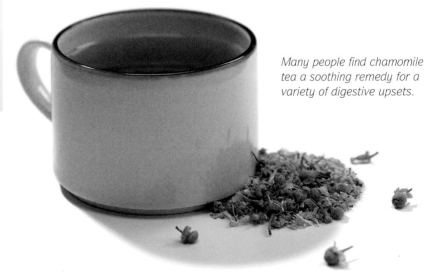

Many people find chamomile tea a soothing remedy for a variety of digestive upsets.

Supplement Recommendations

Vitamin B complex	**Dosage:** 1 pill twice a day for flare-ups; then reduce to 1 pill each morning for maintenance; take with food. **Comments:** Look for a B-100 complex with 100 mcg vitamin B_{12} and biotin; 400 mcg folic acid; and 100 mg all other B vitamins.
PABA	**Dosage:** 1,000 mg 3 times a day for flare-ups. **Comments:** Take 1,000 mg twice a day for maintenance.
Licorice (DGL)	**Dosage:** Chew 2 wafers (380 mg) 3 times a day, between meals. **Comments:** For flare-ups; use deglycyrrhizinated (DGL) form only.
Vitamin E	**Dosage:** 400 IU twice a day for flare-ups or maintenance. **Comments:** Check with your doctor if taking anticoagulant drugs.
Vitamin A	**Dosage:** 50,000 IU a day for flare-ups; reduce to 10,000 IU a day for maintenance. **Comments:** Take only 5,000 IU a day if you may become pregnant.
Essential fatty acids	**Dosage:** 1 tbsp. (14 grams) flaxseed oil or 5,000 mg fish oils a day. **Comments:** Use enteric-coated form of fish oils as maintenance.
Acidophilus	**Dosage:** Take 1 pill twice a day between meals. **Comments:** Get 1-2 billion live (viable) organisms per pill.
Zinc/Copper	**Dosage:** 30 mg zinc and 2 mg copper a day. **Comments:** Add copper only when using zinc longer than 1 month.
Chamomile	**Dosage:** 1 cup of tea up to 3 times a day. **Comments:** Use 2 tsp. dried herb per cup of hot water.

Note: Consider using supplements in **blue** first; those in **black** may also be beneficial. Some dosages may be supplied by supplements you are already taking—see page 39.

Some dosages may be supplied by supplements you are already taking—see page 39.

such as grape seed extract (100 mg once or twice a day) or the amino acid N-acetylcysteine, or NAC (500 mg twice a day). Vitamin C (1,000 mg twice a day) may be an effective—and less costly—alternative to grape seed extract and NAC.

Other supplements are also of value when taken on a regular basis. The **essential fatty acids** found in flaxseed oil or fish oils reduce inflammation and protect and repair the digestive tract. **Acidophilus** helps restore a normal balance of healthy bacteria in the digestive tract. **Zinc** is important because a zinc deficiency is often a complication of IBD; zinc, however, inhibits **copper** absorption, so add extra copper. Finally, **chamomile** tea is a time-honored remedy for easing digestive complaints.

What else you can do

☑ Determine if certain foods trigger flare-ups and then eliminate them.

☑ Apply a hot pack or hot water bottle to the abdomen to prevent cramps.

☑ Minimize stress with yoga, meditation, and regular exercise.

FACTS & Tips

■ The anti-inflammatory drug sulfasalazine, commonly prescribed to treat IBD, depletes folic acid. If you take this drug, ask your doctor about using a folic acid supplement.

■ In addition to chamomile, herbal teas made from flaxseed, slippery elm, or marshmallow aid digestion and soothe the intestines. To make the tea, use 1 or 2 teaspoons of herb per cup of hot water; steep for 10 to 15 minutes, then strain.

LATEST FINDINGS

■ Italian researchers recently found that fish oils reduce the frequency of intestinal attacks in people with Crohn's disease. In patients whose disease was in remission, but who had signs of inflammation, only 28% of those taking enteric-coated fish oil capsules relapsed, as contrasted with 69% of those who were given a placebo.

■ Nicotine patches may help put active cases of ulcerative colitis into remission, according to a small Mayo Clinic study. Of 31 patients who used high-dose nicotine skin patches for four weeks, 12 were significantly better; only 3 of 33 who wore placebo patches showed some improvement. But side effects were common, including dizziness, nausea, and skin rashes. Additional research is needed.

Did You Know?

Nearly 60% of those suffering from Crohn's disease use supplements or alternative therapies to treat their illness. But only a third of them have told their doctors about it.

insect bites and stings

Whether you're picnicking, hiking, or gardening on a summer afternoon, enjoying the outdoors exacts a price in the form of insect bites and stings. Fortunately, nature also provides several antidotes to the itching and swelling that often result.

What it is

During the summer months and in warm climates year-round, people are often bitten by mosquitoes, flies, chiggers, ticks, and spiders or stung by ants, bees, yellow jackets, wasps, and hornets. Although they're not usually serious, insect bites and stings can be itchy and painful and in some cases may need medical attention. Spider bites, for instance, should be watched carefully; severe swelling, pain, or fever can require an emergency medical visit.

You should also see a doctor if you've been bitten by a tick (particularly if a circular red rash develops) and be tested for Lyme disease or Rocky Mountain spotted fever, which are carried by this blood-sucking insect. In addition, approximately one in fifty people has a potentially life-threatening reaction to the venom of bees and other stinging insects; if stung, it is important to get to an emergency room right away.

What causes it

Insect venom contains toxins that cause swelling, burning, and other unpleasant symptoms at the site of the bite or sting. Although mosquitoes, chiggers, and ticks bite to get blood for nourishment, spiders and stinging insects are likely to attack only when threatened, or in the case of bees, if they mistake you for a flower. Your chances of getting stung increase if you sit down on a log where a spider has chosen to live, if you wave your arms wildly when a bee or wasp buzzes around you, or if you wear bright colors or perfume or eat sweet, sticky foods outdoors.

How supplements can help

Before trying any of the supplements in the chart, remove the stinger, if there is one, and wash the area with soap and water. Next, take **bromelain,** a protein-digesting enzyme obtained from pineapple, which can be

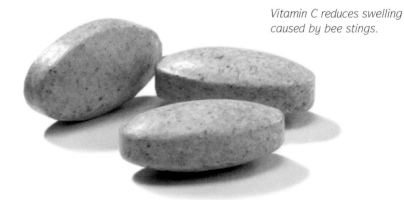

Vitamin C reduces swelling caused by bee stings.

Bromelain	**Dosage:** 500 mg 3 times a day on an empty stomach. **Comments:** Should provide 6,000 GDU or 9,000 MCU daily.
Lavender oil	**Dosage:** Apply a few drops to skin several times a day or as needed. **Comments:** Use 1 or 2 drops every 15 minutes if necessary.
Calendula cream	**Dosage:** Rub small dab into skin several times a day, or as needed. **Comments:** Standardized to contain at least 2% calendula.
Vitamin C	**Dosage:** 1,000 mg 3 times a day. **Comments:** Reduce dose if diarrhea develops.
Quercetin	**Dosage:** 500 mg 3 times a day 20 minutes before meals. **Comments:** Good to take in combination with bromelain.
Tea tree oil	**Dosage:** Apply 1 drop to skin several times a day or as needed. **Comments:** Discontinue use if skin irritation develops.

Note: Consider using supplements in **blue** first; those in **black** may also be beneficial. Some dosages may be supplied by supplements you are already taking—see page 39.

FACTS & Tips

■ Be prepared to treat an insect bite: Whip up a natural insect bite remedy and store it in an oil-resistant plastic bottle with a tight cap. Mix 1 teaspoon lavender oil with 1 tablespoon vegetable oil. Use the mixture as needed by dabbing it directly onto the insect bite. Warning: Keep it away from the eyes.

■ For quick relief for a bite or sting, apply bromelain topically in place of lavender oil. Open two capsules and mix the powder with just enough water to make a paste. Smooth it on the affected area.

LATEST FINDINGS

■ How you remove a bee stinger from your skin is less important than how fast you do it, according to a new study. Conventional thinking holds that pinching the stinger out with your fingers or tweezers causes more venom to be released into the wound, so many experts recommend gently scraping the stinger off the skin. But researchers at the University of California, Riverside, found that the method of removal made no difference in the size of the welt that developed. Simply getting the stinger out as quickly as possible was the key factor.

effective in reducing swelling; use until symptoms subside. Topical treatments can ease pain and itching and also aid healing. **Lavender oil** soothes the itch. Made from a flower in the marigold family, **calendula cream** mitigates swelling and itching and also has an antiseptic effect, which helps prevent infection. **Tea tree oil** can be substituted for calendula, if desired.

If you've been stung by a bee or similar insect, you may need to take additional supplements to control swelling and relieve pain. **Vitamin C** and **quercetin,** a flavonoid, act as antihistamines, which means they can inhibit the release of histamine, an inflammatory compound that the body produces in response to insect venom. Begin taking both as soon as possible after a sting and continue until the symptoms abate.

What else you can do

☑ Use insect repellent before leaving home. Calendula cream and tea tree oil are good natural repellents.

☑ Wear white or khaki-colored clothing when outdoors, as well as long pants and sleeves, to discourage stinging insects and protect your skin from ticks. Light-colored clothing makes ticks easier to spot too.

☑ Do not wear perfume, after-shave lotions, hair spray, or sweet-smelling creams—the scent will attract insects.

☑ Do not swat at an insect. Walk away calmly or lie down and cover your head if insects swarm nearby.

insomnia

Although you might feel as if you're the only one who can't get a good night's sleep, the truth is that one in every three people complains about insomnia. Fortunately, there are a variety of safe, natural "lullabies" that can ease you into dreamland—without the risk of side effects.

SYMPTOMS

- *Difficulty falling asleep.*
- *Inability to sleep all night.*
- *Waking up too early.*

When to Call Your Doctor

- If insomnia lasts a month or more with no obvious cause.
- If sleeping problems follow a traumatic event, such as the loss of a job or a loved one.
- If you feel tired most of the time and frequently doze off during the day.
- If you are so tired that you can't function normally.
- Reminder: If you have a medical or psychiatric condition, talk to your doctor before taking supplements.

What it is

Though many people think of insomnia as the inability to fall asleep, it also involves not being able to stay asleep or continually waking up earlier than planned. Sleep problems that last just a couple of nights or a few weeks are often related to stress, or to excitement. But in some cases, insomnia can become chronic, lasting for months or even years.

What causes it

Insomnia is actually considered a symptom of many underlying and often hard-to-recognize conditions or situations. Dietary and lifestyle factors, physical pain, a major illness, medications, even a bad mattress can all contribute to sleeplessness. For most people, however, tension, anxiety, and depression lie at the root of insomnia. Discovering the basic cause or causes of your sleep problems may take some detective work, but it is ultimately the best way to bring about a cure.

How supplements can help

The supplements listed in the chart may all provide immediate relief from insomnia, but unless otherwise stated, most should be used one at a time, not together. Try one to see whether it works for you. Rotate supplements every couple of weeks, and use only as needed, so you don't become too tolerant of any one.

Numerous studies have found **valerian,** among the most researched of all herbal supplements, to be an effective sleep aid. It works best

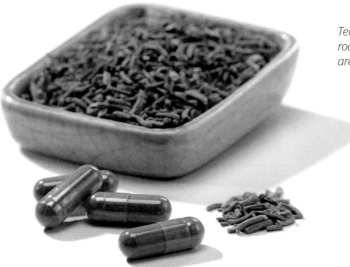

Teas made from dried valerian root—or capsules containing it—are safe, gentle sleep aids.

Supplement Recommendations

Valerian	**Dosage:** 250-500 mg standardized extract before bedtime. **Comments:** Start with the lower dose and increase as needed.
Melatonin	**Dosage:** 1-3 mg before bedtime. **Comments:** Start with the lower dose and increase as needed.
GABA	**Dosage:** 500 mg before bedtime. **Comments:** Alternate with melatonin, valerian, and 5-HTP.
5-HTP	**Dosage:** 100 mg 5-hydroxytryptophan before bedtime. **Comments:** Especially useful when taken with B_6 or magnesium.
Calcium/ Magnesium	**Dosage:** 600 mg calcium and 600 mg magnesium before bedtime. **Comments:** Take with food; sometimes sold in a single supplement.
Vitamin B_6/ Niacinamide	**Dosage:** 50 mg B_6 and 500 mg niacinamide before bedtime. **Comments:** These supplements work well together.
Chamomile	**Dosage:** 1 cup of tea in the evening. **Comments:** Mild enough to use with other sedating supplements.
Kava	**Dosage:** 250 mg before bedtime. **Comments:** Standardized to contain at least 30% kavalactones.

Note: Consider using supplements in **blue** first; those in **black** may also be beneficial. Some dosages may be supplied by supplements you are already taking—see page 39.

when rotated with other sedating herbs, such as **chamomile, kava,** and passionflower. These herbs, taken as pills, teas, or tinctures, promote relaxation and reduce stress, making it easier to fall asleep.

An alternative to valerian is **melatonin,** a synthetic version of the body's own sleep hormone. It may be especially beneficial for people who can't sleep because of chronic pain. Valerian or melatonin can also be rotated with the neurotransmitter **GABA** (gamma-aminobutyric acid), which inhibits nerve impulses and prevents stress-related messages from reaching the brain, or with **5-HTP** (a form of the amino acid tryptophan), which raises levels of the sleep-inducing chemical serotonin.

In some instances, a nutrient deficiency, especially a lack of **calcium, magnesium,** or **vitamin B_6,** can lead to sleep problems; replenishing those nutrients can be beneficial. The B vitamin **niacinamide,** taken with B_6, is useful as well because it helps ease anxiety. It may be especially helpful to try magnesium or B_6 along with 5-HTP.

What else you can do

☑ Stick to a regular sleep schedule, even on weekends.

☑ Use your bed only for sleeping, not for reading or watching television.

☑ Exercise regularly (though not in the evening) to help reduce stress.

☑ Avoid alcohol, tobacco, and caffeine.

irritable bowel syndrome

Though the symptoms of irritable bowel syndrome are very real, tests often show no abnormalities. But doctors who once said, "It's all in your head," now have a better understanding of this frustrating disease, which affects 15% to 20% of adults.

SYMPTOMS

- *Diarrhea, constipation, or alternating bouts of each (usually after meals) for several months.*
- *Abdominal cramping that is often relieved by a bowel movement.*
- *Mucus in the stools.*
- *Gas and bloating.*

When to Call Your Doctor

- If you have abdominal pain accompanied by any changes in bowel patterns or stool consistency.
- If the abdominal pain is continuous, or severe and accompanied by a fever.
- If there is blood in your stools.
- If you lose weight without intending to do so.
- Reminder: If you have a medical condition, talk to your doctor before taking supplements.

What it is

Normally, food is propelled through the digestive tract by rhythmic contractions of the intestinal muscles, a process called peristalsis. In irritable bowel syndrome (IBS), these muscles go into spasm, and the contractions become uncoordinated. This disturbance can cause the intestine's contents to move too fast or too slow, leading to abdominal pain and either diarrhea or constipation. An older term for IBS is "spastic colon."

What causes it

Over the years, researchers have proposed many causes for IBS, none of which has ever been proved. The list of suspects includes a bacterial, viral, or parasitic infection; overuse of antibiotics; lactose intolerance; or adverse reactions to foods (such as wheat or broccoli). Some experts think people with IBS have highly sensitive smooth muscle tissue, not only in the gastrointestinal tract but also elsewhere in the body. Others believe that IBS is the result of an inflammation in the lining of the intestine. One underlying factor in almost all cases of IBS, however, is that stress aggravates the symptoms. Because no one is sure exactly what makes bowel function go awry, doctors tend to diagnose IBS by eliminating other disorders with similar symptoms, such as diverticulitis or inflammatory bowel disease.

How supplements can help

Natural supplements offer a good way to control many IBS symptoms. All those listed here can be combined with one another or with conventional drugs. Enteric-coated **peppermint oil** capsules—which ensure that the oil is released in

The oil from the leaf and stem of the peppermint plant—in pill or liquid form—helps prevent intestinal spasms.

Supplement Recommendations

Peppermint oil
Dosage: 1 or 2 capsules 3 times a day between meals.
Comments: Take enteric-coated capsules with 0.2 ml of oil each; start at lower dose and increase if necessary.

Psyllium
Dosage: 1-3 tbsp. powder dissolved in water or juice a day.
Comments: Be sure to drink extra water throughout the day.

Acidophilus
Dosage: 1 pill a day on an empty stomach.
Comments: Get 1-2 billion live (viable) organisms per pill; also available as a powder; may require refrigeration.

FOS
Dosage: 2,000 mg a day.
Comments: Take in combination with acidophilus; not effective for IBS when used alone.

Some dosages may be supplied by supplements you are already taking—see page 39.

the intestine, not the stomach—are very effective in calming the intestinal spasms that cause abdominal pain, as well as soothing other IBS symptoms. In a study of 110 people with IBS, enteric-coated peppermint oil reduced abdominal pain in 79% of those taking it and eliminated the pain in 56%. Virtually no adverse reactions were seen.

Psyllium, a type of dietary fiber, eases IBS symptoms for many people—although not for all. In most cases, it works to correct constipation and is useful for diarrhea because it absorbs water in the intestine and adds bulk to the stool (bulk also seems to lessen the severity of spasms). Drink at least eight glasses of water a day when using psyllium. If you find that it aggravates your symptoms, stop taking it.

Acidophilus, a type of "good" bacteria that normally inhabits the intestine, helps digest food and prevents the harmful bacteria that cause disease from growing unchecked. **FOS** (fructo-oligosaccharides), sometimes added to acidophilus supplements or available separately, comprises indigestible carbohydrates that feed the friendly bacteria.

What else you can do

☑ Add more high-fiber foods, such as fruits, vegetables, grains, and beans, to your diet. But do it slowly to minimize bloating and gas. Eating lots of these foods may eliminate the need for psyllium.

☑ Eat smaller, more frequent meals. Limit caffeine, alcohol, and foods high in fat. Eliminate certain foods and add them back one at a time over several weeks to find out which, if any, cause symptoms.

☑ Take control of stress. Relaxation techniques or biofeedback may help.

☑ Exercise for at least 20 minutes a day to keep the bowels moving normally and reduce stress.

FACTS
& Tips

■ Lactose intolerance (a sensitivity to the sugars in milk products) may trigger IBS symptoms or even mimic the condition in some people. The ability to digest lactose often declines with age because of a decreased amount of the enzyme lactase in the small intestine. To determine if this is your problem, try drinking two glasses of nonfat milk on an empty stomach. If you notice gas, diarrhea, pain, or bloating within four hours, repeat the test with lactase-treated milk. If no symptoms occur, you probably should be careful with dairy products.

C·a·s·e H·i·s·t·o·r·y

A PROACTIVE APPROACH

Carlos B. woke up one morning and decided he really couldn't accept his doctor's words: "You'll just have to live with it." He was sick and tired of being embarrassed about the unpredictable diarrhea, cramping, and queasiness that alternated with constipation during any stressful period—from a job interview to going out with a new woman.

He decided to work on beating what had been diagnosed as an irritable colon himself. First, he went on a food-sensitivity elimination diet, and discovered that dairy products triggered his symptoms. Then, he made real progress using a combination of high-fiber psyllium and oat bran. Finally, adding peppermint oil capsules seemed to nearly eliminate the problem.

"I'm now convinced anyone can beat IBS," he says. "There are so many options people are unaware of. It's called being 'proactive.' After all, you're the one who should care the most!"

lupus

A butterfly-shaped facial rash may be the first sign of this auto-immune disease, in which the immune system mistakenly attacks healthy cells. The course of lupus is unpredictable, but various forms of therapy can help ease symptoms, delay progression of the disease, and boost overall health.

SYMPTOMS

- *Joint pain and inflammation, skin rashes, fever, fatigue, chest pain or cough, hair loss, strong tendency to sunburn, blurred vision, and swollen glands.*

- *There are many other symptoms, because lupus can affect almost any part of the body. Symptoms typically first appear between the ages of 15 and 35. Proper diagnosis may be difficult.*

When to Call Your Doctor

- If you experience any lingering unexplained illness, especially if symptoms include fever, joint pain, weight loss, rashes, or breathing difficulties. Seek an accurate diagnosis, which may take some persistence, as soon as possible.

- Reminder: If you have a medical condition, talk to your doctor before taking supplements.

What it is

A chronic inflammatory disease marked by flare-ups and remissions, lupus has been called the "great impostor" because it can cause such a wide array of symptoms in almost any part of the body, including the skin, joints, heart, brain, or kidneys. Women are affected eight to ten times more often than men. A quarter-million or more Americans have lupus, though many don't even know it.

What causes it

In lupus, the immune system goes awry and produces abnormal cells that travel through the body, attacking healthy tissues. It's uncertain what causes this condition, though heredity, sex hormones, or infections may play a role. Sunlight, childbirth, stress, or drugs may trigger attacks.

How supplements can help

A wide array of supplements, taken together on a long-term basis, may relieve symptoms, slow disease progression, and lessen the need for conventional drugs, which frequently have serious side effects. All can be used with conventional prescription drugs for lupus, but because lupus is a serious disease, take supplements only under ongoing medical supervision. Benefits may be noticed within a month.

Vitamin B complex works throughout the body to maintain the health of skin, mucous membranes, blood, nerves, and joints. Along with **vitamins C** and **E** and **selenium**—all antioxidants—B-complex vitamins speed healing and help protect the heart and blood vessels, joints, skin, and other areas that can be damaged by the inflammatory process. Vitamin E may be particularly effective for skin and joint problems.

The antioxidant selenium may help protect against lupus-related damage to the joints, nerves, skin, heart, and other parts of the body.

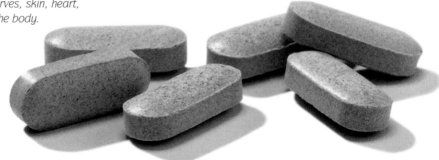

Supplement Recommendations

Vitamin B complex	**Dosage:** 1 pill each morning with food. **Comments:** Look for a B-50 complex with 50 mcg vitamin B_{12} and biotin; 400 mcg folic acid; and 50 mg all other B vitamins.
Vitamin C/ Vitamin E	**Dosage:** 1,000 mg vitamin C 3 times a day; 400 IU vitamin E daily. **Comments:** Vitamin C helps boost the effects of vitamin E.
Flaxseed oil	**Dosage:** 1 tbsp. (14 grams) a day. **Comments:** Can be mixed with food; take in the morning.
Fish oils	**Dosage:** 1,000 mg 3 times a day. **Comments:** Take with food.
Evening primrose oil	**Dosage:** 1,000 mg 3 times a day. **Comments:** Can substitute 1,000 mg borage oil once a day.
DHEA	**Dosage:** 100 mg each morning. **Comments:** Take only under medical supervision. Don't use if you're at risk for hormone-related (breast, prostate, etc.) cancers.
Selenium	**Dosage:** 200 mcg a day. **Comments:** Don't exceed 600 mcg daily; higher doses may be toxic.
Zinc/Copper	**Dosage:** 30 mg zinc and 2 mg copper a day. **Comments:** Add copper only when using zinc longer than 1 month.

Note: Consider using supplements in **blue** first; those in **black** may also be beneficial. Some dosages may be supplied by supplements you are already taking—see page 39.

see page 39.

Essential fatty acids in the form of **flaxseed oil, fish oils,** and **evening primrose oil** may be beneficial as well. These can limit inflammation in the joints, kidneys, skin, and other areas; they may also lower cholesterol levels, which might be elevated. In addition, doctors are finding that the nutritional supplement **DHEA** may reduce a lupus patient's requirements for the prescription steroid drug prednisone. Furthermore, it may relieve symptoms and improve stamina. The recommended doses of DHEA are quite high (100 mg a day), so if you're interested in trying this treatment, talk to a physician experienced with both lupus and DHEA. **Zinc** promotes healing and, along with vitamin C, may help regulate the immune system. Because zinc depletes **copper** stores, it should be taken with that mineral when used over the long term.

What else you can do

☑ Minimize sun exposure and, when outdoors, use high-SPF sunscreens.
☑ Get plenty of rest. Join a support group to help reduce stress.

FACTS & Tips

■ Conventional lupus drugs, including high doses of steroids and cancer medications, can have side effects as bad as the disease itself, causing weakened bones, cataracts, diabetes, and other serious problems. Supplements may allow you to use lower—and therefore safer— doses of such drugs.

LATEST FINDINGS

■ Preliminary studies indicate a connection between lower-than-average blood levels of three nutrients—vitamins A, E, and beta-carotene—and the development, years later, of lupus. Additional studies are needed to determine whether these levels contributed to the onset of lupus or if they were a result of early, undiagnosed disease activity.

Did You Know?

People with lupus may want to avoid alfalfa in any form—including sprouts, seeds, tablets, and tea. It contains a substance called canavanine, which some experts think triggers flare-ups.

macular degeneration

Some 6 million Americans suffer from this eye condition, the most common cause of blindness in those over age 50. Getting plenty of antioxidants—potent protectors of the body's cells—appears to be a key factor in preventing this disorder.

SYMPTOMS

- *A blurry, gray, or blank spot in the center of the field of vision; peripheral vision remains sharp in one or both eyes.*

- *Distorted vision, in which straight lines look wavy, printed words seem blurred, or objects appear to be the wrong size or shape.*

- *Faded or washed-out colors.*

When to Call Your Doctor

- If you're over age 50, see an ophthalmologist yearly to check for macular degeneration.

- If you develop any of the above symptoms, see an ophthalmologist immediately. Prompt diagnosis can minimize vision loss.

- Reminder: If you have a medical condition, talk to your doctor before taking supplements.

What it is

In macular degeneration, the macula—the light-sensitive area in the center of the retina that controls the central visual field and the ability to see colors—breaks down and impairs your eyesight. Though your peripheral vision—the ability to see the outside edges of the scene you are looking at—remains intact, the center of your field of vision is blurry, gray, or filled with a large blank spot. As a result, the condition may make it difficult or impossible to read, drive, watch television, or even recognize someone's face.

There are two forms of this disorder. In age-related, or "dry," macular degeneration, the macula thins and bits of debris gather beneath it. The condition develops slowly and accounts for 90% of all cases. In hemorrhagic, or "wet," macular degeneration, new blood vessels grow underneath the retina, pushing up like the roots of a maple cracking the pavement above. These fragile vessels often leak fluid and blood, causing scar tissue to form and central vision to deteriorate rapidly.

What causes it

Damage from free radicals, the unstable oxygen molecules that can harm cells, is probably the leading cause of macular degeneration. A diet high in saturated fats, cigarette smoke, and exposure to sunlight can lead to the formation of free radicals in the retina. High blood pressure, heart disease, and diabetes may also be contributing factors because they limit blood flow to your eyes.

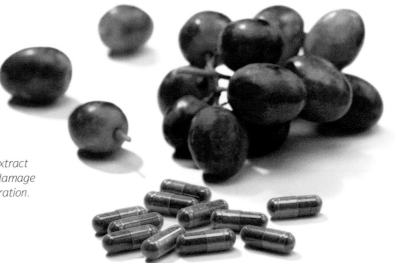

The antioxidants in grape seed extract help protect the retina from the damage that can lead to macular degeneration.

Supplement Recommendations

Vitamin C	**Dosage:** 1,000 mg twice a day. **Comments:** Reduce dosage if diarrhea develops.
Vitamin E	**Dosage:** 400 IU twice a day. **Comments:** Check with your doctor if taking anticoagulant drugs.
Carotenoids	**Dosage:** 2 pills mixed carotenoids a day with food. **Comments:** Each pill should supply 25,000 IU vitamin A activity.
Zinc/Copper	**Dosage:** 30 mg zinc and 2 mg copper a day. **Comments:** Add copper only when using zinc longer than 1 month.
Bilberry	**Dosage:** 80 mg 3 times a day. **Comments:** Standardized to contain 25% anthocyanidins.
Grape seed extract	**Dosage:** 100 mg twice a day. **Comments:** Standardized to contain 92%-95% proanthocyanidins.
Ginkgo biloba	**Dosage:** 40 mg 3 times a day. **Comments:** Standardized to have at least 24% flavone glycosides.
Selenium	**Dosage:** 400 mcg a day. **Comments:** Don't exceed 600 mcg daily; higher doses may be toxic.

Note: Consider using supplements in **blue** first; those in **black** may also be beneficial. Some dosages may be supplied by supplements you are already taking—see page 39.

How supplements can help

Working as antioxidants, **vitamin C, vitamin E,** and different types of **carotenoids** can neutralize the free radicals linked to macular degeneration. The carotenoids lutein and zeaxanthin are especially important—in fact, the macula's yellow color is due to their presence. They protect the macula by filtering out the sun's harmful ultraviolet rays. **Zinc** plays a key role in the functioning of the retina as well. Not only are many older people deficient in this mineral, but some research suggests it can slow the progression of the disorder. You'll also need extra **copper** because zinc inhibits its absorption.

For maximum protection, take all these supplements, plus **bilberry.** This herb contains antioxidant compounds and enhances blood flow to the retina. **Grape seed extract** or **ginkgo biloba** can be substituted for the bilberry. Though neither is as effective as bilberry, grape seed may be a good choice if you have poor night vision, and ginkgo is useful for those who also show signs of memory loss. **Selenium** can be added in an effort to boost the body's overall antioxidant activity.

What else you can do

☑ Wear sunglasses and wide-brimmed hats to protect your eyes.

☑ Stop smoking: It's a major contributor to macular degeneration.

☑ Eat lots of dark green vegetables; they're high in lutein and zeaxanthin.

menopause

Women now have more options to help them deal with this natural change in their lives. Hormone replacement therapy is conventional medicine's answer, but many women are finding natural therapies can also provide relief from symptoms such as hot flashes and night sweats.

SYMPTOMS

- *Hot flashes.*
- *Night sweats.*
- *Menstrual irregularities.*
- *Vaginal dryness.*
- *Irritability or mild depression.*

When to Call Your Doctor

- If you begin to experience changes in your menstrual cycle—find out whether the symptoms are related to menopause or another cause.
- If you are at high risk for heart disease or osteoporosis.
- If you are bothered by symptoms that natural remedies don't relieve.
- Reminder: If you have a medical condition, talk to your doctor before taking supplements.

What it is

Typically, a woman's ovaries stop releasing eggs in her early 50s, and her menstrual cycle ceases. When she hasn't had a period in six months, she is said to have completed menopause. Though not a disease, menopause can have some unpleasant symptoms. For five to ten years before a woman has her last period, she may experience menstrual irregularities, hot flashes, and irritability; after menopause, she faces possible vaginal dryness, a decline in bone mass, and an increased risk of heart disease.

What causes it

As the ovaries gradually stop manufacturing the hormones estrogen and progesterone, menopausal symptoms and the risk of heart disease and osteoporosis increase. To address these concerns, some women opt for hormone replacement therapy (HRT). But worries about links between long-term HRT and breast cancer, or simply a belief that nature should take its own course, motivate other women to try natural remedies. These therapies are also beneficial for the women who experience menopausal symptoms while still menstruating (a stage called perimenopause); most doctors advise against HRT at this stage.

How supplements can help

If you choose not to take HRT, you may want to use the herbs listed in the chart to control hot flashes and other symptoms. Taking them in some combination should work best. First, try **black cohosh** and **chasteberry.** Widely used in Europe, these herbs help stabilize hormone levels, reducing hot flashes and lessening depression and vaginal dryness. **Siberian ginseng** is considered a good female tonic and may have other benefits too.

If this combination doesn't provide relief, add dong quai or licorice root. Some studies suggest that although it's not helpful for menopausal symptoms when used alone, **dong quai** may bolster the effect of other herbs. **Licorice** has plant-based compounds (phytoestrogens) that perform functions similar to those of estrogen produced by a woman's body.

Soy isoflavone supplements may help minimize the side effects of menopause, especially for women who don't regularly eat soy products.

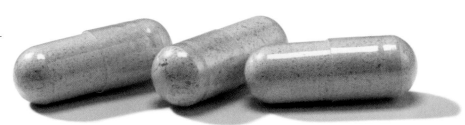

Supplement Recommendations

Black cohosh	**Dosage:** 40 mg twice a day.
	Comments: Standardized to contain 2.5% triterpenes.
Chasteberry	**Dosage:** 225 mg standardized extract twice a day.
	Comments: Also called vitex. Should contain 0.5% agnuside.
Siberian ginseng	**Dosage:** 100-300 mg a day.
	Comments: Standardized to contain at least 0.8% eleutherosides.
Calcium/ Vitamin D	**Dosage:** 600 mg calcium and 200 IU vitamin D a day.
	Comments: Sometimes sold in a single supplement.
Dong quai	**Dosage:** 200 mg, or 30 drops tincture, 3 times a day.
	Comments: Standardized to contain 0.8%-1.1% ligustilide.
Licorice	**Dosage:** 200 mg standardized extract 3 times a day.
	Comments: Can raise blood pressure; see your doctor before taking.
Soy isoflavones	**Dosage:** 50 mg a day.
	Comments: Look for products that contain genistein and daidzein.
Vitamin E	**Dosage:** 400 IU twice a day.
	Comments: Check with your doctor if taking anticoagulant drugs.

Note: Consider using supplements in **blue** first; those in **black** may also be beneficial. Some dosages may be supplied by supplements you are already taking—see page 39.

In addition, some nutrients may be of value in lowering the risk of heart disease and osteoporosis in women after menopause. Studies have shown that soy foods may protect against heart disease. What's more, hot flashes and other menopausal symptoms are rare in countries where soy is a dietary staple. If you don't like the taste of soy, consider supplements with **soy isoflavones,** the compounds thought to be partly responsible for the protective effect of soy. Studies suggest **vitamin E** aids in preventing heart disease by keeping LDL ("bad") cholesterol from adhering to artery walls; some women find high doses of vitamin E also relieve hot flashes. Essential for strong bones, **calcium** helps prevent osteoporosis; combine it with **vitamin D** for proper absorption. (You also might want to take vitamin E, calcium, and vitamin D even if you are using HRT.)

What else you can do

☑ Avoid alcohol, chocolate, coffee, and spicy foods; they can all make hot flashes worse.

☑ Get regular exercise, which can reduce the number of hot flashes and help prevent heart disease. Light weight training may protect the bones.

☑ Soak in a tepid bath for 20 minutes each morning; some women find that this routine prevents hot flashes all day long.

■ Vitamin C and flavonoids may reduce the heavy menstrual bleeding that often appears in perimenopause. These nutrients work by strengthening the capillary walls, which weaken just before and during menstruation. Flavonoids may also control hot flashes and mood swings. Some experts suggest taking 1,000 mg of vitamin C along with 500 mg of flavonoids twice a day.

LATEST FINDINGS

■ In a recent study of soy's effect on menopausal symptoms, researchers found that women who consumed soy daily experienced less severe hot flashes and night sweats. In addition, they had a 10% drop in total cholesterol, a 12% decrease in LDL ("bad") cholesterol, and a 6-point drop in diastolic blood pressure. Test participants added about 2 tablespoons of soy protein powder to their diet each day for six weeks.

■ Whether a woman starts HRT at menopause or waits until her early 60s appears to make no difference in terms of bone density, according to a recent study. This is good news if you're in good general health and want to try natural therapies to control menopausal symptoms. If you wish, you can try HRT later in life to reduce your risk of heart disease and osteoporosis.

menstrual disorders

Though most women experience some discomfort (such as a day or two of mild cramps) during their menstrual periods, a number suffer troublesome irregularities that can cause severe pain or major inconveniences each month.

What it is

Three common menstrual disorders are cramps (dysmenorrhea), heavy bleeding or prolonged periods (menorrhagia), and irregular or absent periods (amenorrhea). These conditions usually affect women in times of hormonal change, such as adolescence or the years shortly before menopause, but they may occur anytime during the reproductive years.

What causes it

Menstrual cramps are triggered by prostaglandins—hormonelike substances released during menstruation by cells in the lining of the uterus (endometrium). Women who bleed so heavily that they have to change a tampon or pad every hour or so, and those whose periods last longer than seven days, are considered to have menorrhagia. Though the most common causes of this condition are hormonal or nutritional imbalances, an abnormal growth in the uterus (fibroid) can induce heavy bleeding. In addition, blood vessels in the uterus tend to be weak and rupture easily. Hormonal imbalances as well as extreme exercise or diet regimens can lead to amenorrhea.

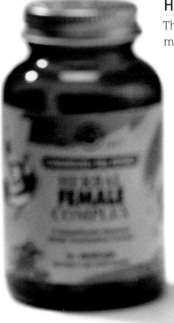

How supplements can help

The menstrual disorder you experience determines the supplements you should use. All those recommended can be combined with over-the-counter or prescription drugs.

To combat menstrual cramps, the **essential fatty acids** in evening primrose and flaxseed oils help block prostaglandin

Chasteberry, dong quai, and other herbs such as black cohosh that ease menstrual disorders are often sold in a single "female" formula.

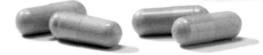

Supplement Recommendations

Essential fatty acids	**Dosage:** 1,000 mg evening primrose oil 3 times a day; 1 tbsp. (14 grams) flaxseed oil a day. **Comments:** Or use 1,000 mg borage oil once a day for primrose oil.
Chasteberry	**Dosage:** 225 mg standardized extract a day. **Comments:** Also called vitex. Should contain 0.5% agnuside.
Dong quai	**Dosage:** 200 mg, or 30 drops tincture, 3 times a day. **Comments:** Standardized to contain 0.8%-1.1% ligustilide.
Shepherd's purse	**Dosage:** 3 ml tincture (about 60 drops) 3 times a day. **Comments:** Good for heavy periods and spotting between periods.
Iron	**Dosage:** 100 mg a day for 6 weeks. **Comments:** Have your blood iron measured by your doctor after 6 weeks to determine how long iron supplements are needed.
Vitamin A	**Dosage:** 25,000 IU a day for 3 weeks, then 10,000 IU daily. **Comments:** Women who are pregnant or considering pregnancy should not exceed 5,000 IU a day.
Vitamin C/ Flavonoids	**Dosage:** 1,000 mg vitamin C and 500 mg flavonoids twice a day. **Comments:** Sometimes sold in a single supplement.

Note: Consider using supplements in **blue** first; those in **black** may also be beneficial. Some dosages may be supplied by supplements you are already taking—see page 39.

see page 39.

production. The herb **chasteberry** eases PMS-like symptoms by balancing hormone levels and is quite useful if you also have breast tenderness; add another herb, **dong quai,** to enhance its benefits. These three supplements may reduce the need for pain relievers, such as ibuprofen.

To help relieve amenorrhea, first make sure you are not pregnant, and then try chasteberry and dong quai to restore normal periods. These herbs may correct hormonal imbalances and may regulate the menstrual cycle. However, six months of treatment may be needed before you see any beneficial effect.

To treat menorrhagia, take the herb **shepherd's purse** together with essential fatty acids to reduce the bleeding. Some women may also need extra **iron,** because heavy blood flow depletes stores of this mineral, and paradoxically, low iron levels may promote abnormal menstrual bleeding. Always check with your doctor before self-treating with iron, however. **Vitamin A** levels are also often low in women with menorrhagia. If this is the case, use a supplement. **Vitamin C** and **flavonoids** strengthen capillaries—the tiniest blood vessels—in the uterus, so they are less likely to rupture and cause additional bleeding.

What else you can do

☑ Take a hot bath or use a heating pad to relax the uterus to relieve cramps.

☑ Exercise—activity releases endorphins, the body's natural painkillers.

FACTS & Tips

■ Different herbal teas can help ease menstrual disorders. For cramps, try chamomile or cramp bark tea; for excessive bleeding, sip either shepherd's purse, red raspberry, or lady's mantle tea; for missed periods, drink squawvine tea. To brew, use 1 teaspoon of your herb of choice for each cup of hot water, steep for 10 to 15 minutes, strain, and drink.

LATEST FINDINGS

■ In a recent study designed to determine the effect of vitamins on birth defects, women who took a daily multivitamin had more regular menstrual cycles than those given a placebo.

■ Fish oil supplements may lessen menstrual cramps. In a study of adolescent girls—prone to painful cramps because of high hormone levels—those who took fish oil supplements needed less painkilling medication to control their cramps than those who didn't use the supplements. Further study is needed to confirm these results.

migraine

For the estimated 10% of the population who suffer from migraines, there is good news. A growing body of research suggests that certain supplements may be as effective as—or even superior to—conventional medicine in the prevention and treatment of these debilitating headaches.

SYMPTOMS

- *Intense, throbbing pain, first near one eye or temple, then throughout one or both sides of the head.*
- *Nausea and vomiting.*
- *Painful aversion to light.*
- *Loss of appetite.*
- *Early warning signs include visual disturbances (flashing lights or wavy lines) called an aura; tingling sensations, dizziness, and ringing in the ears; sweating, chills, fatigue; swelling of the face; and irritability.*

When to Call Your Doctor

- If you have a sudden onset of severe headaches, especially if they first appear after age 35.
- If intense headaches occur after physical exertion.
- If a headache is accompanied by a fever, stiff neck, confusion, loss of speech, or weakness on one side of the body.
- If migraines become more severe or more frequent.
- Reminder: If you have a medical or psychiatric condition, talk to your doctor before taking supplements.

What it is

A migraine is a severe, throbbing headache that usually begins on one side of the head (hence the name "migraine"—from the Greek *hemikrania*, or "half the skull"), but may affect the whole head. Attacks can last for hours or days and may be preceded by warning signs.

What causes it

The precise underlying cause of migraines is unknown. The prevailing theory is that they are sparked by spasms in the arteries that supply blood to the brain. Some researchers believe a low level of the brain chemical serotonin is the reason the blood vessels constrict and widen abnormally.

A variety of triggers can precipitate an attack in those susceptible to migraines. These initiators include certain foods, stress, lack of sleep, changes in the weather, bright light, fluctuations in blood sugar levels, liver problems, dental pain, hormonal swings that occur with the menstrual cycle or the use of birth control pills, environmental chemicals, and exposure to cigarette smoke. Migraines run in families, and women are more susceptible than men.

How supplements can help

The recommended supplements are useful in preventing migraines and may be used in place of prescription drugs. (Don't stop taking them, however, without your doctor's approval.) You'll probably still need prescription medication to combat a migraine headache that has already begun.

Feverfew supplements may prevent migraine attacks.

Supplement Recommendations

Magnesium/ Calcium	**Dosage:** 400 mg magnesium and 100 mg calcium twice a day. **Comments:** Take with food; sometimes sold in a single supplement.
Feverfew	**Dosage:** 250 mg every morning. **Comments:** Standardized to contain at least 0.4% parthenolide.
5-HTP	**Dosage:** 100 mg 3 times a day. **Comments:** Consult doctor if taking a prescription antidepressant.
Riboflavin	**Dosage:** 400 mg every morning. **Comments:** Best used for chronic migraines. Also called vitamin B_2.
Vitamin C	**Dosage:** 1,000 mg 3 times a day. **Comments:** Reduce dose if diarrhea develops.
Pantothenic acid	**Dosage:** 400 mg twice a day. **Comments:** Take with meals.

Note: Consider using supplements in **blue** first; those in **black** may also be beneficial. Some dosages may be supplied by supplements you are already taking—see page 39.

see page 39

Everyone who gets migraines should take **magnesium** and **calcium** long term. These minerals help maintain healthy blood vessels, and low levels of magnesium are common in people who have migraines.

In addition, two natural remedies are beneficial in preventing some migraines. Widely used in Europe and approved by health authorities in Canada, the herb **feverfew** can reduce the intensity and frequency of migraines when taken over several months. Or try **5-HTP** (5-hydroxy-tryptophan), a form of the amino acid tryptophan and a basic building block of serotonin. Some studies show it can prevent migraines as effectively as drugs—with only minor side effects, primarily nausea. The side effects tend to disappear in about two weeks. But several months of therapy may be needed to derive the maximum benefit.

If your migraines are ongoing, the B vitamin **riboflavin** may reduce the number of times they occur more effectively than feverfew or 5-HTP. At high doses, riboflavin seems to increase energy reserves in brain cells. If none of these work, consider adding **vitamin C** and **pantothenic acid.** Both boost the production of hormones that assist the body in dealing with the adverse effects of stress; pantothenic acid is also important for serotonin production.

What else you can do

☑ Identify and eliminate your migraine triggers.
☑ Try biofeedback or relaxation training to help you cope with stress.
☑ Drink at least 48 ounces of water a day and exercise regularly.

FACTS & Tips

■ Certain foods and beverages— especially those containing compounds known as amines— are notorious migraine triggers. If you're a migraine sufferer, try to avoid the following: aged cheeses, onions, pickles, cured meats, red wine, beer, sour cream, nuts, freshly baked yeast products, eggs, tomatoes, citrus fruits, and caffeinated drinks. Although chocolate is often implicated as a migraine trigger, some new studies indicate that this connection may be a misconception.

■ Eating fish rich in omega-3 fatty acids, such as salmon and tuna, may help prevent migraines. Omega-3s seem to alter blood chemicals, reducing the risk of blood vessel spasms associated with migraines.

LATEST FINDINGS

■ According to a recent Belgian study, 400 mg a day of the B vitamin riboflavin reduced the frequency (but not the severity or duration) of migraine attacks in chronic sufferers by about a third. The study suggests that people who average about four migraines a month may benefit from riboflavin.

multiple sclerosis

This disabling nerve disorder can cause fatigue, impair vision, and hamper mobility in previously healthy people. Conventional drugs are only partially successful against it, prompting interest in supplements to help slow the disease's progress.

SYMPTOMS

- *Early signs mimic those of many other conditions. They include blurred or double vision; tingling in the arms or legs; clumsiness or unsteadiness; and other motor, visual, and sensory problems.*

- *The disease's course varies greatly. Depending on its severity, a person with MS may experience severe fatigue; muscle stiffness and tremors; poor coordination; impaired speech; and continence difficulties. Symptoms often come and go.*

When to Call Your Doctor

- If vision or motor skills become impaired with no known cause—your doctor can rule out other neurological conditions, such as a brain tumor.
- If you suffer an acute attack.
- Reminder: If you have a medical condition, talk to your doctor before taking supplements.

What it is

Multiple sclerosis (MS), a progressive and degenerative nerve disorder that strikes young adults, follows a highly variable course. In some people, damage to the optic nerve or nerves in the brain and spinal cord may lead to difficulty seeing or walking, slurred speech, loss of bowel or bladder function, clouded thinking, and paralysis. But many of those with MS experience years' long remissions and minimal disability.

What causes it

Many experts believe MS is an autoimmune disorder, in which the body's immune system attacks its own nerve tissue. What triggers this reaction is unknown. It may be a virus—perhaps even a common one, such as measles or herpes simplex—that's been dormant for years.

How supplements can help

Supplement therapy should start as soon as possible. It has several goals: to enhance antioxidant activity and protect nerve cells from the highly reactive chemicals called free radicals; to boost the production of fatty acids and other substances that build up nerves; and to decrease nerve inflammation. All the supplements can be taken together, and with conventional prescription drugs. It may take a month to notice benefits.

Vitamins C and **E** are valuable in treating MS because of their antioxidant properties. **Vitamin B complex,** plus extra **vitamin B$_{12}$** and **folic acid,** are important as well because they play a role in maintaining nerve structure and function. Some studies show MS patients have low levels of vitamin B$_{12}$ or have problems processing it well.

Flaxseeds are the source of a nutty-tasting oil that is rich in nerve-protecting essential fatty acids.

Supplement Recommendations

Vitamin C/ Vitamin E	**Dosage:** 2,000 mg of vitamin C and 400 IU of vitamin E a day. **Comments:** Vitamin C helps boost the effects of vitamin E.
Vitamin B complex	**Dosage:** 1 pill twice a day for flare-ups; then reduce to 1 pill each morning as maintenance. **Comments:** Look for a B-100 complex with 100 mcg vitamin B_{12} and biotin; 400 mcg folic acid; and 100 mg all other B vitamins.
Vitamin B_{12}/ Folic acid	**Dosage:** 1,000 mcg of vitamin B_{12} and 400 mcg folic acid a day. **Comments:** Take sublingual form for best absorption.
NAC	**Dosage:** 500 mg 3 times a day, every other day. **Comments:** Take between meals. Alternate with zinc/copper.
Zinc/Copper	**Dosage:** 30 mg zinc and 2 mg copper every other day. **Comments:** Add copper only when using zinc longer than 1 month.
Flaxseed oil	**Dosage:** 1 tbsp. (14 grams) a day. **Comments:** Can be mixed with food; take in the morning.
Evening primrose oil	**Dosage:** 1,000 mg 3 times a day. **Comments:** Can substitute 1,000 mg borage oil once a day.
Ginkgo biloba	**Dosage:** 40 mg 3 times a day. **Comments:** Standardized to have at least 24% flavone glycosides.

Note: Consider using supplements in **blue** first; those in **black** may also be beneficial. Some dosages may be supplied by supplements you are already taking—see page 39.

Another supplement that may help is the amino acid-like substance **NAC** (N-acetylcysteine), an antioxidant that may protect nerve cells; every other day, alternate NAC with a combination of **zinc** and **copper** to help reduce inflammation. It's also important to get extra essential fatty acids, such as **flaxseed oil** and **evening primrose oil;** they reduce inflammation and, over time, help build healthy nerves. Finally the herb **ginkgo biloba** may be beneficial because it acts as an antioxidant and improves blood flow to the nervous system.

What else you can do

☑ Avoid overheating. Sunbathing, heavy exertion, and very hot baths can all make symptoms worse.

☑ Ask your doctor about nutritional therapies. Some special diets have been developed that may slow the progress of MS.

☑ Exercise gently to improve muscle strength and flexibility—but not during an attack.

☑ Investigate telecommuting or part-time status if your full-time work schedule is physically difficult.

FACTS & Tips

■ Counseling may be beneficial for patients, as well as family members, who are coping with the illness. Physical and occupational therapy may also help.

LATEST FINDINGS

■ Too much stress is not good for anyone; it's especially harmful if you have MS. A study of people with MS found a connection between increased levels of stress (both simple hassles and major life events) and new nerve damage in the brain.

■ A recent study discovered a previously unknown facet of MS: It kills brain cells in a fashion similar to that seen in Alzheimer's or Parkinson's disease. Experts are looking into applying therapies that have shown promise in treating those conditions to MS patients.

■ Animal research has uncovered a potential link between high vitamin D levels and immunity to MS. This theory may partially explain why MS is so rare in the tropics (where the sun boosts vitamin D levels) and in coastal Norway (where fish rich in vitamin D are a diet staple). But don't start popping extra vitamin D: It can be toxic, and more study is needed.

Did You Know?

Some people with MS swear by bee venom and regularly arrange to be stung by bees to relieve their symptoms. This therapy should be pursued only under the care of a doctor experienced with its use—and those with a bee allergy should certainly avoid it.

muscle aches and pains

Though not serious, muscle cramps or the muscle soreness that comes from overextending yourself can be very uncomfortable. And the weekend gardener is just as likely to be affected as the world-class athlete.

SYMPTOMS

- *Sudden tightening of the muscles during physical activity.*
- *Soreness and stiffness in the muscles after activity, often not beginning until 24 to 48 hours later.*
- *Muscle spasms occurring at night, usually in the calf muscle.*
- *A muscle that feels hard to the touch, called a knot.*
- *In severe cases, visible twitching of the affected muscle.*

When to Call Your Doctor

- If tightness or cramping occurs in the chest muscle—this may be a sign of a heart attack.
- If pain causes numbness or radiates down arms or legs.
- If muscle aches and pains begin to occur frequently.
- If nighttime calf cramps are interfering with sleep.
- Reminder: If you have a medical condition, talk to your doctor before taking supplements.

What it is

There are two common types of muscle pain. The first is soreness and stiffness that develop as the result of overdoing some physical activity—whether running a marathon, digging in the yard, or simply carrying a heavy bag of groceries. This kind of pain, which doctors call delayed-onset muscle soreness (DOMS), typically begins a day or two after the activity and can last up to a week.

When a muscle suddenly contracts and can't relax, the result is the second type of muscle pain, known as a cramp. Most common in the thigh, calf, or foot, cramps can strike at any time, even during sleep.

What causes it

Even if you are in good shape, any new physical activity can cause muscle soreness. For example, if you are a runner, helping a friend move furniture will probably make your arms and shoulders ache. Most experts think the pain is a symptom of microscopic tears in the muscles, which rebuild themselves in a matter of days. Activities that require lengthening a muscle against force—such as running downhill or lowering a weight—are most likely to produce this kind of injury. Almost any kind of exercise or activity involves this type of movement.

In contrast, muscle cramps are not the result of an injury—though no one knows exactly why they occur. The cause may be an imbalance in the minerals that govern muscle contraction and relaxation—calcium, magnesium, potassium, and sodium—or a lack of fluid. Exercising too strenuously during the day may lead to calf cramps painful enough to wake you from a sound sleep, as can wearing high heels, or sleeping with your toes pointed or with bedding wrapped too tightly around your legs.

The white willow tree yields an herbal pain reliever that is helpful for muscle aches.

Supplement Recommendations

Calcium/ Magnesium	**Dosage:** 250 mg calcium and 500 mg magnesium twice a day. **Comments:** Take with food; sometimes sold in a single supplement.
Vitamin E	**Dosage:** 400 IU a day. **Comments:** Check with your doctor if taking anticoagulant drugs.
Bromelain	**Dosage:** 500 mg 3 times a day on an empty stomach. **Comments:** Should provide 6,000 GDU or 9,000 MCU daily.
White willow bark	**Dosage:** 1 or 2 pills 3 times a day as needed for pain (follow package directions). **Comments:** Standardized to contain 15% salicin.
Creatine	**Dosage:** 1 tsp. (5 grams) creatine monohydrate powder a day. **Comments:** Powdered form is common; can be mixed with juice.
Valerian	**Dosage:** 250-500 mg standardized extract at bedtime. **Comments:** Start with the lower dose and increase as needed.

Note: Consider using supplements in **blue** first; those in **black** may also be beneficial. Some dosages may be supplied by supplements you are already taking—see page 39.

How supplements can help

To balance the minerals needed for proper muscle contraction, take supplemental **calcium** and **magnesium** on a routine basis. (Most people get enough potassium and sodium from their diet.) Add **vitamin E** daily if you are prone to exercise-related cramps or nighttime calf cramps.

For soreness, consider the herbs bromelain and white willow bark, which have the same benefits as—and can be substituted for—over-the-counter (OTC) pain medications, such as aspirin or ibuprofen. In fact, they are gentler on your system and help the muscles heal themselves. **Bromelain** (an enzyme derived from pineapple) has an anti-inflammatory effect on the muscles and helps excess fluid drain from the site of a muscle injury. Often called "nature's aspirin," **white willow bark** comes from the inner bark of white willow trees and is an effective pain reliever.

Body-builders use the nutritional supplement **creatine** to improve strength, and there's good evidence that it aids in repairing microscopic tears following a strenuous workout or injury. The herb **valerian** is a natural sleep aid that can be useful if soreness interferes with sleep. Take these supplements in any combination you like until the soreness goes away. Except for willow bark, they can also be combined with OTC drugs.

What else you can do

☑ Drink a lot of fluids before, during, and after exercise.

☑ Warm up before exercise and stretch afterward to help muscles relax.

☑ Apply ice to sore muscles, if pain is severe, to reduce inflammation.

FACTS & Tips

■ An herbal oil massage can soothe muscle soreness. Blend ½ ounce of a neutral oil, such as almond oil, with a few drops of any of the following botanical oils: birch, borage, eucalyptus, evening primrose, ginger, lavender, peppermint, or wintergreen. Gently rub the oil mixture into sore muscles.

■ To ease a cramp in your calf muscle, flex your foot, grab your toes and the ball of your foot, and gently pull toward your knee as you lie down. Massage your calf at the same time to relax the muscle. People also get relief by standing up, putting their full weight on the affected leg, and bending the knee slightly.

■ Stretching exercises can reduce the risk of postexercise muscle soreness. One recommended exercise is to stand about three feet from a wall, step one foot forward, and lean against the wall with your forearms. Keeping your back heel on the ground, hold the stretch for 15 to 20 seconds to loosen the calf. Repeat with the other foot.

Did You Know?

Pregnant women should take care during exercise, because they are at higher risk of muscle cramps. The metabolic needs of the developing baby affect the normal balance of body fluids, making cramps more likely.

nail problems

Nails protect both the fingertips and toes, are extremely helpful when peeling off price tags, and are often considered a sign of beauty. They can even provide clues about your overall health and any underlying diseases. Good nutrition is the key to nail vitality.

SYMPTOMS

- *Dry, brittle nails that split and grow slowly could be caused by nutritional deficiencies.*
- *Thick, yellowed nails (often the toenails) may be harboring a fungus. Debris collecting under the nail may cause it to peel away from the nail bed below.*
- *Changes in nail color, shape, or texture may indicate an underlying illness.*

When to Call Your Doctor

- Nail irregularities may signal a more serious medical disorder. For example, white streaks running the length of the nail may indicate heart disease, a bluish tint under the nails (rather than a healthy pink) could be a sign of asthma or emphysema.
- Reminder: If you have a medical condition, talk to your doctor before taking supplements.

What it is

Composed mainly of a fibrous protein called keratin, nails are one of the body's strongest tissues. But they can grow slower than normal, become weakened, or break for a number of reasons. One of the most common problems is a fungal infection: As many as one in 25 people has this ornery, unsightly nail disorder.

What causes it

Nutrition plays a key role in nail growth and appearance. An insufficient intake of the B vitamins, for example, can produce ridges in the nail, and a lack of calcium can cause dryness and brittleness. And too little vitamin C or folic acid may be partially responsible for the development of hangnails. In addition, nails can change color when the blood doesn't get enough oxygen because of an underlying illness (such as asthma). Also, exposure to chemicals can dry them out, making them weak and brittle.

The fungus that causes athlete's foot may infect toenails as well. It thrives in sweaty shoes and socks and can enter any tiny breaks in nails caused by strenuous physical activities such as jogging.

How supplements can help

Various supplements can be used as general nail strengtheners. About eight weeks of therapy may be required to notice results. **Biotin** and other **B vitamins,** taken together with an **amino acid complex** and **vitamins C** and **E,** have a synergistic effect that helps the body build keratin and other proteins that it needs to make nails strong. A mixed amino acid complex also contains sulfur, which is necessary for nail growth.

Vitamin C, shown below in timed-release capsule form, helps build strong, healthy nails.

Supplement Recommendations

Biotin	**Dosage:** 600 mcg twice a day for 8 weeks. **Comments:** Take with meals.
Vitamin B complex	**Dosage:** 1 pill each morning with food. **Comments:** Look for a B-50 complex with 50 mcg vitamin B_{12} and biotin; 400 mcg folic acid; and 50 mg all other B vitamins.
Amino acid complex	**Dosage:** 1 pill twice a day. **Comments:** For best absorption, take on an empty stomach.
Vitamin C/ Vitamin E	**Dosage:** 1,000 mg vitamin C 3 times a day; 400 IU vitamin E daily. **Comments:** Vitamin C helps boost the effects of vitamin E.
Bone-building formula	**Dosage:** Follow package instructions. **Comments:** Supplement should supply at least 600 mg calcium, 250 mg magnesium, and 200 IU vitamin D a day.
Flaxseed oil	**Dosage:** 1 tbsp. (14 grams) a day. **Comments:** Can be mixed with food; take in the morning.
Evening primrose oil	**Dosage:** 1,000 mg 3 times a day. **Comments:** Can substitute 1,000 mg borage oil once a day.
Tea tree oil	**Dosage:** For fungal infections, rub into affected nails twice a day. **Comments:** Use pure tea tree oil. Should never be ingested.

Note: Consider using supplements in blue first; those in **black** may also be beneficial. Some dosages may be supplied by supplements you are already taking—see page 39.

Besides strengthening the skeleton, a **bone-building formula** supplies calcium and other minerals that benefit the nails. As for **flaxseed oil** and **evening primrose oil,** they are rich in two different types of essential fatty acids, both of which nourish nails and prevent them from cracking.

Nails infected with a fungus, unfortunately, are harder to treat. Oral vitamin C, taken with vitamin E, remains a good option, because it boosts immunity and may aid the body in fighting off the infection. In addition, try rubbing **tea tree oil,** garlic oil, or calendula ointment onto affected nails twice a day for several months.

What else you can do

☑ Don't trim cuticles. They protect nails from fungi and bacteria.

☑ Wear gloves if you're doing household chores or if you're using any type of chemical. Apply petroleum jelly to nails after your hands have been in water.

☑ Keep nails short. Long nails break easily. Soak nails before trimming to prevent splitting and peeling.

FACTS & Tips

■ A daily cup of tea made from oat straw, horsetail, or nettle may improve nail health. These herbs are rich in silica and other minerals necessary for nail growth.

■ Tea tree oil is much cheaper and has fewer side effects than prescription antifungal drugs— but it doesn't always work. Ask your doctor about alternatives to high-priced prescription anti-fungals: Some pharmacists will prepare inexpensive formulas that can be highly effective.

■ Despite claims to the contrary, gelatin will not strengthen nails or help them grow. The protein in gelatin does not contain the right mixture of amino acids needed for nail formation.

LATEST FINDINGS

■ In a head-to-head study, tea tree oil and a popular antifungal medication (clotrimazole) performed equally well in people with nail fungus. After six months of therapy, 60% in each treatment group experienced partial or full resolution.

■ Swiss researchers discovered that people with thin, weak, and split nails who took 2,500 mcg of biotin daily experienced a 25% increase in nail thickness.

Did You Know?

Veterinarians have long used biotin to strengthen horses' hooves, which are composed primarily of keratin. Medical researchers subsequently found that it strengthens human nails too.

nausea and vomiting

It happens to paupers and presidents and it's probably happened to you too. Nausea and vomiting are natural, possibly lifesaving, reactions to eating something dangerous or to illness. But occasionally they occur even when there's no risk to health.

SYMPTOMS

- *Sweating and chills.*
- *Excessive salivation.*
- *Dizziness.*
- *Weakness.*
- *Shortness of breath.*
- *Abdominal pain.*
- *Loss of appetite.*

When to Call Your Doctor

- If you vomit several times over a 24-hour period.
- If you vomit blood or black, grainy-looking matter.
- If you have nausea and a fever.
- If you suspect a medication is making you nauseated.
- If you become nauseated and vomit often.
- If morning sickness prevents you from eating properly.
- Reminder: If you have a medical condition, talk to your doctor before taking supplements.

What it is

Often described as "coming in waves," nausea is an overall uncomfortable, woozy feeling. It's frequently accompanied by sweating, chills, or increased saliva production. Sometimes nausea ends in what doctors refer to as emesis (most people call it "throwing up"). In this process, your stomach muscles relax, and the normal rhythmic contractions that propel food through your small intestine shift into reverse, sending the contents back into the stomach. The stomach then contracts and pushes the contents upward through the esophagus. Though unpleasant, vomiting is actually valuable because it enables the body to rid itself of toxic matter—and most people feel much better afterward.

What causes it

Spoiled food (which may contain bacteria), illnesses such as the flu, some medications (even those that are helpful in other ways, such as chemotherapy drugs used to treat cancer), and too much alcohol can induce nausea and vomiting. Additional causes include overindulging or eating rich foods, strong smells (from smoke, perfume, food odors), stress and anxiety, and motion sickness.

In other cases, the nerves in the stomach just get confused and transmit warning signals to the brain, even when no real threat to health exists. For example, the high levels of hormones released during pregnancy are beneficial, but they are also thought to be the cause of morning sickness. And elevated hormone levels may be the reason nausea is one symptom of premenstrual syndrome (PMS).

Goldenseal in either tea or tablet form can help quell nausea.

178

Supplement Recommendations	
Ginger	**Dosage:** 200 mg every 4 hours as needed.
	Comments: Standardized to contain gingerols.
Peppermint oil	**Dosage:** 1 enteric-coated capsule 3 times a day.
	Comments: Each capsule should contain 0.2 ml peppermint oil.
Goldenseal	**Dosage:** 125 mg standardized extract every 4 hours as needed.
	Comments: Don't use during pregnancy or with high blood pressure.

Note: Consider using supplements in **blue** first; those in **black** may also be beneficial. Some dosages may be supplied by supplements you are already taking—see page 39.

How supplements can help

When you are nauseated and feel the urge to vomit, there is almost nothing you can do to stop it. In fact, if you have eaten something foul, it's better not to fight this powerful reflex because the offending food needs to be purged from your system. But when nausea persists or is the result of pregnancy, motion sickness, stress, essential medications, or strong odors, natural remedies can provide welcome relief.

Your first choice should be **ginger,** in capsule form or as a tea. The herb's restorative powers originate in its volatile oils, which enhance digestion, soothe irritated membranes, and tone the muscles of the digestive tract. In addition, ginger stimulates the liver to produce bile, which helps digest fats; this action is especially useful in cases of over-eating. To combat motion sickness, take your first dose of ginger three to four hours before traveling. If you're pregnant, you can probably use ginger safely for morning sickness as long as you don't take too much; check with your doctor. If you are trying to relieve the nausea of chemotherapy, consult your doctor; avoid ginger if your blood platelet count is low—high doses may interfere with blood clotting.

Because it helps ease spasms in the digestive tract, **peppermint oil** or tea may be worthwhile for nausea accompanied by intestinal cramping. Peppermint oil is fairly powerful when taken internally, so peppermint tea is probably a better choice for any nausea associated with pregnancy. If ginger and peppermint don't work (and your nausea is not caused by pregnancy), try **goldenseal.** Taken in pill or tea form, this herb increases digestive secretions and soothes the stomach and liver.

What else you can do

☑ Lie down with a cool cloth on your forehead to relieve nausea. Focus on your breathing to prevent thinking about how you feel.

☑ Avoid exposure to strong, unpleasant odors that can trigger nausea, such as tobacco smoke, chemical preparations, cleaning supplies, or perfume.

☑ Don't eat food for two hours after vomiting, but drink as much as you can to replenish lost fluids. (Water, juice, and noncaffeinated beverages in small sips are best.) If you vomit again, suck on ice cubes.

FACTS & Tips

■ Herbal teas that calm a queasy stomach can do double duty by providing much-needed fluids after vomiting. Try a tea of ginger, goldenseal, or peppermint; drink three or four cups a day. Or steep ⅛ teaspoon nutmeg and 1 teaspoon ground cumin in very hot water for 10 minutes, strain, and drink. Sweeten with honey, if you wish.

■ Acupressure may halt nausea in its tracks. Place your right thumb on the inside of your left forearm, about two thumb-widths from the crease of your wrist. Press firmly with your thumb for about a minute, then move your thumb half a finger-width closer to the wrist crease. Apply firm pressure for about one minute more. Repeat on the right forearm.

LATEST FINDINGS

■ A review of studies assessing natural remedies for morning sickness concluded that ginger and vitamin B_6 are effective, but warned that little is known about their effect on the developing baby. In doses of 25 to 50 mg a day, vitamin B_6 is both safe and beneficial. Ginger is safe too, as long as you don't overdo it. Still, pregnant women should always check with their doctor before using supplements.

numbness and tingling

The tingling of a foot or hand that "falls asleep" comes from temporary nerve compression. But this feeling, along with pain, numbness, or weakness, can be a constant companion for people affected by disorders that damage the nerves.

SYMPTOMS

- *A feeling of numbness, tingling, pain, or weakness, usually in the feet, hands, or legs.*

When to Call Your Doctor

- Frequent or persistent bouts of numbness, tingling, or weakness in your hands or feet require a doctor's visit. They may be the first signs of a more serious underlying condition.
- Seek emergency help if numbness or tingling comes on suddenly and lasts longer than a half hour. Get help sooner if accompanied by weakness, particularly along one side of the body, which could be a sign of a stroke.
- Reminder: If you have a medical condition, talk to your doctor before taking supplements.

What it is

Much like individual wires wrapped in a single electrical cable, nerves are grouped in bundles and encased in a fatty coating called a myelin sheath. Numbness, tingling, and pain that don't go away can usually be traced to a damaged sheath, or to inflammation, compression, or an injury to the nerves themselves—particularly to the peripheral nerves, which lead from the spinal cord to the arms and legs.

What causes it

Though a variety of disorders can contribute to numbness and tingling, frequently there is no apparent cause. When a medical condition can be identified, often it is progressive nerve damage associated with poor blood sugar control called diabetic neuropathy, which primarily affects the feet. Numbness and pain in the hands may be related to carpal tunnel syndrome, which occurs when the median nerve in the wrist is inflamed or compressed. And a severe, jabbing pain on the trunk of the body along a nerve can linger for months after a bout of shingles, a viral illness that is related to herpes and chicken pox. Numbness and pain running down the thigh and leg may be caused by a herniated disk or other spinal problem in which the main nerve to the legs (the sciatic) is compressed. In multiple sclerosis, the myelin sheath is gradually destroyed, which may result in numbness and tingling. And sometimes a nutritional deficiency is responsible for this sensation.

How supplements can help

Whatever the underlying causes of numbness and tingling, the same nutrients are useful. Except for cayenne, they help heal the nerves, not simply mask the pain. Results may take three to six months.

It is safe to take all the recommended supplements together. The **vitamin B complex** promotes a healthy, functioning nervous system

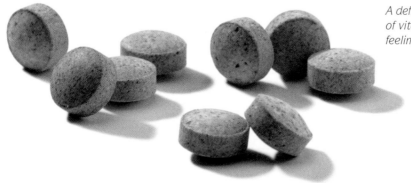

A deficiency of B vitamins, especially of vitamin B_{12}, may contribute to feelings of numbness and tingling.

Supplement Recommendations

Vitamin B complex	**Dosage:** 1 pill twice a day with food. **Comments:** Look for a B-50 complex with 50 mcg vitamin B_{12} and biotin; 400 mcg folic acid; and 50 mg all other B vitamins.
Vitamin B_{12}/ Folic acid	**Dosage:** 1,000 mcg vitamin B_{12} and 400 mcg folic acid a day. **Comments:** Sometimes sold in a single supplement. Take sublingual form for best absorption.
Thiamin	**Dosage:** 50 mg at bedtime. **Comments:** Also called vitamin B_1.
Flaxseed oil	**Dosage:** 1 tbsp. (14 grams) twice a day. **Comments:** Can be mixed with food.
Evening primrose oil	**Dosage:** 1,000 mg 3 times a day. **Comments:** Can substitute 1,000 mg borage oil once a day.
Alpha-lipoic acid	**Dosage:** 200 mg twice a day. **Comments:** May affect blood sugar levels; use with care in diabetes.
Cayenne cream	**Dosage:** Apply cream topically 3 or 4 times a day. **Comments:** Standardized to contain 0.025%-0.075% capsaicin.

Note: Consider using supplements in **blue** first; those in **black** may also be beneficial. Some dosages may be supplied by supplements you are already taking—see page 39.

see page 39.

FACTS & Tips

- Try to eat fish and nuts at least twice a week. Both foods are high in essential fatty acids and may have a healing effect on the nerves.

LATEST FINDINGS

- Alpha-lipoic acid may reverse diabetic nerve damage, according to a recent German study. Researchers gave 73 patients with damage to the nerves that control involuntary body functions (such as heartbeat) either 800 mg a day of alpha-lipoic acid or a placebo. After four months, those taking alpha-lipoic acid showed improvement in nerve function, whereas the condition in those receiving the placebo worsened. More study is needed to confirm these findings, and also to determine whether the same results can be obtained with lower doses.

(vitamin B_6 is especially important for people with diabetic neuropathy or carpal tunnel syndrome). Extra **vitamin B_{12}** and **thiamin** are needed for a variety of functions throughout the body; depletions of these vitamins are common in older people. (**Folic acid** should always be taken with high doses of vitamin B_{12}.) The different essential fatty acids in **flaxseed oil** and **evening primrose oil** foster proper communication between the brain and nerve cells and play a role in maintaining the myelin sheaths. The gamma-linolenic acid found in evening primrose oil (and borage oil) is valuable in treating diabetic neuropathy.

Because of its potent antioxidant effect, **alpha-lipoic acid** is believed to protect nerve cells from damage. Studies have shown that this vitamin-like substance is effective for diabetic neuropathy, although whether it is better than other, less expensive antioxidants, such as vitamin E, is not clear. **Cayenne cream** provides relief from any type of nerve pain. Its active ingredient, capsaicin, is thought to work by blocking substance P, a chemical messenger that transmits pain signals from the injury site to the brain.

What else you can do

- ☑ Exercise regularly to increase blood flow to the nerves and extremities.
- ☑ Don't sit still for long periods of time; inactivity makes numbness and tingling worse. Walk around and flex your fingers and ankles.

osteoporosis

Resulting in millions of bone fractures each year, osteoporosis, which is characterized by a loss of bone density, can be prevented. The earlier in life you begin to address the problem, the better your chances of avoiding broken bones and pain later on.

SYMPTOMS

- *The first sign can be dramatic: a severe backache or a fracture (often of the spine, hip, or wrist).*
- *Other classic symptoms include a gradual loss of height accompanied by the initially subtle development of a stooped posture (dowager's hump).*
- *Dental X rays may detect early osteoporosis by revealing bone loss in the jaw.*

When to Call Your Doctor

- If you suspect you've fractured a bone.
- If you have sudden, severe back pain, which may indicate a spinal compression fracture.
- If you experience any significant bone pain (in the spine, ribs, or feet) after an injury.
- If you have no symptoms but have significant risk factors—consider a painless 10-minute DEXA (dual-energy X ray absorptiometry) test that your doctor can perform to measure bone density.
- Reminder: If you have a medical condition, talk to your doctor before taking supplements.

What it is

Osteoporosis, derived from the Latin for "porous bones," is a progressive condition that diminishes the mass (mineral content) of bones and weakens their structure, making them highly susceptible to fracture. Half of postmenopausal women, and up to one in eight older men, will suffer a fracture as a result of osteoporosis. No single measure is sufficient to prevent the disorder, but a combination of supplements and lifestyle changes can be effective in limiting damage.

What causes it

The decline in estrogen after menopause is directly related to the dramatic rise of osteoporosis in older women. This hormone assists the body in absorbing calcium and keeps the bones strong. (Older men experience osteoporosis as well; but because they have denser bones, bone loss is generally less severe.) Lack of regular weight-bearing exercise is another risk factor, as is a diet low in calcium and other nutrients necessary for optimal bone production. Your risk of osteoporosis is also higher if you're small boned (white and Asian women tend to be small boned), underweight, or postmenopausal; if you have a family history of osteoporosis; or if you've taken steroids or anticonvulsants for long periods.

How supplements can help

The supplements in the chart—taken for at least six months—can help strengthen bones. They are safe to use together and with prescription osteoporosis drugs and estrogen therapy. Bone-building combination products may be a convenient and less expensive way to get many of

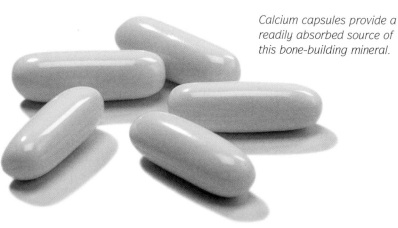

Calcium capsules provide a readily absorbed source of this bone-building mineral.

Supplement Recommendations

Calcium	**Dosage:** 600 mg twice a day. **Comments:** Take with food.
Vitamin D	**Dosage:** 200 IU twice a day. **Comments:** Crucial in the winter, when sun exposure is limited.
Magnesium	**Dosage:** 250 mg twice a day. **Comments:** Take with food.
Boron	**Dosage:** 3 mg a day. **Comments:** Reduces calcium loss; may enhance estrogen's effects.
Vitamin C	**Dosage:** 1,000 mg twice a day. **Comments:** Reduce dose if diarrhea develops.
Zinc/Copper	**Dosage:** 30 mg zinc and 2 mg copper a day. **Comments:** Add copper only when using zinc longer than 1 month.
Manganese	**Dosage:** 10 mg twice a day. **Comments:** Helps metabolize other minerals.

Some dosages may be supplied by supplements you are already taking—see page 39.

these supplements, but take care if you're on anticoagulants because many contain vitamin K, which can enhance the blood's clotting ability.

Calcium is vital for maintaining bone strength, **vitamin D** ensures that calcium is well absorbed, and the minerals **magnesium** and **boron** help convert vitamin D into a usable form. Recent research links the antioxidant **vitamin C** to greater bone mass and improved formation of collagen, a protein that strengthens the bones and connective tissue. Also important for mineral absorption and bone health are **zinc, copper,** and **manganese.** Adding other key vitamins and minerals, such as silicon, vitamin B$_6$, and folic acid provides further protection.

What else you can do

☑ Perform regular weight-bearing exercise (such as walking or lifting weights), in which the legs or other parts of the body meet resistance.

☑ Quit smoking. It not only helps the bones but general health as well

☑ Limit your alcohol intake to no more than one or two drinks a day.

☑ Consider hormone replacement therapy if you're menopausal.

☑ Eat calcium-rich foods such as low-fat dairy products, canned salmon (include the soft bones), collard greens, broccoli, and almonds.

overweight

Losing weight is hard. Fad diets promising quick success without effort don't make it any easier. Truth is, no herb, vitamin, or special food will magically melt away the pounds. But some nutritional and herbal supplements may enhance a healthy diet and exercise program.

Symptoms

- *Body weight exceeds by 20% or more the recommended ideal.*
- *Excess weight affects energy level and the ability to carry out a daily routine.*
- *Fatigue and/or shortness of breath during normal activity.*

When to Call Your Doctor

- If you gain weight suddenly.
- If weight gain is the result of taking medication.
- If you need help changing your eating or exercise habits.
- If you are unable to lose weight despite exercise and calorie reduction.
- Reminder: If you have a medical condition, talk to your doctor before taking supplements.

What it is

Being overweight becomes a medical concern when you weigh more than 20% over the ideal for your height. According to government statistics, more than a third of Americans fit into this category and are defined as obese. Though not a disease, obesity is a risk factor for serious medical conditions, including diabetes, heart disease, high blood pressure, and certain types of cancer. Excessive body weight also puts great stress on joints and so increases a person's chance of developing arthritis.

What causes it

Everyone's metabolism (the rate at which the body burns calories) is different and is influenced by many factors, including genetics. Regularly eating even a few more calories than your body needs can lead to weight gain. By consuming only 100 extra calories a day, for example, you'll gain a pound in approximately a month (a pound of body fat equals 3,500 calories). Some experts think a sedentary lifestyle influences weight gain even more than eating too many calories. Exercise burns calories and builds muscle. And the more muscle mass you have, the greater number of calories your body burns at rest.

How supplements can help

Although supplements are not "magic bullets," they may be effective in suppressing the appetite or easing weight loss. Do not exceed the dosages listed—larger amounts will not produce quicker results and instead may cause unpleasant side effects.

St. John's wort should be used along with ephedra to aid weight loss only if other measures—including diet and exercise—have not produced results.

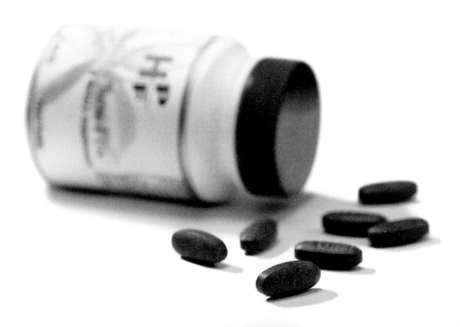

Supplement Recommendations

Chromium	**Dosage:** 200 mcg twice a day. **Comments:** Take with food or a full glass of water.
Psyllium	**Dosage:** 1-3 tbsp. powder dissolved in water or juice 3 times a day. **Comments:** Take half an hour before meals; drink plenty of water.
Garcinia cambogia	**Dosage:** 500 mg 3 times a day. **Comments:** Hydroxycitric acid, or HCA, is the active ingredient.
St. John's wort/ Ephedra	**Dosage:** 300 mg St. John's wort and 130 mg ephedra twice a day. **Comments:** Do not use if you have glaucoma, high blood pressure, heart disease, anxiety, or insomnia; or if you take prescription antidepressants or the supplement 5-HTP.
Essential fatty acids	**Dosage:** 1,000 mg evening primrose oil 3 times a day; 1,000 mg (1 capsule) flaxseed oil twice a day. **Comments:** Or use 1,000 mg borage oil once a day for primrose oil.
Chitosan	**Dosage:** 1,000 mg 3 times a day. **Comments:** Take with food; avoid if you have a shellfish allergy.
5-HTP	**Dosage:** 100 mg 3 times a day. **Comments:** Take half an hour before meals. After two weeks, increase dose to 200 mg 3 times a day.

Note: Consider using supplements in **blue** first; those in **black** may also be beneficial. Some dosages may be supplied by supplements you are already taking—see page 39.

Chromium helps the body use fat for energy and build muscle. It won't lead to dramatic weight loss, but may give you a slight edge. **Essential fatty acids** may block excessive accumulation of body fat. Use them together with **psyllium,** a type of fiber that adds "fullness," and/or **chitosan,** a substance that slows the absorption of fat in the intestine.

If you need help controlling your appetite, rotate the following supplements in month-long cycles, so your body doesn't accustom itself to any particular one. **Garcinia cambogia,** the extract of a fruit grown in India, may quell hunger pangs. Because low levels of the brain chemical serotonin may be linked to overeating, try either **St. John's wort** or **5-HTP** (5-hydroxytryptophan), a form of the amino acid tryptophan. Both boost serotonin production and also have antidepressant effects (some experts think overweight and depression may be linked). Only the seriously obese should consider using **ephedra** with St. John's wort.

What else you can do

☑ Center your diet on fruits, vegetables, whole grains, and beans.

☑ Eat slowly. When you eat too fast, your brain doesn't get the message that you're full—until you've had too much.

☑ Exercise regularly and find new ways to increase your daily activity, such as using the stairs instead of an elevator.

parkinson's disease

Although there's still no cure for this slowly progressive brain disorder, advances that can greatly improve the quality of life for those affected continue to be made. Prompt treatment may help ease tremors, stiffness, and other disabling symptoms.

SYMPTOMS

■ *Shaking or trembling limbs and rigid muscles.*

■ *Slow and shuffling walk.*

■ *Stooped posture.*

■ *Drooling, inexpressive face, and infrequent blinking.*

■ *Trouble swallowing or talking.*

■ *Incontinence and constipation.*

■ *Anxiety, depression, and in severe cases, confusion and memory loss.*

When to Call Your Doctor

■ If you have any symptoms of Parkinson's disease.

■ If you've been diagnosed with Parkinson's and note new symptoms—these may be easily remedied side effects of prescription Parkinson's drugs.

■ Reminder: If you have a medical condition, talk to your doctor before taking supplements.

What it is

Parkinson's disease, named for the English doctor who identified it nearly 200 years ago, is the most common degenerative disorder of the nervous system. It usually strikes after age 60, with more than 15% of people over age 65 showing some symptoms of the disease. It is more common in men than in women. Though they are usually very mild at first, symptoms generally worsen over time.

What causes it

In Parkinson's disease, cells in an area of the brain called the basal ganglia gradually die and no longer produce the chemical dopamine, which transmits impulses from nerve to nerve. Lack of dopamine produces the progressive stiffness, shaking, and loss of muscle coordination typical of the disorder. Though viral brain infections, antipsychotic drugs, and exposure to herbicides or toxins are responsible for a small number of cases, most of the time no underlying cause can be determined.

How supplements can help

Anyone suffering from this serious ailment should be under a doctor's care. The array of supplements here can help temper or slow the progression of symptoms, particularly if they are taken in the early years of the disease. Results may be noticed within about eight weeks, but supplements usually must be continued long term. You can try them separately or in combination, but always discuss their use with your doctor. Some, such as vitamin B_6, can interact adversely with drugs for this condition.

Most of the supplements, including **vitamin B_6,** work to increase production of the brain chemical dopamine; levels of this B vitamin are

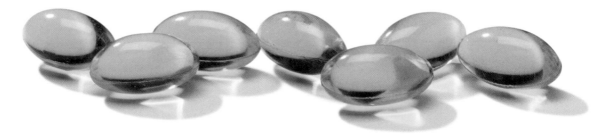

Vitamin E is one of several antioxidants that can help temper the progression of Parkinson's disease.

Supplement Recommendations

Vitamin B₆	**Dosage:** 50 mg 3 times a day.
	Comments: People taking the common prescription drug levodopa (L-dopa) without a companion drug, carbidopa, should not take B₆.
Coenzyme Q₁₀	**Dosage:** 50 mg 3 times a day.
	Comments: For best absorption, take with food.
NADH	**Dosage:** 5 mg a day.
	Comments: Best taken in the morning or between meals.
Vitamin E	**Dosage:** 400 IU a day.
	Comments: Check with your doctor if taking anticoagulant drugs.
Amino acids	**Dosage:** 1,000 mg tyrosine; 1,000 mg methionine; 500 mg acetyl-L-carnitine; 100 mg phosphatidylserine, twice a day without food.
	Comments: Discontinue after 8 weeks if you see no benefits. If you improve after 8 weeks, add a mixed amino acid complex as well.
Ginkgo biloba	**Dosage:** 80 mg 3 times a day.
	Comments: Standardized to have at least 24% flavone glycosides.
Vitamin C	**Dosage:** 1,000 mg twice a day.
	Comments: Reduce dose if diarrhea develops.
Flaxseed oil	**Dosage:** 1 tbsp. (14 grams) a day.
	Comments: Can be mixed with food; take in the morning.

Note: Consider using supplements in **blue** first; those in **black** may also be beneficial. Some dosages may be supplied by supplements you are already taking—see page 39.

often depleted in those with Parkinson's. **Coenzyme Q₁₀, NADH** (nicotinamide adenine dinucleotide, related to the B vitamin niacin), **vitamin E,** and **vitamin C** are all antioxidants that help protect cells, including the dopamine-producing ones in the brain. Vitamins C and E may be especially effective in those who have not yet started taking conventional medications for the disease. The various **amino acids** and **flaxseed oil** have nerve-nourishing effects that can boost dopamine levels; the **amino acid phosphatidylserine** may also improve mental function and combat depression. To this regimen, the herb **ginkgo biloba** can be added. It increases blood circulation in the brain, so dopamine is more likely to reach the sites that can use it.

What else you can do

☑ Walk every day and stretch to keep muscles toned and strong.

☑ Keep your mind stimulated with new interests and challenges. Recent studies suggest daily "mental exercise" may diminish symptoms.

☑ Get physical and speech therapy. Counseling may also help you manage stress. Join a local support group.

☑ Ask your doctor about new drugs or, for severe cases, surgery.

premenstrual syndrome

Many women are all too familiar with the often unpleasant symptoms of PMS. Affecting both body and emotions, this condition can be difficult to diagnose—except that it begins a week or so before menstruation and then disappears.

What it is

Before their periods, many women experience crying jags, cravings for sweets, and outbursts of anger. These, as well as some 200 other symptoms including fatigue, depression, bloating, headaches, and breast pain, characterize the condition known as premenstrual syndrome (PMS). Typically, these monthly symptoms vary in number and severity. Most women experience few of them or are mildly inconvenienced by them. However, for 5% to 10% of women, PMS can be so severe that it interferes with their ability to live a full and rich life.

What causes it

Just why some women suffer from PMS and others don't is not known. Some experts believe PMS may stem from an imbalance of the female hormones estrogen and progesterone during the second half of the menstrual cycle, after ovulation. Too much estrogen, along with too little progesterone, limits the production of the brain chemicals that control mood and pain; this hormonal abnormality can lead to mood changes and carbohydrate cravings. The imbalance also triggers increased levels of the hormone prolactin, which results in breast tenderness and prevents the liver from working as well as it should in clearing excess estrogen from the body.

Another theory is that PMS symptoms are caused by low levels of serotonin, a brain chemical (neurotransmitter) that sends signals from nerve cell to nerve cell. Although the results of studies examining the connection between serotonin and PMS are inconsistent, many women report that their PMS symptoms improve when they undergo treatment designed to return serotonin levels to normal. Improving the body's production and use of serotonin is particularly helpful in lifting depression.

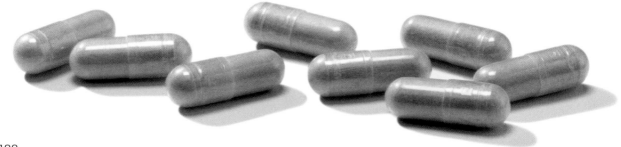

Chasteberry may help correct the hormonal imbalances that are thought to contribute to PMS.

Supplement Recommendations

Chasteberry	**Dosage:** 225 mg a day. **Comments:** Also called vitex. Choose a product standardized to contain 0.5% agnuside. Take when not menstruating.
Vitamin B$_6$	**Dosage:** 50 mg twice a day. **Comments:** 200 mg daily over long term can cause nerve damage.
Evening primrose oil	**Dosage:** 1,000 mg 3 times a day. **Comments:** Can substitute 1,000 mg borage oil once a day.
Magnesium	**Dosage:** 250 mg twice a day. **Comments:** Take with food.
St. John's wort	**Dosage:** 300 mg 3 times a day. **Comments:** Standardized to contain 0.3% hypericin.

Some dosages may be supplied by supplements you are already taking—see page 39.

How supplements can help

A combination of nutrients, taken for part or all of the menstrual cycle, can relieve PMS symptoms. If you use conventional medications for this problem, check with your doctor before adding these supplements.

Chasteberry is a leading PMS remedy in Europe. It acts on the pituitary gland in the brain (which controls the production of estrogen and progesterone in the body) and may be useful in correcting hormonal imbalances. The herb dong quai (200 mg three times a day) may enhance chasteberry's effectiveness; combination products with additional herbs such as black cohosh are often available.

In place of chasteberry, try **vitamin B$_6$.** It assists the liver in processing estrogen, increases progesterone levels, and enables the brain to make serotonin. (Some practitioners recommend combining chasteberry and vitamin B$_6$.) **Evening primrose oil,** with its essential fatty acids, may help ease breast tenderness and control carbohydrate cravings. Many women with PMS have been found to be deficient in **magnesium** and may benefit from supplements of it.

Begin taking chasteberry and/or vitamin B$_6$ in combination with evening primrose oil at ovulation and continue until your period begins; have magnesium every day. If your primary PMS symptom is depression, or if the other supplements are not effective, add **St. John's wort** to your program.

What else you can do

☑ Exercise several times a week to lift your spirits and help your body release fluids that cause bloating and breast tenderness.

☑ Cut back on caffeine, alcohol, and salt, which can contribute to PMS.

☑ Keep a symptom diary; it can give you a sense of control and a better understanding of your physical and emotional feelings, aid in proper diagnosis, and help determine which treatment works for you.

FACTS & Tips

■ PMS may have certain positive effects. Some researchers say that women who have PMS are very attuned to their surroundings and have a sharp memory, not just in the days or weeks immediately before their period but all month long.

LATEST FINDINGS

■ Chasteberry may be a more effective treatment for PMS than vitamin B$_6$, according to a recent German study. Women who took chasteberry had a greater reduction in typical PMS symptoms—breast tenderness, swelling, tension, headache, and depression—than those consuming B$_6$. Overall, 36% of those in the chasteberry group were free of symptoms compared with 21% of participants in the vitamin B$_6$ group.

■ In a Columbia University study of 500 women, researchers found that taking 1,200 mg of calcium a day reduced PMS symptoms by more than 50%. Compared with women given a placebo, those using calcium showed improvement in mood swings, food cravings, bloating, and menstrual pain. The researchers now believe that low calcium levels may contribute to the hormonal imbalance thought to be a factor in PMS.

Did You Know?

Americans have been slow to try herbal cures for PMS. Evening primrose oil, chasteberry, and St. John's wort are widely used in Europe and have withstood the test of time.

prostate problems

If you're a man over age 50, you probably have a prostate problem—usually a benign enlargement of the gland. Herbal and nutritional therapies can help ease discomfort and even preclude or delay the need for conventional drugs or surgery.

SYMPTOMS

- *Frequent, urgent need to urinate, particularly at night.*
- *Difficulty or hesitancy in urinating; inability to empty the bladder.*
- *A weak urine stream or dribbling.*
- *Burning during urination, fever, chills, pain behind the scrotum, or painful ejaculation.*

When to Call Your Doctor

- If you have any symptoms of a prostate condition—a simple PSA blood test can help distinguish a benign prostate disorder from cancer.
- If you have blood in the urine or semen.
- Reminder: If you have a medical condition, talk to your doctor before taking supplements.

What it is

These disorders typically cause urinary complaints because they affect the prostate, the walnut-size gland that is located below the bladder and surrounds the urethra (the tube that transports urine out of the bladder). By far, the most common problem is BPH (benign prostatic hyperplasia, or hypertrophy), a noncancerous enlargement of the prostate that occurs in more than half of men over age 50. The condition can progress for many years, with few or no symptoms at first; it is not a risk factor for developing prostate cancer. But a doctor should evaluate your condition to rule out cancer and prostate inflammation (prostatitis), which are more serious.

What causes it

As men age, the prostate typically enlarges. No one is sure why this happens, though male sex hormones may play a role. Depending on the degree of enlargement, the prostate can press against the urethra and impede the flow of urine, causing the symptoms of BPH. Less often, men develop prostatitis, which is usually caused by a bacterial infection that begins elsewhere in the urinary tract, or cancer. In these conditions, swelling of the prostate or growth of a tumor can disrupt urine flow.

How supplements can help

The supplements recommended here are best for mild to moderate BPH and may take a month or longer to produce results. They can be safely used long term, along with any conventional drugs your doctor has prescribed. See your doctor every six months to check whether they are working. Supplements may also help some cases of mild prostatitis, but prostate infections and cancer require prompt medical intervention.

Saw palmetto, derived from a dwarf palm tree, is among the most widely used herbs for prostate complaints.

Supplement Recommendations

Zinc/Copper	**Dosage:** 30 mg zinc and 2 mg copper a day. **Comments:** Add copper only when using zinc longer than 1 month.
Vitamin E	**Dosage:** 400 IU a day. **Comments:** Check with your doctor if taking anticoagulant drugs.
Saw palmetto	**Dosage:** 160 mg twice a day between meals. **Comments:** Standardized for 85%-95% fatty acids and sterols.
Pygeum africanum	**Dosage:** 100 mg twice a day between meals. **Comments:** Standardized to contain 13% sterols.
Flaxseed oil	**Dosage:** 1 tbsp. (14 grams) a day. **Comments:** Can be mixed with food; take in the morning.
Nettle	**Dosage:** 250 mg twice a day. **Comments:** Standardized to contain at least 1% plant silica.
Amino acids	**Dosage:** 500 mg each of glycine, glutamine, and alanine daily. **Comments:** After 1 month, add a mixed amino acid complex.

Note: Consider using supplements in **blue** first; those in **black** may also be beneficial. Some dosages may be supplied by supplements you are already taking—see page 39.

One of the key nutrients for prostate health, **zinc** has been shown to reduce the size of the gland and relieve BPH symptoms. Because zinc interferes with copper absorption, it is important to take **copper** too. Extra **vitamin E** can aid in preserving prostate health: As an antioxidant, it scavenges free radicals that can damage DNA and lead to cancer.

Herbs may also help relieve symptoms of BPH and slow prostate growth. **Saw palmetto,** the best researched and most popular of these, can be very effective, partly by altering hormone levels; it may be useful as well in curbing inflammation and swelling in chronic cases of prostatitis. If saw palmetto alone is not sufficient, try adding the herb **pygeum africanum,** which may be beneficial for BPH or prostatitis because of its anti-inflammatory properties. Either can be combined with **nettle,** which may boost their ability to ease symptoms and slow BPH progression.

Additional nutrients are recommended. The essential fatty acids in **flaxseed oil** help prevent the swelling and inflammation of the prostate in BPH and prostatitis. In addition, the **amino acids** glycine, alanine, and glutamine, taken together each morning on an empty stomach, may aid in relieving symptoms, though they do not slow prostate growth.

What else you can do

☑ Don't take decongestants or other over-the-counter cold remedies; they can make symptoms worse.

☑ To help reduce urinary complaints, avoid caffeinated and alcoholic beverages, especially beer. Reduce consumption of liquids in the evening.

FACTS & Tips

- Check the label carefully when buying so-called "Prostate Formulas" and other commercial supplement mixtures. Many contain only insignificant amounts of specific prostate-healthy vitamins, minerals, herbs, and other nutritional supplements.
- Foods rich in soy may benefit men with prostate problems. Tofu, miso, and other soy products contain healing substances called isoflavones that may help protect against prostate enlargement and prostate cancer.
- When taken with saw palmetto, pumpkin seeds (high in zinc and amino acids) have aided in the treatment of BPH.

LATEST FINDINGS

- A report in the medical journal *Urology* concluded that saw palmetto can significantly ease symptoms of BPH. Symptoms improved dramatically in 21% of men after two months, in 30% after four months, and in 46% after six months.
- Several recent reports show that supplements may help prevent prostate cancer. A study of 30,000 male Finnish smokers discovered that those who took vitamin E daily were almost a third less likely to develop prostate cancer. Another study confirmed earlier reports that high selenium intakes may reduce prostate cancer risk.

Did You Know?

A recent survey found a third of those with serious prostate disease spent at least $25 a month on alternative therapies—though most failed to mention it to their urologist. It's essential to discuss supplement use with your doctor.

psoriasis

Although not life-threatening, psoriasis can be very painful. This persistent skin condition affects about 6 million people in the United States, flaring up and retreating in cycles. Though it can't be prevented and there's no cure, nutritional and herbal supplements may help control it.

SYMPTOMS

- *Patches of raised, inflamed red skin with white flaking scales.*
- *Itching.*
- *Loosened, pitted, discolored fingernails or toenails.*
- *Cracked or blistered skin, with pain in severe cases.*
- *Joint pain and stiffness.*

When to Call Your Doctor

- If home treatments don't control the rash.
- If the rash spreads or emerges in new areas.
- If a widespread rash develops, with or without fatigue, fever, or joint pain—call a doctor immediately.
- Reminder: If you have a medical condition, talk to your doctor before taking supplements.

What it is

Characterized by raised, inflamed red patches that are usually covered with whitish or silvery scales, psoriasis is a noncontagious chronic skin condition. It typically emerges between ages 10 and 30, although it can occur at any time. In most people, the rash is confined to the scalp, elbows, knees, lower back, or buttocks. Fingernails and toenails can become yellow or pitted. Though flare-ups are unsightly, most cases are not itchy or particularly painful. However, about 15% of people with psoriasis have such a severe, widespread rash that they suffer great discomfort and may be unable to perform daily activities. In about 5% of cases, joint pain and swelling similar to symptoms of rheumatoid arthritis develop.

What causes it

The rash itself occurs because skin cells replicate much faster than normal. Skin cells originate in the deep layers of the skin and usually take about 28 days to come to the surface, where they are sloughed off. However, in areas affected by psoriasis, this process takes only eight days. Because these new cells accumulate so quickly, they never have a chance to mature and cannot be shed. As a result, the skin becomes red and inflamed and develops overlapping white scaly patches.

No one knows why skin growth is accelerated in areas where psoriasis lesions form. Because one in three psoriasis sufferers has a family history of the disorder, some experts think there is a genetic link. Certain stimuli—alcohol, stress, sunburn, cold temperatures, dry air, skin injury, throat infection, and some medications—may also trigger the onset of psoriasis or worsen existing lesions.

How supplements can help

All the supplements in the chart may help control flare-ups of psoriasis, and can be taken in combination. Most people experience improvement in about a month. Found in fish oils and flaxseed oil, the omega-3

Studies show the essential fatty acids in fish oils, available in softgel form, can help control outbreaks of psoriasis.

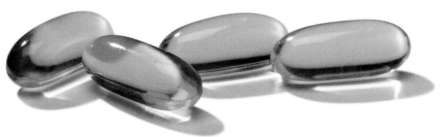

Supplement Recommendations

Essential fatty acids	**Dosage:** 1,000 mg fish oils 3 times a day; 1 tbsp. (14 grams) flaxseed oil each morning. **Comments:** People with diabetes should take less than 2,000 mg of fish oils a day; higher doses can worsen blood sugar control.
Grape seed extract	**Dosage:** 100 mg twice a day. **Comments:** Standardized to contain 92%-95% proanthocyanidins.
Alpha-lipoic acid	**Dosage:** 150 mg each morning. **Comments:** Can be taken with or without food.
Vitamin A	**Dosage:** 25,000 IU a day for 1 month, then 10,000 IU daily. **Comments:** Women who are pregnant or considering pregnancy should not exceed 5,000 IU a day.
Zinc/Copper	**Dosage:** 30 mg zinc and 2 mg copper a day. **Comments:** Add copper only when using zinc longer than 1 month.
Milk thistle	**Dosage:** 150 mg twice a day. **Comments:** Standardized to contain at least 70% silymarin.

Some dosages may be supplied by supplements you are already taking—see page 39.

Some dosages may be supplied by supplements you are already taking—see page 39.

LATEST FINDINGS

■ Difficulty expressing anger may trigger the onset of psoriasis, according to a recent study at the University of Michigan. Researchers took psychological profiles of 137 individuals and found that those who buried their anger were more likely to develop psoriasis before age 40. Anger and stress may also be linked to flare-ups in people who already have the disease.

■ Antioxidants might be valuable in preventing psoriasis. In an Italian study of about 600 people (half with psoriasis and half with other skin problems), researchers discovered a link between a high intake of carrots, tomatoes, and fresh fruit—all excellent sources of antioxidants—and a reduced chance of developing psoriasis.

essential fatty acids block the action of arachidonic acid, a substance made by the body that causes inflammation. (Indeed, low levels of omega-3s are common in those with psoriasis.) The nutritional supplements **grape seed extract** and **alpha-lipoic acid** are powerful antioxidants that may prevent damage to skin cells. Both contain flavonoids, which reduce inflammation.

Vitamin A is necessary for maintaining healthy skin and nails and **zinc** promotes healing. (The extra **copper** is important because long-term zinc use interferes with copper absorption.) **Milk thistle,** an herb with anti-inflammatory properties, may control the rash and slow the abnormal skin cell proliferation. For outbreaks, apply a fumaric acid cream (available in health-food stores) to skin lesions three times a day to reduce their size and provide relief from pain and itching.

What else you can do

☑ Get some sun. Just 15 to 30 minutes of sunlight a day may improve psoriasis lesions in three to six weeks. Apply a sunscreen with an SPF of 15 or greater to nonaffected areas to guard against sunburn.

☑ Use a humidifier in the winter. Dry indoor air may cause lesions.

☑ Apply moisturizer all over your body—and especially on lesions—to prevent dry skin and reduce itching. Aloe vera gel is a good choice.

☑ Eat fatty fish often. (Good choices include mackerel, sardines, tuna, salmon, and herring.) Or get your fish oil in capsule form.

Did You Know?

People who smoke 20 cigarettes or more a day (especially women) are twice as likely to develop psoriasis as nonsmokers. A quarter of all psoriasis cases may be related to smoking.

raynaud's disease

Imagine that your fingers quickly go numb when you step outside on a winter day, or even when you accept a cold drink at a summer picnic. This often happens to people who have Raynaud's disease, a little-understood circulatory disorder.

What it is

First identified in 1862 by Maurice Raynaud, a French physician, Raynaud's disease affects the tiny arteries (arterioles) that deliver blood to the skin of the fingers, toes, nose, and ears. In some people, cool temperatures prompt spasms in these blood vessels, reducing blood flow and depriving the area of oxygen. As a result, the skin changes color and may tingle or go numb. Although it can be annoying and uncomfortable, in most cases Raynaud's disease is not associated with more serious circulation problems.

What causes it

The cause of Raynaud's is not known. However, some experts believe that the blood vessels of people with Raynaud's overreact to the cold, possibly from an instability in the nerves of the affected areas. More women than men are affected by the disorder. Raynaud's can occur by itself or accompany other medical conditions, such as migraine headaches, rheumatoid arthritis, lupus, atherosclerosis, or an underactive thyroid. (When an underlying cause can be found, the disorder is called Raynaud's phenomenon.) Going outside in winter, reaching into a refrigerator, or even entering an air-conditioned room often produces symptoms that can last from minutes to hours. Stress is also a trigger. Raynaud's symptoms may be a side effect of decongestants and some heart or migraine medications.

How supplements can help

Because Raynaud's is often chronic, these supplements may be most helpful when used over the long term. **Vitamin E** improves blood flow through the arteries. The mineral **magnesium** has many beneficial effects on the cardiovascular system. One of these—its ability to relax constricted blood

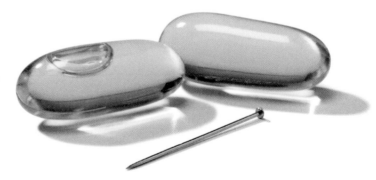

Use a pin to prick open an evening primrose capsule. Then massage the oil into your fingers or toes to relieve the symptoms of Raynaud's.
.

Supplement Recommendations

Vitamin E	**Dosage:** 400 IU a day. **Comments:** Check with your doctor if taking anticoagulant drugs.
Magnesium	**Dosage:** 400 mg twice a day. **Comments:** Take with food; reduce dose if diarrhea develops.
Inositol hexaniacinate	**Dosage:** 500 mg 3 times a day. **Comments:** This form of niacin does not cause flushing.
Ginkgo biloba	**Dosage:** 40 mg 3 times a day. **Comments:** Standardized to have at least 24% flavone glycosides.
Evening primrose oil	**Dosage:** 1 or 2 capsules, applied topically, each day. **Comments:** Can substitute capsules of borage oil.
Fish oils	**Dosage:** 1,000 mg 3 times a day. **Comments:** People with diabetes should take less than 2,000 mg of fish oils a day; higher doses can worsen blood sugar control.

Note: Consider using supplements in blue first; those in black may also be beneficial. Some dosages may be supplied by supplements you are already taking—see page 39.

LATEST FINDINGS

■ Women with Raynaud's were found to have low levels of vitamin C and selenium in their bloodstream, according to a recent study. In addition, vitamin C levels were especially low in smokers. More research is needed, though, before these nutrients can be recommended as a treatment for this condition.

C·a·s·e H·i·s·t·o·r·y

REMEDY FOR RAYNAUD'S

Until a magazine article alerted her to ginkgo biloba, winter was Ann D.'s least favorite season. Even though she wore heavy gloves to combat the cold, her fingers still changed color— going from healthy pink to dead white. Her doctor determined that it was Raynaud's disease, but he wasn't optimistic about treating it. "I could tell that he gave me a prescription just to give me something," Ann recalls.

"But then I tried ginkgo!" she says. "What a finger saver, especially when I added a little vitamin E every day." Though she had to wait a month for results, her patience paid off. Today, while remaining wary of excessive cold, she's a champion of supplements, and enjoys sharing her success with others.

"Raynaud's is pretty common," Ann notes, "but not too many people who have it realize what it is. Those who do, often just suffer. I can honestly recommend ginkgo for safe, natural— and very effective—relief."

vessels—makes it useful for Raynaud's. In addition to these nutrients, you might consider **inositol hexaniacinate,** a form of the B vitamin niacin that enhances blood flow in the extremities. Or take **ginkgo biloba,** an herb that's especially effective in widening small blood vessels. When massaged into the fingertips, the gamma-linolenic acid (GLA) in **evening primrose oil** was shown to improve Raynaud's symptoms in one study. The oil can be used alone or with the other supplements. (Borage oil is a good substitute; it also contains GLA and is generally less expensive.)

If these treatments don't help, try **fish oil** supplements. In a double-blind, placebo-controlled study of 32 patients with Raynaud's, fish oil supplementation delayed the onset of symptoms by an average of 15 minutes.

What else you can do

☑ Avoid nicotine and caffeine, which cause blood vessels to contract.

☑ Practice biofeedback and relaxation techniques.

☑ Take precautions to prevent injuring affected areas.

☑ Protect yourself from the cold by wearing mittens—which keep fingers warmer than gloves—and heavy socks in winter. Use gloves when reaching even briefly into the freezer or supermarket frozen food case.

☑ Don't take decongestants and ask your doctor if any other medications you're taking can trigger your symptoms.

rheumatoid arthritis

The inflamed joints of rheumatoid arthritis can cause even the simplest movements to be difficult and painful. A number of natural remedies, combined with conventional medications as needed, may make many regular activities easier.

SYMPTOMS

Early signs

- *Fatigue; weakness; weight loss; low-grade fever; and joint stiffness (often in the morning), followed several weeks later by joint pain and inflammation.*
- *Red, painful, swollen joints that may be warm to the touch. Typically affects the wrists, fingers, knees, ankles, and feet, on both sides of the body.*
- *Painless red lumps (nodules) on the elbows, ears, nose, knees, toes, or scalp.*

Long-term effects

- *Chest pain, breathing difficulties.*
- *Joints that become shapeless, bent, or gnarled.*

When to Call Your Doctor

- If you have the early symptoms of the disease.
- If new symptoms appear.
- Reminder: If you have a medical condition, talk to your doctor before taking supplements.

What it is

Rheumatoid arthritis is a chronic disorder in which the cartilage and tissues in and around the joints become inflamed and damaged. Scar tissue replaces the damaged tissue, narrowing the spaces in the joints and limiting movement. Some people experience only mild joint stiffness, punctuated by periodic inflammatory flare-ups. In others, however, symptoms are persistent and worsen over time, causing deformities of the hands and feet. In very severe cases, rheumatoid arthritis can also affect the heart, lungs, muscles, and skin.

What causes it

In rheumatoid arthritis, the immune system, for unknown reasons, attacks its own joints and surrounding tissues. Experts don't completely understand why this so-called autoimmune reaction occurs, but they think that some people have a genetic predisposition to rheumatoid arthritis and that its onset can be triggered by an infection, an inadequate diet, or emotional stress. This chronic inflammatory condition can begin at any age but most often appears between the ages of 20 and 40.

How supplements can help

There's no cure for rheumatoid arthritis, but any of the remedies listed in the chart may alleviate chronic pain, reduce inflammation, or help slow joint damage. They can be used alone or together, as well as with conventional drugs. Effects may take several weeks to be felt.

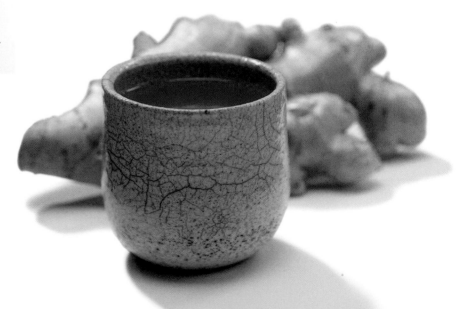

Many arthritis sufferers find ginger tea a refreshing way to reduce joint inflammation.

Supplement Recommendations

Vitamin C	**Dosage:** 1,000 mg 3 times a day. **Comments:** Reduce dose if diarrhea develops.
Vitamin E	**Dosage:** 400 IU twice a day. **Comments:** Check with your doctor if taking anticoagulant drugs.
Zinc/Copper	**Dosage:** 30 mg zinc and 2 mg copper twice a day. **Comments:** Add copper only when using zinc longer than 1 month.
Fish oils	**Dosage:** 2,000 mg 3 times a day. **Comments:** Check with your doctor if taking anticoagulant drugs.
Evening primrose oil	**Dosage:** 1,000 mg 3 times a day. **Comments:** Can substitute 1,000 mg borage oil once a day.
Glucosamine	**Dosage:** 500 mg glucosamine sulfate 3 times a day. **Comments:** Take with food to minimize stomach upset.
Ginger	**Dosage:** 100 mg 3 times a day. **Comments:** Standardized to contain gingerols. Can also drink up to 4 cups a day of ginger tea.
Cat's claw	**Dosage:** 250 mg standardized extract twice a day. **Comments:** Take between meals. Don't use if pregnant.
Cayenne cream	**Dosage:** Apply topically to affected joints 3 or 4 times a day. **Comments:** Standardized to contain 0.025%-0.075% capsaicin.

Some dosages may be supplied by supplements you are already taking—see page 39.

Because they're powerful antioxidants, **vitamins C** and **E** work to protect cells, including those in the joints, from damage. Also acting as an antioxidant, **zinc** is important because those who are afflicted with rheumatoid arthritis are often deficient in it. Taking zinc with **copper** helps maintain a proper balance of these minerals; and, as an added benefit, copper also has an anti-inflammatory effect. **Fish oils** combat stiffness, **evening primrose oil** helps control inflammation, and the nutritional supplement **glucosamine** aids in building healthy cartilage. The herbs **ginger** and **cat's claw** may relieve inflammation; topical **cayenne cream** can dramatically reduce arthritic pain.

Other good inflammation reducers include the Indian herb boswellia (take 150 mg boswellic acid three times a day) and the pineapple-based enzyme bromelain (take 500 mg three times a day between meals). Even homemade, cartilage-rich chicken soup may be beneficial.

What else you can do

☑ Perform gentle non-weight-bearing exercises, such as swimming.

☑ Try physical therapy; massage, heat, or cold packs may help too.

☑ Get plenty of rest—10 to 12 hours or more a night if needed.

FACTS & Tips

■ Many patients who take supplements are able to reduce or even eliminate the need for arthritis medications. Although they are often essential in the management of rheumatoid arthritis, aspirin, ibuprofen, and other pain relievers can cause stomach bleeding and other serious side effects. It's always a good idea to minimize their use.

LATEST FINDINGS

■ Several recent studies confirm that people with rheumatoid arthritis who take daily fish oil supplements have fewer tender joints and less morning stiffness. Most participants took fish oil for at least 12 weeks before noticing an improvement, and benefits increased after 18 to 24 weeks of treatment. In addition, their symptoms were relieved for up to eight weeks after stopping the supplement.

■ Rheumatoid arthritis sufferers who took capsules containing gamma-linolenic acid (GLA), the active ingredient in evening primrose and borage oils, for six months had less pain and fewer signs of inflammation than those who received a placebo, according to a University of Pennsylvania study.

Did You Know?

Many people with arthritis wear copper bracelets, an old folk remedy. Though some copper in the bracelets is absorbed through the skin, taking copper supplements (along with zinc) assures a steadier supply of this anti-inflammatory mineral.

rosacea

The ruddy complexion of many fair-skinned people may not always be a healthy glow, but a sign of rosacea, a common skin problem. Even though there is no cure, symptoms of this chronic condition can often be controlled and skin damage prevented.

SYMPTOMS

- *Frequent, prolonged redness and flushing of the cheeks, nose, forehead, and chin.*
- *Feeling that skin is being pulled tightly across the face.*
- *The appearance of tiny red spots and bumps in the affected area.*
- *Bumpiness, redness, and swelling on the nose.*
- *Bloodshot, burning, or itchy eyes.*

When to Call Your Doctor

- If you develop any of the symptoms listed above.
- If your skin does not promptly return to its normal complexion color after blushing.
- Reminder: If you have a medical condition, talk to your doctor before taking supplements.

What it is

The first signs of rosacea (rose-AY-shah) are recurrent patches of redness on the cheeks, nose, forehead, and chin, and the appearance of tiny blood vessels just under the skin. As the disorder progresses, the skin on the face becomes ruddier and then permanently inflamed; bumps may also form. The eyes may be affected too, resulting in burning or itching. In severe rosacea, the nose may develop excess tissue.

About one in 20 adults has rosacea, with fair-skinned people at the highest risk. Although women develop the condition three times more often than men, the latter have more severe symptoms. Smokers are vulnerable because nicotine impairs circulation. Without treatment, rosacea may worsen; conventional therapy often includes long-term use of antibiotics.

What causes it

Rosacea occurs when unknown genetic and/or environmental factors cause blood vessels in the skin to lose elasticity and dilate easily, sometimes permanently. Blood vessel abnormalities are one possible cause. Episodes can be triggered by any stimulus that leads to flushing, including hot or spicy foods or beverages; alcohol or caffeine; stress; weather; vigorous exercise; hormonal changes (especially at menopause); and certain medications (especially niacin and some blood pressure drugs).

How supplements can help

Because rosacea is a chronic condition, supplements should be continued indefinitely; it may take about a month before initial improvements are obvious. Begin with vitamin A and the B vitamins. Then add vitamin C, the minerals, and the essential fatty acids, if necessary. All can be used with the conventional antibiotics that are often prescribed for rosacea.

Vitamin A is important for healthy skin and may help minimize rosacea flare-ups.

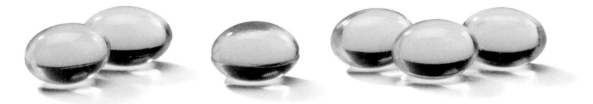

Supplement Recommendations

Vitamin A	**Dosage:** 25,000 IU a day for 2 months, then 15,000 IU a day. **Comments:** Women who are pregnant or considering pregnancy should not exceed 5,000 IU a day.
Vitamin B complex	**Dosage:** 1 pill each morning with food. **Comments:** Look for a B-50 complex with 50 mcg vitamin B_{12} and biotin; 400 mcg folic acid; and 50 mg all other B vitamins.
Riboflavin	**Dosage:** 50 mg a day in addition to that in B complex (above). **Comments:** Also called vitamin B_2. May darken the urine.
Vitamin B_{12}	**Dosage:** 1,000 mcg a day in addition to that in B complex (above). **Comments:** Sublingual form best for absorption. Always take with 400 mcg folic acid, such as in vitamin B complex.
Vitamin C	**Dosage:** 1,000 mg 3 times a day. **Comments:** Reduce dose if diarrhea develops.
Zinc/Copper	**Dosage:** 30 mg zinc and 2 mg copper a day. **Comments:** Add copper only when using zinc longer than 1 month.
Essential fatty acids	**Dosage:** 1,000 mg evening primrose oil 3 times a day; 1 tbsp. (14 grams) flaxseed oil a day. **Comments:** Or use 1,000 mg borage oil once a day for primrose oil.

Some dosages may be supplied by supplements you are already taking—see page 39.

Some dosages may be supplied by supplements you are already taking—see page 39.

FACTS & Tips

■ To soothe inflamed skin, splash your face with a strong chamomile and calendula tea. To prepare it, pour 2 cups of very hot water over 1 tablespoon of each herb. Let sit, covered, for 20 minutes, then strain, cool, and use it to wash your face.

■ Women who wear makeup may be able to hide persistent redness with a sheer green base applied under a foundation that matches their normal skin tone.

■ Men with rosacea may minimize flare-ups by using an electric razor instead of a blade.

Did You Know?

Everyone has tiny skin mites living in their hair follicles, but some rosacea sufferers have exceptionally high numbers of them. A breakdown of the immune system is the probable cause. The B vitamins, especially riboflavin, may help control mite growth.

Without enough **vitamin A,** skin cells can harden, and the protective effect of mucus (which some skin cells produce) declines. A deficiency of B vitamins is common in people with rosacea, so **vitamin B complex** is beneficial. It's important to take extra **riboflavin** and **vitamin B_{12}** in addition to the amounts found in a B-complex supplement. Riboflavin improves mucus secretion and promotes elimination of cellular waste; vitamin B_{12} plays a central role in cell growth, reproduction, and repair.

As for **vitamin C,** it strengthens the membranes that line the blood vessels and the connective tissue between skin cells. It also minimizes the release of histamine, a chemical that widens blood vessels in response to an allergic substance. **Zinc** helps heal the top layer of the skin (epidermis) and regulates blood levels of vitamin A. (Add **copper** for long-term use.) And the **essential fatty acids** in flaxseed oil and evening primrose oil reduce inflammation, control the cell's use of nutrients, and produce hormonelike substances called prostaglandins, which stimulate contraction of blood vessels.

What else you can do

☑ Use fragrance-free, greaseless makeup and facial cleansers. Never use astringents on your skin.

☑ Gently blot—never rub—your face dry after washing.

☑ Wear a sunscreen with an SPF of at least 15 when you are outdoors.

shingles

Remember chicken pox? Its virus is still lurking in your nerve cells and can flare up at any time during your adult years, causing the intensely painful blisters known as shingles. The good news is that natural remedies can often help ease this sometimes lingering condition.

SYMPTOMS

- *Intense burning and tingling in an isolated area of the body one to three days prior to reddening of the skin. May be accompanied by fever and headache.*
- *Clusters of fluid-filled, bubblelike blisters that form on an inflamed band of skin, usually on the torso or buttocks, but sometimes on the face or arms. Blisters cause intense pain and itching and form scabs after 10 days.*
- *Pain typically subsides after two or three weeks but sometimes persists for months or years (postherpetic neuralgia).*

When to Call Your Doctor

- If you develop shingles symptoms. To be effective, antiviral drugs must be taken early on.
- If you have a bruised sensation on one side of the face or body.
- If facial skin lesions spread close to your eyes.
- If an inflamed area is infected or lasts more than 10 days without real improvement.
- If you are unable to endure the pain.
- Reminder: If you have a medical condition, talk to your doctor before taking supplements.

What it is

Shingles, known medically as herpes zoster, is a form of the same herpes virus infection that causes chicken pox. After a childhood attack of chicken pox, the virus doesn't die but lies dormant in nerve cells. Later, it can be reactivated, producing intensely painful clumps of skin blisters. Shingles itself is not contagious, though open sores can transmit the chicken pox virus to young children or others who've never been infected.

What causes it

The virus responsible for shingles is thought to become revitalized when the immune system is weakened by age, stress, the flu, or certain immune-impairing drugs or illnesses. But no one knows for sure what causes the virus to resurface and produce symptoms.

How supplements can help

Therapies for shingles are designed for acute flare-ups (and are taken until lesions heal) and for post-shingles pain, which can persist for months or even years. The supplements for an acute shingles attack—which should be taken together—can be further divided into two main groups: topical therapies applied directly to skin lesions and supplements ingested to boost the immune system and help heal inflamed skin and nerves.

Topical treatments, such as **aloe vera gel** combined with **vitamin E** oil, may provide immediate relief. They act as soothing emollients,

Applied gently to the skin, liquid vitamin E helps heal painful outbreaks of shingles.

Supplement Recommendations

Aloe vera gel	**Dosage:** Apply gel liberally to the skin as needed.
	Comments: Use fresh aloe leaf or store-bought gel.
Vitamin E	**Dosage:** Apply topical oil for acute attacks.
	Comments: For post-shingles pain, take 400 IU orally twice a day.
Vitamin C/ Flavonoids	**Dosage:** 1,000 mg vitamin C and 500 mg flavonoids 3 times a day.
	Comments: Reduce vitamin C dose if diarrhea develops.
Vitamin A	**Dosage:** 25,000 IU twice a day for acute attacks (up to 10 days).
	Comments: Women who are pregnant or considering pregnancy should not exceed 5,000 IU a day.
Echinacea/ Goldenseal	**Dosage:** 200 mg echinacea and 125 mg goldenseal 4 times a day.
	Comments: Use only during acute stage; available as combination.
Lysine	**Dosage:** 1,000 mg L-lysine 3 times a day only during acute stage.
	Comments: Take on an empty stomach; don't take with milk.
Selenium	**Dosage:** 600 mcg a day only during acute stage.
	Comments: Don't exceed 600 mcg daily; higher doses may be toxic.
Flaxseed oil	**Dosage:** 1 tbsp. (14 grams) a day for flare-ups.
	Comments: Can be mixed with food; take in the morning.

Note: Consider using supplements in **blue** first; those in **black** may also be beneficial. Some dosages may be supplied by supplements you are already taking—see page 39.

relieve pain and itching, enhance healing, and reduce the likelihood that shingles lesions will become infected. In addition, a cream of melissa or licorice applied to the affected areas of the skin may be effective.

For internal treatment during flare-ups, **vitamin C, flavonoids,** and **vitamin A** are antioxidants that help protect against cell damage. Along with the herbs **echinacea** and **goldenseal,** they boost immune function, assisting in the fight against the herpes virus and bacterial skin infections. In addition, the amino acid **lysine,** as well as **selenium** and **flaxseed oil,** promote healthy skin growth and speed healing.

For lingering post-shingles pain, stick with what worked for you during the acute phase while adding vitamin E (400 IU twice a day) to protect against cell damage and vitamin B_{12} (1,000 mcg with 400 mcg of folic acid every morning) to nourish the sheath that covers and protects the nerves. Also try topical cayenne (capsaicin) cream to dull the pain.

What else you can do

☑ Keep affected areas clean and dry. Never scratch or try to burst blisters, which can cause a bacterial infection.

☑ Use cool, wet compresses or ice packs to soothe the area and reduce pain. You can also apply calamine lotion to the skin.

FACTS & Tips

■ Natural supplements can safely be used along with prescription medicines (such as acyclovir), which also promote healing.

■ Colloidal oatmeal, a form of finely ground oatmeal that is sold in pharmacies, can be added to baths to help relieve itching. You can also make your own blend by grinding oatmeal in a food processor and adding several cups to bath water. Be careful when leaving the tub, though: Oatmeal makes smooth surfaces very slippery.

LATEST FINDINGS

■ Capsaicin, the element responsible for the hotness of cayenne peppers, is available in an ointment formula for topical application. Studies in pain clinics have found that it helps reduce the lingering nerve pain that afflicts some people with shingles (a condition called postherpetic neuralgia); but always check with your doctor before using it. Don't apply it to active shingles infections: It can cause intense burning on open skin wounds. Instead, use it only for long-term pain, after shingles lesions have completely healed.

Did You Know?

Shingles strikes hundreds of thousands of people every year, most of them over the age of 50—though younger people can also be afflicted with the disease.

sinusitis

Each year about 35 million Americans develop sinus trouble. The sinus cavities produce mucus to help keep the respiratory system free of debris. When the sinuses become inflamed or blocked, the flow of mucus is hindered, and a number of painful symptoms can result.

What it is

The sinuses are four pairs of openings in the bones at the front of the skull, located above the eyes, on either side of the nose, behind the bridge of the nose, and behind the cheekbones. They are lined with a thin membrane that secretes mucus, which passes into the nose through small openings in the sinuses. Mucus sweeps away inhaled dust, pollen, germs, and other matter, then drains into the back of the throat, where it is swallowed. (Most dangerous germs are destroyed by stomach acid.)

Normally, the work of the sinuses is so subtle you don't even notice it. But the membrane can become irritated or inflamed, producing more (or thicker) mucus and blocking the tiny sinus openings. When this occurs, the sinuses cannot drain properly, which can cause headaches, a feeling of fullness in the face, and excessive postnasal drip. The mucus buildup also provides a breeding ground for bacteria.

What causes it

Sinusitis may occur as a complication of an upper respiratory infection, such as a cold or the flu. The linings of the sinuses can be irritated by smoke, air pollution, or allergies as well. In addition, those who have a deviated septum or nasal polyps may also be prone to sinusitis.

How supplements can help

Some cases of sinusitis—a bacterial infection, for instance—require treatment with antibiotics. However, even conventional medicine is beginning to question the universal application of these drugs, especially for people with chronic sinus conditions, which may not stem from bacteria. In addition, antibiotics don't help the body prevent future sinus infections. Supplements can be used to help clear up an acute sinus infection, even if you're on antibiotic drugs. The recommended vitamins and herbs are

Vitamin C builds the immune system and fights inflammation—both valuable properties when treating sinusitis.

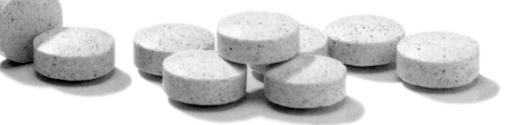

Supplement Recommendations

Echinacea	**Dosage:** 200 mg 4 times a day. **Comments:** Standardized to contain at least 3.5% echinacosides.
Astragalus	**Dosage:** 200 mg twice a day between meals. **Comments:** Supplying 0.5% glucosides and 70% polysaccharides.
Cat's claw	**Dosage:** 250 mg standardized extract twice a day. **Comments:** Take between meals. Don't use if pregnant.
Reishi/Maitake mushrooms	**Dosage:** 500 mg reishi and/or 200 mg maitake 3 times a day. **Comments:** Avoid reishi mushrooms if you're on anticoagulants.
Vitamin C/ Flavonoids	**Dosage:** 1,000 mg vitamin C and 500 mg flavonoids 3 times a day. **Comments:** Reduce vitamin C dose if diarrhea develops.
Ephedra	**Dosage:** 130 mg standardized extract 3 times a day. **Comments:** May cause insomnia. Don't use if you have high blood pressure, heart disease, or anxiety or take an MAO inhibitor.

Note: Consider using supplements in **blue** first; those in **black** may also be beneficial. Some dosages may be supplied by supplements you are already taking—see page 39.

Some dosages may be supplied by supplements you are already taking—see page 39.

particularly valuable for people who have recurring sinus problems. None of these cause the side effects (such as dry mouth) that decongestants or other conventional medicines prescribed for this condition do.

One of the best ways to prevent and treat sinusitis is to strengthen the body's defenses against germs. Start off by choosing one of the following immune-boosting herbs: **echinacea, astragalus, cat's claw, reishi** or **maitake mushrooms.** For acute sinus attacks, take just one of these herbs until the infection clears up. For chronic sinusitis, try alternating each one in two-week rotations to build and then maintain immunity.

Vitamin C and **flavonoids,** also immune strengtheners, offer an additional benefit for people whose allergy attacks develop into full-blown sinusitis. Both can minimize the effect of histamine—an inflammatory substance produced by the cells in response to pollen or other allergens.

A natural decongestant, the herb **ephedra** *(Ma huang)* widens the blood vessels in the respiratory tract, relieving congestion and swelling. However, it should be used only for stubborn acute attacks that don't respond to other treatments, because its side effects may include nervousness, trembling, insomnia, and heart palpitations.

What else you can do

☑ Avoid cigarette smoke and excess dust.

☑ Drink plenty of fluids to thin mucus.

☑ Use a humidifier or cool-mist vaporizer to keep indoor air moist.

☑ Place warm compresses on your face to help open up your sinuses.

☑ Consider using a sinus irrigator, a device found in health-food stores and pharmacies, that uses saltwater to flush out mucus.

smoking

It's never too late to quit smoking, but unfortunately a tobacco addiction is one of the most difficult habits to overcome. A number of natural supplements can boost your chances of success by helping you cope with cravings and reducing the anxiety that often accompanies quitting.

SYMPTOMS

Smoking
- *Persistent cough or recurring bouts of bronchitis or pneumonia.*
- *Hoarseness, sore throat, bad breath, yellowed teeth.*
- *Premature graying, balding, wrinkling of the skin.*
- *Impotence and many additional complaints.*

Quitting smoking
- *Anxiety, depression, craving for cigarettes, compulsive eating, nervousness, irritability.*
- *Drowsiness, fatigue, headaches, productive cough, constipation.*

When to Call Your Doctor

- If you develop symptoms of a serious smoking-related illness: pains in your chest or upper back; chronic wheezing or coughing; pink or blood-tinged mucus; or persistent sores or white patches on the mouth, tongue, or throat.
- If you need help quitting.
- Reminder: If you have a medical condition, talk to your doctor before taking supplements.

What it is

Though not considered an illness per se, smoking is a habit with serious health consequences. Within minutes of lighting a cigarette or cigar, blood pressure and pulse rate rise, and oxygen levels in the body drop. After several months of smoking, cough, sinus congestion, fatigue, shortness of breath, and other symptoms can appear. Over the long term, smoking can lead to cancer, chronic lung disorders, heart disease, and stroke.

What causes it

Why do so many people continue to smoke despite the health risks? Because smoking is an extremely powerful addiction. Not only does nicotine, the addictive drug in tobacco, cause physical effects throughout the body, but it goes almost straight to the brain, where it temporarily lifts spirits and soothes anxiety. The social rituals associated with lighting up also work to calm anxieties. When you stop smoking, nicotine levels drop, and jittery feelings accompany a range of physical complaints.

How supplements can help

Various supplements may help soothe the frazzled nerves and powerful cravings that afflict those trying to kick the smoking habit. Used for several weeks or months, they can help smokers through this difficult time. All can be taken with other stop-smoking aids, such as a nicotine patch or gum, and under your doctor's supervision, with antidepressant drugs.

Begin by increasing your intake of B vitamins and vitamin C—which are depleted in smokers. **Vitamin B complex** promotes healthy nerves and can lessen anxiety; if you still remain unusually anxious, also take **niacinamide,** a form of the B vitamin niacin. The antioxidant **vitamin C** mops up excess free radicals generated by cigarette smoke and can work to ease cravings and other withdrawal symptoms.

A number of additional nutrients—used singly or together—may also lessen cravings. **Baking soda** (sodium bicarbonate) might provide short-term relief. Studies show it reduces the desire to smoke by

The B vitamin pantothenic acid can help you cope with the stress of quitting smoking.

Supplement Recommendations

Vitamin B complex
Dosage: 1 pill twice a day with food.
Comments: Look for a B-50 complex with 50 mcg vitamin B_{12} and biotin; 400 mcg folic acid; and 50 mg all other B vitamins.

Vitamin C
Dosage: 2,000 mg 3 times a day.
Comments: Will likely loosen stools at this dosage. Use buffered powder form for reduced stomach irritation and for convenience.

Baking soda
Dosage: 1 tsp. in a glass of water twice a day.
Comments: Don't take if you must restrict sodium or have an ulcer.

Oat extract
Dosage: ½ tsp. tincture 4 times a day.
Comments: An alcohol-based extract, also called *Avena sativa.*

Kava
Dosage: 250 mg 3 times a day.
Comments: Standardized to contain at least 30% kavalactones.

Niacinamide
Dosage: 500 mg twice a day between meals.
Comments: Long-term use can cause liver damage and other serious side effects; physician monitoring is necessary during treatment.

Pantothenic acid
Dosage: 500 mg twice a day.
Comments: Use calcium pantothenate, the least expensive form.

Note: Consider using supplements in **blue** first; those in **black** may also be beneficial. Some dosages may be supplied by supplements you are already taking—see page 39.

increasing the pH of the urine, thereby slowing the elimination of any nicotine stored in the body. **Oat extract,** which healers in India have used to treat opium addiction for centuries, presents another intriguing possibility. In one study, it significantly reduced the craving for cigarettes, even two months after people stopped taking it, possibly by affecting levels of the brain chemicals responsible for addiction.

The anti-anxiety herb **kava** may also be effective in calming the jitters of nicotine withdrawal, which typically dissipate within a month or so. In addition, everyone trying to kick the smoking habit may benefit from the antistress B vitamin **pantothenic acid,** which boosts production of stress hormones by the adrenal gland.

What else you can do

☑ Consider nicotine gums or patches, the antidepressant drug bupropion, acupuncture treatment, or hypnosis. All can reduce cravings.

☑ Exercise to cut down on stress. A brisk walk can also help overcome an intense craving, which usually lasts only a few minutes.

FACTS & Tips

■ The "up" feeling smoking produces comes from nicotine and other compounds that mimic the effects of the brain chemical acetylcholine, which plays a vital role in mental alertness and memory. Eating a well-balanced diet and taking a high-potency multivitamin daily can help boost your natural production of acetylcholine and reduce your need to smoke.

■ Many people put off quitting for fear of gaining weight. To help keep pounds off (and stay off cigarettes), exercise regularly and keep your hands busy. Try munching on healthy "rabbit food"—carrots, celery, cucumbers, and the like. In addition, pursue hobbies such as painting, knitting, or woodworking.

LATEST FINDINGS

■ Researchers have long known that drinkers tend to smoke more than nondrinkers and that drinking often serves as a social cue to smoke. Now, a Purdue University study shows that in smokers, alcohol can actually increase the craving to smoke.

■ The *Journal of the National Cancer Institute* reports that people who quit smoking for longer than three months are much less likely to relapse than those who quit for less time—which is another reason to try supplements and other strategies to get you over the hump.

Did You Know?

Within 3 months of quitting smoking, lung capacity increases. After about 15 years, most of the elevated health risks return to normal.

sore throat

Whatever the cause, a sore throat can make life unpleasant, particularly if you need to use your voice a lot. Fortunately, this ailment responds exceptionally well to natural treatments: Not only do they alleviate the pain and discomfort, but they also reduce throat inflammation.

Symptoms

- *Pain or burning in throat and sometimes ears; redness.*
- *Difficulty swallowing.*
- *A lumplike feeling in the throat.*
- *Hoarseness.*
- *Swollen lymph glands under jaw.*

When to Call Your Doctor

- If your sore throat is severe and comes on suddenly—you could have strep throat.
- If you have a fever over 101°F and no symptoms of a cold.
- If you have extreme difficulty swallowing.
- If you develop a rash.
- If a mild sore throat persists for more than a week.
- Reminder: If you have a medical condition, talk to your doctor before taking supplements.

What it is

It has been described as a scratchy feeling, a tickle, or even a burning pain. Still, a sore throat by any other name is just that—a feeling of soreness that begins at the back of the mouth and extends to the middle of the throat. Usually the result of inflammation, a sore throat is not an illness but a symptom. When the throat is infected or otherwise irritated, the body responds by sending more blood to the area. It carries white blood cells and other substances to fight the infection—and these actually cause the redness, swelling, and pain in the throat.

What causes it

Allergies, bacterial or viral infections, and environmental triggers (dust, low humidity, smoke) are the most common causes of a sore throat. In the case of an allergy or viral infection, a sore throat is often the result of postnasal drip, the draining of excessive mucus from the nose or sinuses down the back of the throat. In addition, the viruses that cause colds often attack throat tissue directly. Usually a viral sore throat develops slowly over the course of several days. It lasts longer but is milder than a bacterial infection (such as strep throat), which often strikes quite suddenly—sometimes in a matter of hours—inducing severe throat pain, difficulty in swallowing, and fever.

How supplements can help

The remedies listed here will strengthen your immune system, help heal inflamed throat tissue, and ease pain. Unless otherwise noted, use them together for the duration of your symptoms. These supplements can be

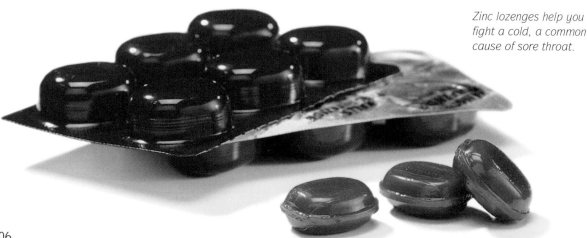

Zinc lozenges help you fight a cold, a common cause of sore throat.

206

Supplement Recommendations

Vitamin C	**Dosage:** 1,000 mg 3 times a day. **Comments:** Reduce dose if diarrhea develops.
Vitamin A	**Dosage:** 50,000 IU twice a day until symptoms improve; if needed after 7 days, reduce to 25,000 IU a day. **Comments:** Women who are pregnant or considering pregnancy should not exceed 5,000 IU a day.
Echinacea	**Dosage:** 200 mg 4 times a day. **Comments:** Standardized to contain at least 3.5% echinacosides.
Garlic	**Dosage:** 400-600 mg 4 times a day with food. **Comments:** Each pill should provide 4,000 mcg allicin potential.
Zinc	**Dosage:** 1 lozenge every 3 or 4 hours as needed. **Comments:** Do not exceed 150 mg zinc a day from all sources.
Slippery elm	**Dosage:** As a tea, 1 tsp. per cup of hot water as needed. **Comments:** May substitute or combine with marshmallow root.

Some dosages may be supplied by supplements you are already taking—see page 39.

see page 39

FACTS & Tips

■ Gargling several times a day reduces sore throat pain. Two gargles to try: a tea of equal parts slippery elm, raspberry leaf, goldenseal, and licorice, cooled to lukewarm; or ½ teaspoon salt and 1 teaspoon turmeric mixed into 8 ounces of warm water.

■ Before you take antibiotics for a sore throat, have your doctor perform a simple in-office test to determine whether your problem is indeed related to a bacterial infection. If you do have strep throat, antibiotics are necessary, but they may destroy the "friendly" bacteria that keep your digestive system functioning well. Replenish your internal supply with acidophilus.

combined with over-the-counter or prescription medications for colds or allergies or with antibiotics for strep throat.

Vitamin C assists the body in fighting the upper respiratory infections that often cause sore throat. As a natural antihistamine, it can also reduce inflammatory compounds that the body produces in people with allergies. **Vitamin A** speeds healing of mucous membranes, such as those in the throat. The herbs **echinacea** and **garlic** have antiviral and antibacterial properties; begin taking them at the first sign of throat irritation.

In addition, try **zinc** lozenges to help prevent a sore throat caused by a cold; studies have shown that they may shorten the duration of the illness. If you dislike the taste of zinc or don't have a cold, drink a tea of **slippery elm** or marshmallow root. These herbs coat the throat, making swallowing easier and relieving pain. Slippery elm also contains compounds known as procyanidolic oligomers (PCOs), which fight infection and allergic reactions. For an extra immunity boost, add a few drops of goldenseal tincture to your tea—it is especially effective against bacterial infections because it contains berberine, an antibacterial compound. If you are congested as well, you can add licorice (in dried herb or tincture form), but don't take it if you have high blood pressure.

What else you can do

☑ Use a humidifier or cool-mist vaporizer to keep the throat lubricated.

☑ Don't smoke and stay out of smoke-filled rooms.

☑ Drink eight or more cups of liquids daily. Warm liquids, such as soup or tea, may be especially helpful.

LATEST FINDINGS

■ Although zinc lozenges have proved effective in reducing the duration of cold viruses in adults, new research shows they do not have the same effect in children. The study involving 249 school-age children found that those using zinc lozenges took just as long to get over their colds as children taking a placebo (nine days on average). Other studies in adults have shown that zinc lozenges cut the duration of the cold almost in half. It is not clear why zinc works for adults, but not for children.

sprains and strains

Whether caused by overzealous "weekending," slipping on a patch of ice, or stepping off a curb the wrong way, sprains and strains can affect anyone. Whatever the reason, it's surprising how much a natural therapy program can help.

SYMPTOMS

Sprains

- *Mild to severe pain at time of injury; tenderness and swelling of the joint; bruising.*
- *Lack of, or very painful, motion in injured joint.*

Strains

- *Stiff, sore muscles; tenderness and swelling.*
- *Slight skin discoloration, which may appear after several days.*

When to Call Your Doctor

- If swelling is severe or gets worse, or an injured joint becomes conspicuously misshapen—it may be a fracture.
- If pain continues to be extreme despite self-treatment, or if pain spreads to other parts of the injured area.
- If severe bruising or skin discoloration occurs.
- If the injured area cannot sustain movement or bear weight.
- Reminder: If you have a medical condition, talk to your doctor before taking supplements.

What it is

Strains are minor injuries to the muscles. They occur most often in the calf, thigh, groin, or shoulder, causing soreness and stiffness. Sprains are similar to strains, but are more serious and painful, and take longer to heal. They can entail damage to ligaments, tendons, or muscles—usually those surrounding a joint.

What causes it

Strains and sprains result from physical stress to the muscles and other tissues. Lifting a heavy object, overswinging your nine iron, or overstretching before a workout can lead to a strain. Sprains, on the other hand, are the result of a sudden force to a muscle, tendon, or ligament. Any unexpected movement, such as a fall or a twisting motion, can yank and tear these structures.

How supplements can help

Along with self-care measures, supplements—taken internally or applied externally—promote tissue repair, strengthen injured areas, and reduce inflammation. They can be very effective for sprains or strains, and most need only be used for a week or so, or until the injury begins to feel better.

Various oral supplements can speed the healing process; they can all be taken in combination and with conventional painkillers. Try **vitamin A** in high doses for five days; it helps the body use protein and repair tissue. The antioxidants **vitamin C** and **flavonoids** aid in healing and in limiting further injury to connective tissues and muscles. A builder of cartilage (the "shock absorber" of the body), **glucosamine** serves to strengthen and protect the joints and ligaments. **Bromelain,** an enzyme derived from the pineapple plant, may prevent swelling and reduce inflammation, thereby relieving pain; it also promotes blood circulation and speeds recovery. Although most people don't need **manganese**

Glucosamine strengthens and protects joints, helping sprains and strains to heal faster.

Supplement Recommendations

Vitamin A	**Dosage:** 25,000 IU twice a day for 5 days.
	Comments: Women who are pregnant or considering pregnancy should not exceed 5,000 IU a day.
Vitamin C/ Flavonoids	**Dosage:** 1,000 mg vitamin C and 500 mg flavonoids 3 times a day.
	Comments: Reduce vitamin C dose if diarrhea develops.
Glucosamine	**Dosage:** 500 mg glucosamine sulfate 3 times a day.
	Comments: Take with food to minimize digestive upset.
Bromelain	**Dosage:** 500 mg 3 times a day on an empty stomach.
	Comments: Should provide 6,000 GDU or 9,000 MCU daily.
Manganese	**Dosage:** 100 mg a day for 7 days.
	Comments: Helps heal ligaments, tendons, and cartilage.
Arnica ointment	**Dosage:** Apply ointment to painful area 4 times a day.
	Comments: Don't put on broken skin; never ingest arnica.
Sweet marjoram oil	**Dosage:** Add a few drops to a basin of cold water.
	Comments: Soak towel in mixture, wring it out, then apply.
Rosemary oil	**Dosage:** Add a few drops to a basin of cold water.
	Comments: Soak a towel in mixture, wring it out, then apply.

Note: Consider using supplements in **blue** first; those in **black** may also be beneficial. Some dosages may be supplied by supplements you are already taking—see page 39.

see page 39.

supplements on a regular basis, those with sprains or strains may benefit from a one-week course of this mineral, which plays a role in keeping tendons and ligaments healthy.

Topical therapies may also work. Apply creams or ointments containing the plant extract **arnica** to sore muscles or joints to reduce pain and swelling and encourage healing. Compresses soaked in a mixture of either **sweet marjoram oil** or **rosemary oil** and water can produce a soothing, pain-relieving effect and are useful in decreasing swelling.

What else you can do

☑ Follow the RICE acronym: **R**est the injured part; **I**ce the painful area; **C**ompress the injury with an elastic support bandage; and **E**levate the injured area above the level of the heart. Apply ice for 10 to 20 minutes at a time; reapply it every two or three hours for one to two days following the injury. A bag of frozen vegetables—peas work best—is a good substitute for ice and it can be easily molded around the injured area.

☑ Once the swelling subsides, use a hot compress or heating pad on the area to increase blood circulation.

FACTS & Tips

■ Nonsteroidal anti-inflammatory drugs (NSAIDs), such as ibuprofen, aspirin, and naproxen, are treatment mainstays for various sprains and strains. However, supplements are actually safer alternatives because they have very few of the drugs' dangerous side effects, such as stomach bleeding.

■ Although scientists have found no evidence to confirm that magnets have any benefits, some people insist that applying magnets to painful areas can speed healing. Magnet therapy is especially popular in Japan.

LATEST FINDINGS

■ A recent study of 59 people with strains and torn ligaments who were given 500 mg of bromelain three times a day for one to three weeks found that the supplement caused a marked reduction in swelling, tenderness, and pain, at rest and during movement. The results were comparable to those in people taking NSAIDs such as aspirin.

Did You Know?

Sprains can weaken ligaments and lead to recurring injuries. Be sure to warm up before exercising and adapt your exercise regimen accordingly. An elastic support bandage may help protect weakened joints.

stress

An inevitable part of modern life, stress can exhaust natural defenses, leaving the body susceptible to a wide range of health problems. Certain nutrients can help you cope, and various herbs and other nutritional supplements can calm the mind and restore equanimity.

SYMPTOMS

- *Fatigue, insomnia, or difficulty in concentrating.*
- *Nervousness, agitation, or unusual excitability.*
- *Loss of appetite, nausea, upset stomach, diarrhea, or constipation.*
- *Headaches.*
- *Loss of sexual interest.*
- *Irritability, anger, resentment, apathy, or pessimism.*

When to Call Your Doctor

- If you have prolonged or pronounced symptoms of stress. These weaken your immune system and increase your risk of medical problems—heart disease, high blood pressure, digestive disorders, ulcers, migraines, and possibly cancer.
- If stress symptoms (changes in appetite, mood, and sleep patterns) lead to problems with work, relationships, or everyday activities, or to substance abuse—you may need to be treated for depression.
- Reminder: If you have a medical or psychiatric condition, talk to your doctor before taking supplements.

What it is

Stress is simply an individual's response to taxing physical, emotional, or environmental demands. Though the body is equipped to deal with brief episodes, high-level stress on a regular basis can eventually take a heavy toll on your physical and mental health.

What causes it

A variety of predicaments can produce stress: job pressures, family discord, financial problems, traumatic events, injuries, illness. The body's initial reaction to stress, called the "fight or flight" response, is a natural and healthy reaction in which the adrenal glands prepare the body for impending danger. These two small glands, one atop each kidney, release adrenaline and other so-called stress hormones that provide an instant burst of energy and strength—allowing the body to confront an enemy or escape to safety.

Problems arise, however, if stress persists. Over time, chronically high levels of stress hormones deplete both nutrient and energy reserves, creating an overall state of exhaustion. What's more, blood pressure and cholesterol levels increase (sometimes damaging heart and blood vessels); the stomach secretes too much acid; sex hormones diminish; and the brain becomes starved for glucose (its only energy source), impairing mental ability. All these effects take an additional toll on the immune system, which can become so weakened that the body can muster little resistance to infection and illness.

How supplements can help

Because many nutrients are crucial to the body's natural ability to cope, a daily multivitamin and mineral is especially important during times of stress. Take **vitamin B complex** as well; the extra B vitamins it supplies

The dried root of Panax ginseng, which is often packaged in capsule form, helps combat stress.

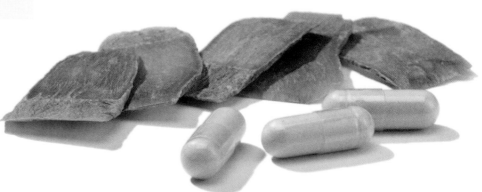

Supplement Recommendations

Vitamin B complex	**Dosage:** 1 pill twice a day with food. **Comments:** Look for a B-50 complex with 50 mcg vitamin B_{12} and biotin; 400 mcg folic acid; and 50 mg all other B vitamins.
Calcium/ Magnesium	**Dosage:** 250 mg calcium and 250 mg magnesium twice a day. **Comments:** Take with food; sometimes sold in a single supplement.
Siberian ginseng	**Dosage:** 100-300 mg 3 times a day. **Comments:** Standardized to contain at least 0.8% eleutherosides.
Panax ginseng	**Dosage:** 100-250 mg twice a day. **Comments:** Standardized to contain at least 7% ginsenosides.
Kava	**Dosage:** 250 mg 3 times a day. **Comments:** Standardized to contain at least 30% kavalactones.
Melatonin	**Dosage:** 1-3 mg before bedtime. **Comments:** Start with the lower dose and increase as needed.
St. John's wort	**Dosage:** 300 mg 3 times a day. **Comments:** Standardized to contain 0.3% hypericin.

Note: Consider using supplements in **blue** first; those in **black** may also be beneficial. Some dosages may be supplied by supplements you are already taking—see page 39.

promote the health of the nervous and immune systems and can counteract fatigue. **Calcium** and **magnesium** are worthwhile too, because they can relieve muscle tension and strengthen the heart. Both **Siberian** and **Panax ginseng,** which bolster the adrenal glands, may also be effective. These stress-fighting herbs are sometimes called "adaptogens" (because they help the body "adapt" to challenges) or "tonics" (because they "tone" the body, making it more resilient). All can be safely taken together.

Other herbs and nutritional supplements, used singly or together or combined with the supplements above, may be of value in special circumstances. For stress-induced anxiety, try **kava,** which is best reserved for high-stress periods lasting up to three months. Take **melatonin** if worry is keeping you up at night, and **St. John's wort** if stress is accompanied by mild depression.

What else you can do

☑ Exercise regularly. In addition, try breathing exercises, yoga, t'ai chi, meditation, massage, biofeedback, and other relaxation techniques.

☑ Eliminate or restrict your intake of caffeine and alcohol. They can contribute to jitteriness and keep you from sleeping.

☑ Consider psychological counseling and therapy, which can help increase your coping skills.

☑ Maintain social ties. A close network of family and friends—or even a cherished pet—is vital to good health.

FACTS & Tips

■ Adrenal formulas, found in health-food stores, may be a convenient addition to a stress-management program. They contain B vitamins, licorice, Siberian ginseng, or other stress-fighting substances and can be taken along with other supplements.

■ Check the label carefully when buying ginseng in tincture form. Some formulas contain as much as 27% alcohol—that's about 54 proof, the same strength as many liqueurs. The extra alcohol can aggravate stress.

LATEST FINDINGS

■ A University of Utah study found that high altitudes and extremes in temperature—which exerted physical stress on the body comparable to the effect of emotional stress—increased the body's needs for nutrients and calories, especially antioxidant vitamins (such as vitamin C) and minerals. That's one more reason to get plenty of vitamins and minerals when you're under stress.

■ Researchers report that being highly stressed for more than a month doubles your chances of catching a cold, compared with only routine stress. Work-related stress and problems with personal relationships had the greatest impact on who got sick.

Did You Know?

In 1984, the Russian Ministry of Health reported that job performance among telegraph operators improved when they took Siberian ginseng. Workers were able to transmit text faster while making fewer mistakes and were generally better able to cope with job-related stress.

sunburn

A round of golf or an outing at the beach may be a warm-weather treat, but even if you protect yourself from the sun's rays, your skin can sometimes burn. A number of healing supplements that can relieve the pain and help prevent long-term skin damage are readily available.

SYMPTOMS

- **Mild** *Pink or reddish skin that is hot to the touch.*
- **Moderate** *Red skin with small blisters filled with fluid; blisters may itch or break.*
- **Severe** *Deep red to purplish skin, with or without blisters, accompanied by chills, fever, headache, nausea, or dizziness.*

When to Call Your Doctor

- If you experience chills, fever, headache, nausea, or dizziness.
- If large blisters form, which can become infected.
- If you experience unusually severe itching or pain.
- Reminder: If you have a medical condition, talk to your doctor before taking supplements.

What it is

Sunburn is the reddening and inflammation of the skin's outer layers, which occurs in response to overexposure to the sun. It may be mild with some redness; moderate, with small blisters; or severe, with purple skin, chills, and fever. Symptoms appear gradually and may not peak until 24 hours after exposure. Sunburn is best avoided, and not just because it may hurt: It speeds up the aging of your skin and increases your risk of skin cancers later in life.

What causes it

The amount of sun exposure needed to produce a sunburn varies with an individual's skin pigmentation, the geographic location, the season, the time of day, and the weather conditions. Melanin, a skin pigment that absorbs the sun's ultraviolet (UV) rays, is the body's natural defense against sunburn. Fair-haired people with light eyes have less melanin than darker-skinned people and are more prone to sunburn. Some antibiotics and other drugs can also make the skin more sensitive to the sun.

How supplements can help

Supplements cannot prevent sunburn, but applied to the skin and taken orally, they can lessen the discomfort and damage that it causes.

Topical treatments may provide immediate soothing relief. For a mild sunburn, add 10 drops each of **chamomile oil** and **lavender oil** to a cool

The clear gel found in the aloe leaf provides a soothing balm for sunburned skin.

Supplement Recommendations

Chamomile oil	**Dosage:** Add to a cool bath or mix with ½ ounce almond oil (or other neutral oil) and apply to skin twice a day. **Comments:** Use with lavender oil; chamomile or calendula ointment applied several times a day also promotes healing.
Lavender oil	**Dosage:** Add to a cool bath or mix with ½ ounce almond oil (or another neutral oil) and apply to skin twice a day. **Comments:** Use with chamomile oil.
Aloe vera gel	**Dosage:** Apply gel to affected areas of skin as needed. **Comments:** Use fresh aloe leaf or store-bought gel.
Vitamin C	**Dosage:** 1,000 mg 3 times a day. **Comments:** Reduce dose if diarrhea develops.
Vitamin E	**Dosage:** 400 IU twice a day, or topical cream applied as needed. **Comments:** Don't use orally if taking an anticoagulant drug.
Flaxseed oil	**Dosage:** 1 tbsp. (14 grams) twice a day. **Comments:** Can be mixed with food. Use until fully healed.

Some dosages may be supplied by supplements you are already taking—see page **39**.

bath and soak for 30 minutes or more to relieve discomfort and moisturize the skin; alternatively, soak in a lukewarm bath containing a cup of dissolved baking soda. If the burn is more serious, prepare a topical remedy using a few drops of chamomile oil or lavender oil, or both, and half an ounce of a neutral oil, such as almond oil, and apply it gently to the affected areas twice a day. **Aloe vera gel** and chamomile or calendula cream (available in health-food stores) also soothe the skin and help speed healing.

Because sun exposure releases free radicals that can damage the skin, oral supplementation with the antioxidants **vitamin C** and **vitamin E** (used long term, if needed) may also be beneficial. For bad burns, vitamin E cream is very useful and should be applied to aid the skin in healing and to prevent scarring. Or try **flaxseed oil,** which is rich in fatty acids that reduce inflammation and promote skin healing.

What else you can do

☑ Use a sunscreen with a sun protection factor (SPF) of at least 15. Avoid the sun between 10 A.M. and 3 P.M., when rays are strongest, and cover up with clothing and wide-brimmed hats.

☑ Relieve severe sunburn pain by soaking a cotton-flannel towel or shirt, or a gauze pad, in cold milk and placing it gently on the affected areas. Or place cooled, used tea bags on the affected areas. The tannins in the tea may be effective in easing the sunburn pain.

☑ Add a cup of finely ground oatmeal (sold as colloidal oatmeal in pharmacies) to the bath. It can help relieve the pain and itching of sunburn.

FACTS
& Tips

■ To help speed healing, make your own vitamin E cream by breaking open a capsule and squeezing the oil into about a tablespoon of moisturizing cream. Mix well and apply to the sunburned skin as needed.

■ Aloe vera is an old, time-tested remedy for sunburn. Grow your own aloe plant on an indoor windowsill. It can provide a convenient and inexpensive source of the healing gel. Many sunburn products also include aloe vera as a key ingredient. Look for preparations that contain at least 20% aloe vera to be sure you're getting the benefits of this healing herb.

LATEST FINDINGS

■ Scientists in Munich, Germany, have discovered that taking vitamins C and E in combination reduces the body's reaction to sunburn damage. This, they believe, may also lower the risk of long-term skin damage, such as wrinkling and skin cancer.

■ Though some healers recommend taking beta-carotene supplements to protect against sunburn, doctors at Tufts University in Boston have found that these do not afford any detectable protection against sunburn damage.

Did You Know?

Sunlight reflected off water, sand, and snow—or even passing through clouds on an overcast day—can be as harmful to your skin as direct sunlight.

thyroid disease

An estimated one in every twenty Americans—or more than 13 million people in this country—has a thyroid disorder, and yet, alarmingly, millions of cases go undiagnosed. Fortunately, once identified, thyroid disease is readily treatable.

SYMPTOMS

Hyperthyroidism

- *Mood changes; restlessness; anxiety; sleeping difficulty.*
- *Weight loss despite increased appetite; diarrhea; rapid heartbeat; increased sweating and intolerance to heat.*
- *Goiter (painless swelling in the throat); bulging, irritated eyes; muscle weakness; light or no menstrual periods.*

Hypothyroidism

- *Fatigue, lethargy, or slowed movement; mental depression; memory problems.*
- *Weight gain; constipation; intolerance to cold.*
- *Dry hair and skin; goiter; puffiness around the eyes; heavier menstrual periods.*

When to Call Your Doctor

- If you have any of the above symptoms—a blood test will confirm the diagnosis.
- Reminder: If you have a medical condition, talk to your doctor before taking supplements.

What it is

The thyroid gland, consisting of two large lobes at the base of the throat, produces hormones essential for the proper functioning and maintenance of all the cells in the body. If it releases too much thyroid hormone—a condition known as hyperthyroidism—the body runs too fast, comparable to an overheated engine. Conversely, if it secretes too little—a disorder called hypothyroidism—the body metabolism can become sluggish. Symptoms of either condition can appear very quickly, or they may develop gradually, often mimicking long-term mild depression.

What causes it

Most cases of thyroid disease result from an autoimmune disorder, in which the body's immune system attacks the thyroid gland. Genetic factors, hormonal disturbances elsewhere in the body, surgery, radiation, or medications are other possible causes. Insufficient amounts of iodine in the diet (uncommon in this country) can also lead to hypothyroidism.

How supplements can help

The supplements listed here may be beneficial for those with thyroid disorders, including people already taking conventional drugs. But always check with your doctor first, because some of these nutrients may alter your prescription drug dose. It may take a month or so to notice benefits.

   Vitamin C and the **B-complex vitamins** are important in the treatment of hyperthyroidism and hypothyroidism. They play key roles in improving the overall function of the immune system and thyroid gland.

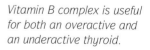

Vitamin B complex is useful for both an overactive and an underactive thyroid.

Supplement Recommendations

Vitamin C	**Dosage:** 1,000 mg a day. **Comments:** Useful for both hyperthyroidism and hypothyroidism.
Vitamin B complex	**Dosage:** 1 pill each morning for hyperthyroidism or hypothyroidism. **Comments:** Look for a B-100 complex with 100 mcg vitamin B_{12} and biotin; 400 mcg folic acid; and 100 mg all other B vitamins.
Kelp	**Dosage:** 10 grains of powdered kelp a day. **Comments:** Should supply 300 mcg iodine.
Tyrosine	**Dosage:** 1,000 mg L-tyrosine a day. **Comments:** After 1 month, add a mixed amino acid complex.
Zinc/Copper	**Dosage:** 30 mg zinc and 2 mg copper a day. **Comments:** Add copper only when using zinc longer than 1 month.
Forskolin	**Dosage:** 50 mg twice a day. **Comments:** May lower blood pressure; don't use with prescription blood pressure drugs. Standardized to contain 18% forskolin.

Note: Consider using supplements in **blue** first; those in **black** may also be beneficial. Some dosages may be supplied by supplements you are already taking—see page 39.

Individuals with a sluggish thyroid may need additional supplements, but only under a doctor's supervision. If the condition is caused by an iodine deficiency, which is very rare in the United States, **kelp** (which contains a good amount of iodine) can be used as a complement to conventional treatment. Your doctor may also recommend the amino acid **tyrosine;** like iodine, it is another key component of thyroid hormone. Extra **zinc** (take with **copper** when using long term, because zinc inhibits copper absorption) may be necessary as well to help boost thyroid function. Those with hypothyroidism may also benefit from long-term use of **forskolin,** an extract of *Coleus forskohlii,* an herb used in traditional Indian medicine that stimulates the release of thyroid hormone.

What else you can do

☑ Regularly check the area of your neck just below the Adam's apple for any bulging, which may be a sign of thyroid problems.

☑ If you have an overactive thyroid, eat plenty of raw cruciferous vegetables, such as broccoli, cauliflower, brussels sprouts, kale, cabbage, and collard greens, which contain a natural thyroid blocker. Avoid iodized salt and iodine-containing foods, including saltwater fish and shellfish.

☑ If you have an underactive thyroid, stay away from cruciferous vegetables and eat iodine-rich foods.

FACTS & Tips

■ If you have hypothyroidism, ask your doctor about natural thyroid hormone. Most doctors prescribe a synthetic thyroid hormone because dosages are well standardized; it consists of a single hormone, known as T4, that is converted in the body to its active form, called T3. But not everyone has adequate amounts of an enzyme needed for this conversion. Natural thyroid (extracted from cows) may be superior for some people because it contains both T4 and T3. Though dosage strength may vary from batch to batch, many patients, especially older ones, improve significantly when switched from the synthetic to the natural form.

■ Some doctors are concerned about the safety of natural thyroid hormone because they think it may be contaminated with harmful viruses. Although there's no clinical evidence that natural thyroid hormone has caused disease, a synthetic thyroid hormone called liotrix, containing both T4 and T3, may be an acceptable alternative.

LATEST FINDINGS

■ Smokers take heed: A team of Swiss researchers found smoking can significantly increase the severity of hypothyroidism.

Did You Know?

Hypothyroidism is at least four times more prevalent among women than it is among men. Women over age 50 are especially at risk.

tinnitus

It may be all in your head, but it's nonetheless very real—a persistent buzzing, humming, whistling, or plain old ringing in the ears that afflicts many older Americans. And though there's no outright cure, treatment is at hand in the form of vitamins, minerals, and herbs.

SYMPTOMS

■ *Persistent ringing, buzzing, or humming in one or both ears.*

■ *Possible hearing loss.*

■ *Sleep disturbances, distress, or anxiety.*

When to Call Your Doctor

■ If you experience unusual or unrelenting noise in one or both ears that persists and interferes with daily tasks or sleep.

■ If ringing is accompanied by facial numbness, dizziness, nausea, or loss of balance.

■ If ringing affects only one ear for an extended period.

■ Reminder: If you have a medical condition, talk to your doctor before taking supplements.

What it is

The medical name for persistent ringing in the ears is *tinnitus*—which is a Latin word meaning "ringing." As many as 36 million Americans experience some form of this condition, and nearly a third of them seek medical help for it. In certain people (usually those over age 60), the ringing may become so intrusive it interferes with sleep or leads to depression and anxiety. About 80% of sufferers also have some degree of hearing loss.

What causes it

Most cases of tinnitus probably stem from repeated exposure to loud noises (rock music, gunshots, industrial machinery), which can damage the nerves and tiny hairs in the inner ear that detect sound. Other causes, some of which are easily remedied, include excess earwax, ear infections, too much alcohol, poor blood circulation, and the side effects of certain medications, especially antibiotics or aspirin. Recent research indicates that the ringing probably involves some sort of nerve malfunction in the brain—not simply problems within the ear.

How supplements can help

For the many chronic cases with no readily treatable cause, supplements may be effective. Those listed can be safely used together and usually need to be taken long term, though benefits may be noticed within a month.

Because poor blood circulation to certain parts of the brain may affect the inner ears and cause ringing, the herb **ginkgo biloba** may relieve some cases, though its benefits may take weeks or months to be felt. For the same reason, the B-vitamin **inositol hexaniacinate** may be useful because it dilates blood vessels in the brain.

The herb ginkgo biloba, shown here in tablet form, may help relieve annoying ringing in the ears.

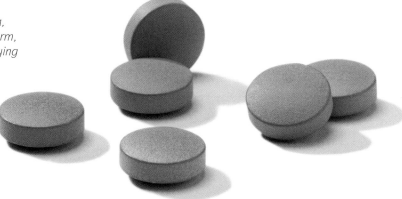

Supplement Recommendations

Ginkgo biloba	**Dosage:** 40 mg 3 times a day.
	Comments: Standardized to have at least 24% flavone glycosides.
Inositol hexaniacinate	**Dosage:** 500 mg 3 times a day.
	Comments: This form of niacin does not cause flushing.
Vitamin B$_6$	**Dosage:** 50 mg 3 times a day.
	Comments: 200 mg daily over long term can cause nerve damage.
Vitamin B$_{12}$/ Folic acid	**Dosage:** 1,000 mcg vitamin B$_{12}$ and 400 mcg folic acid a day.
	Comments: Take sublingual form for best absorption.
Magnesium	**Dosage:** 400 mg twice a day.
	Comments: Take with food; reduce dose if diarrhea develops.
Zinc/Copper	**Dosage:** 30 mg zinc and 2 mg copper a day.
	Comments: Add copper only when using zinc longer than 1 month.

Some dosages may be supplied by supplements you are already taking—see page 39.

Some dosages may be supplied by supplements you are already taking—see page 39.

Other supplements may help by improving the health of the nerves—including those that lead to the inner ear. **Vitamin B$_6$** has beneficial effects on nerve function, as does **vitamin B$_{12}$,** which the body uses to make myelin, a fatty substance that covers and protects the nerves and enables them to function efficiently. (Vitamin B$_{12}$ should be taken with **folic acid** to prevent deficiencies of either B vitamin.) If your symptoms don't improve after three months, discontinue the regimen of vitamins B$_6$ and B$_{12}$, folic acid, and inositol hexaniacinate.

Magnesium also plays an important role in maintaining nerve function and hearing. Low magnesium levels can cause the blood vessels to constrict, inhibiting circulation in the brain. Because the inner ear has a higher concentration of **zinc** than most other parts of the body, insufficient zinc might contribute to tinnitus. Indeed, even a slight deficiency can worsen the hearing loss associated with aging. Zinc interferes with **copper** absorption, so be sure to take supplemental copper as well.

What else you can do

☑ Cut back on caffeine, alcohol, nicotine, and aspirin; they can make ringing in the ears worse.

☑ Have your hearing checked. A properly adjusted hearing aid may diminish or even eliminate the ringing.

☑ Ask your doctor about ear devices that cover up, or mask, tinnitus. Low-volume white noise, such as television or radio static, may also help.

☑ Exercise to improve circulation and possibly ease symptoms.

☑ Consider acupuncture to relieve the buzzing.

FACTS & Tips

- Aspirin, especially if it's overused, can cause ringing in the ears—and so can the aspirin-like herb white willow bark. Avoid both of them if ringing in the ears is a problem.

- Because it often begins with isolated incidents and becomes chronic with age, tinnitus has been described as "listening to old age sneak up on you." Taking supplements may keep it from sneaking up so quickly.

- Loud noises may be the prime contributing factor to tinnitus. To help prevent further damage to the ears, wear earplugs. They are a boon if you're often exposed to noisy machinery, music, or explosives.

LATEST FINDINGS

- A Japanese study found zinc useful in treating some people suffering from tinnitus. The researchers administered zinc to people who had low levels of the mineral in their blood. After two weeks, their zinc levels were significantly elevated, and their symptoms had improved.

- Researchers in Buffalo, New York, recently pinpointed precise areas of the brain responsible for ringing in the ears—which may help them develop new therapies in the future.

Did You Know?

Vitamin B$_{12}$ supplements may be especially important for treating tinnitus in older people, because many of them have trouble absorbing this vitamin.

ulcers

One in ten people will develop an ulcer during his lifetime. These painful and occasionally life-threatening erosions in the lining of the stomach or intestine can often be quickly and effectively treated with both conventional drugs and a number of useful natural remedies.

SYMPTOMS

Typical symptoms
- *A gnawing or aching pain in the stomach, either just before or several hours after a meal. The pain may feel like heartburn or be accompanied by indigestion, nausea, vomiting, or weight loss. Pain may be relieved by antacids, bland foods, or milk and crackers during the night.*

Emergency symptoms
- *Passing black or bloody stools, or vomiting blood or particles that look like coffee grounds, may indicate internal bleeding. Sudden, severe abdominal pain could mean a perforated intestinal wall. These are life-threatening emergencies.*

When to Call Your Doctor

- If you have ulcer symptoms.
- If you experience any signs of internal bleeding or perforation (blood in vomit, black and tarlike stools, or severe pain in the abdomen)—these require immediate medical attention.
- Reminder: If you have a medical condition, talk to your doctor before taking supplements.

What it is

An ulcer is a craterlike erosion in the protective lining of the stomach or the duodenum, a part of the small intestine. Normally, glands in the stomach secrete substances that aid digestion, including acids and the enzyme pepsin. At the same time, the stomach and duodenum secrete mucus, which protects the lining from damage by these digestive juices. An ulcer is formed when this balance breaks down, causing the juices to begin literally digesting the stomach or intestinal lining.

What causes it

Until recently, conventional wisdom held that a stressful lifestyle and a diet rich in fats and spicy foods lead to an ulcer. Now researchers have discovered that most ulcers are actually caused by a bacterium named *Helicobacter pylori*. Once the digestive tract is infected, the protective mucous membrane is weakened, and even small amounts of digestive juices can eat into the intestinal wall. After an ulcer appears, such secondary influences as stress, diet, alcohol, caffeine, and smoking can aggravate it. Other factors contributing to ulcers include heredity—ulcers often run in families—and long-term use of aspirin, ibuprofen, or other nonsteroidal anti-inflammatory drugs (NSAIDs).

How supplements can help

If you have an ulcer, your doctor will likely give you a blood test for *H. pylori* and prescribe antibiotics and other medications if the test comes back positive. Whether or not bacteria are present, taking the various natural remedies listed (all of which are safe to use together and with

Aloe vera juice contains the astringent but ulcer-healing gel from the leaf of the aloe vera plant.

Supplement Recommendations	
Vitamin A	**Dosage:** 100,000 IU daily for 7 days, then 10,000 IU a day. **Comments:** Women who are pregnant or considering pregnancy should not exceed 5,000 IU a day.
Vitamin C	**Dosage:** 1,000 mg twice a day. **Comments:** Take in a buffered form to reduce gastric irritation.
Zinc/Copper	**Dosage:** 30 mg zinc and 2 mg copper a day. **Comments:** Add copper only when using zinc longer than 1 month.
Licorice (DGL)	**Dosage:** Chew 1 or 2 deglycyrrhizinated licorice (DGL) wafers of 380 mg each 3 times a day. **Comments:** Take 30 minutes before meals.
Glutamine	**Dosage:** 500 mg L-glutamine 3 times a day for 1 month. **Comments:** Take on an empty stomach.
Gamma-oryzanol	**Dosage:** 150 mg 3 times a day for 1 month. **Comments:** Also known as rice bran oil. Take on an empty stomach.
Aloe vera juice	**Dosage:** ½ cup juice 3 times a day for 1 month. **Comments:** Containing 98% aloe vera and no aloin or aloe-emodin.

Some dosages may be supplied by supplements you are already taking—see page 39.

conventional drugs) can help speed healing. Pain usually diminishes in about a week, although the ulcer can take up to eight weeks to heal.

Vitamin A helps protect the lining of the stomach and small intestine, allowing ulcers to heal. **Vitamin C** may directly inhibit the growth of the *H. pylori* bacterium. Substances that foster healing include **zinc** (take it with **copper** because zinc inhibits copper absorption) and deglycyrrhizinated **licorice (DGL)** wafers. The wafers, which don't raise blood pressure as regular licorice does, should be used for three months to maximize healing. **Glutamine,** an amino acid, promotes healing by nourishing the cells that line the digestive tract; **gamma-oryzanol,** an extract of rice bran oil, also seems to be beneficial.

Other research has shown that juice from the **aloe vera** plant may reduce stomach acid secretions and relieve ulcer symptoms in some people; this popular herb also contains astringent compounds that may help prevent internal bleeding. And, it may be worthwhile to try herbal teas made from marshmallow, slippery elm, meadowsweet, or calendula; these botanicals all work to soothe irritated mucous linings.

What else you can do

☑ Eat a sensible diet rich in fiber and avoid foods that cause discomfort.

☑ Refrain from alcohol, coffee, caffeinated soda, and acidic fruit juices, which can irritate the lining of the digestive tract.

☑ Don't smoke. It can delay ulcer healing.

FACTS & Tips

■ Antibiotics are probably your best bet for eliminating *H. pylori*, the bacterium that causes most ulcers. But natural supplements offer a safer alternative to most of the other conventional ulcer drugs. The supplements recommended (see chart) provide relief and hasten the healing process. And most have few, if any, known adverse effects.

LATEST FINDINGS

■ Several studies have shown DGL (deglycyrrhizinated licorice) is more effective than antacids for both short-term and maintenance ulcer therapy. And at about $15 for a month's supply, licorice is no more expensive— and sometimes far cheaper— than most over-the-counter antacids or prescription drugs.

■ Test tube and animal studies suggest that vitamin C may directly inhibit the ulcer bacterium *H. pylori*—giving this vitamin a potentially important role in both the prevention and treatment of ulcers.

■ A large study of doctors ages 40 to 75 found that those who got the most vitamin A—from a combination of diet, supplements, and multivitamins— were least likely to get ulcers of the duodenum. Those who ate high-fiber diets were also less likely to suffer from ulcers.

Did You Know?

Folk healers have long recommended cabbage juice for people with ulcers. It's good advice—cabbage is rich in the healing amino acid glutamine.

urinary tract infection

Modern science has proved what folk healers have long claimed: These bothersome and potentially serious infections, one of the most common health problems for women, can often be relieved with some of nature's own remedies.

SYMPTOMS

- *Frequent urge to urinate.*
- *Voiding a small amount of urine despite frequent urges.*
- *Burning sensation or searing pain when urinating.*
- *Foul-smelling, cloudy, or unusually dark urine.*
- *Cramps or a heavy feeling in the lower abdomen.*

When to Call Your Doctor

- **If you've tried self-treatment for 24 to 36 hours and a burning sensation, pain, or other symptoms persist.**
- **If a burning sensation is accompanied by a vaginal or penile discharge.**
- **If fever, chills, or back pain are present.**
- **If there is blood in your urine.**
- **Reminder: If you have a medical condition, talk to your doctor before taking supplements.**

What it is

Also known as cystitis or a bladder infection, a urinary tract infection (UTI) inflames the bladder or urethra (the tube that transports urine out of the bladder). The problem most frequently affects females; in fact, one in five women suffers from a UTI at least once a year. These infections are best treated promptly—and antibiotics may be necessary—because recurring UTIs can lead to potentially serious kidney infections.

What causes it

Essentially, all UTIs result from a bacterial infection. Normally, urine is sterile (germ free) when it is excreted by the kidneys and stored in the bladder; it washes out the small amount of bacteria in the urethra as it passes to the outside. But sometimes, bacteria in the urinary tract overwhelm the body's immune defenses and multiply, causing an infection. Ignoring the urge to urinate may increase the likelihood of UTIs. In addition, improper hygiene may be a factor, as well as pregnancy (the bladder can be compressed by the fetus and is unable to empty completely).

How supplements can help

Take the recommended supplements at the first hint of burning during urination. Start with **vitamin C** and **cranberry.** Vitamin C helps acidify urine, making the bladder a less inviting environment for harmful bacteria to colonize; it strengthens the body's immune defenses as well. Cranberry also acidifies the urine, but more important, it prevents infectious bacteria from adhering to the lining of the urinary tract. Less is known about how **uva ursi** works, though for some people this herb is a very effective alternative to vitamin C and cranberry (it should not be taken with those

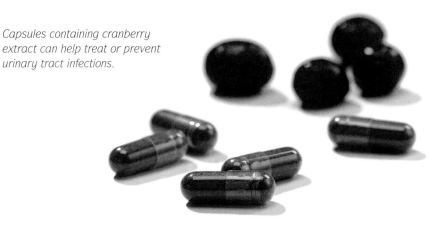
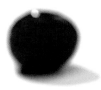

Capsules containing cranberry extract can help treat or prevent urinary tract infections.

Supplement Recommendations

Vitamin C	**Dosage:** 500 mg every other hour, as tolerated.
	Comments: Stop using if bowel movements become loose.
Cranberry	**Dosage:** 400 mg twice a day.
	Comments: Or drink 16 ounces of pure, unsweetened juice a day.
Goldenseal	**Dosage:** 1 cup goldenseal tea several times a day.
	Comments: Avoid if you're pregnant. Goldenseal can also be blended with echinacea or nettle tea.
Acidophilus	**Dosage:** 1 pill (1-2 billion live organisms) twice a day.
	Comments: Take if your doctor has also prescribed antibiotics.
Uva ursi	**Dosage:** 500 mg, or ½ tsp. tincture, 4 times a day for 1 week.
	Comments: Buy extract standardized to contain 20% arbutin. Don't take with vitamin C or cranberry. Avoid if pregnant.
Echinacea	**Dosage:** 1 cup echinacea tea several times a day.
	Comments: You can blend this herb with goldenseal or nettle.
Nettle	**Dosage:** 1 cup nettle tea several times a day.
	Comments: You can blend this herb with echinacea or goldenseal.

Note: Consider using supplements in **blue** first; those in **black** may also be beneficial. Some dosages may be supplied by supplements you are already taking—see page 39.

acidifying substances or for longer than a week). Any of these supplements can be used along with various anti-inflammatory and immune-boosting herbal teas made from **goldenseal, echinacea,** and **nettle;** in addition, the extra fluids help wash bacteria away.

Because some UTIs can progress to more serious kidney infections, it is important that these natural therapies be tried for only 24 to 36 hours before seeking professional advice. If an infection is confirmed, your doctor will likely prescribe antibiotics. Unfortunately, antibiotics kill harmful as well as healthy bacteria, which normally help to protect the digestive and urinary tracts. **Acidophilus** (which may be combined with another source of "friendly" bacteria, bifidus) is helpful specifically for those taking antibiotics because it reintroduces healthy bacteria. The other supplements can also be continued while taking antibiotics.

What else you can do

☑ Drink at least one 8-ounce glass of water every hour. Lots of water increases urine flow, improving the likelihood that harmful substances will be flushed from your system. If you have to urinate, don't "hold it in."

☑ Keep genital and anal areas clean and dry. Wash before and after intercourse. After eliminating, wipe from front to back; wear cotton (breathable) underwear; change into dry clothing quickly after exercising or swimming.

FACTS & Tips

■ To make a UTI-fighting herbal tea, pour a cup of very hot water over 2 teaspoons of goldenseal, echinacea, or nettle (or a combination). Steep for 15 minutes and strain. Sweeten to taste with honey.

■ In addition to their use in teas, goldenseal and echinacea can be employed as cleansers to help prevent recurrences in women who are prone to bladder infections. Prepare a cup of tea using either herb (or a blend) and let it cool. Then swab the genital area with the cooled solution.

■ If you're considering uva ursi, you'll need to make your urine alkaline. To do so, drink plenty of citrus fruit juices, such as orange or grapefruit, as well as milk. You can also add a small amount of baking soda to foods so you get about 2 teaspoons a day. Avoid baking soda, however, if you're watching your salt.

■ Avoid using scented douches and feminine hygiene sprays. These products can irritate the urinary tract.

LATEST FINDINGS

■ Harvard researchers found that among elderly women who had high levels of bacteria in their urine, those who routinely drank 10 ounces of cranberry juice a day significantly reduced their risk of getting a UTI over a six-month period.

Did You Know?

A home-testing kit sold in drugstores will help determine if you have a UTI. But always see your doctor if symptoms persist beyond 24 to 36 hours.

varicose veins

The bulging, bluish blood vessels that can pop up on the legs are often unsightly and painful. You may avoid invasive surgery by eating the right diet, making a few lifestyle changes, taking an adequate supply of vitamins, and using some helpful herbs.

SYMPTOMS

- *Swollen, snakelike purple veins, usually on the calf, behind the knee, or inside the thigh.*
- *Painful, aching legs, especially after long periods of standing.*
- *In severe cases, swollen ankles.*

When to Call Your Doctor

- If the area around the varicose veins turns red—this could be a sign of vein inflammation, which can be serious.
- If pain makes it hard to walk.
- If skin around the vein is discolored or peels.
- If a small, persistent sore develops over a varicose vein.
- If ankles are swollen—a possible sign you're retaining water.
- Reminder: If you have a medical condition, talk to your doctor before taking supplements.

What it is

Normal veins—the vessels that carry blood to the heart—contain valves that open and close to permit blood to flow in only one direction. If these valves become weak and don't fully close, blood flows backward and collects, resulting in bulging veins. Commonly referred to as varicose veins, they almost always develop in the legs (although hemorrhoids are actually varicose veins in the anus).

In most people, varicose veins produce only mild discomfort. In severe cases, however, blood and other fluids leak out of the veins into the surrounding tissue, causing scaly, itchy skin or swelling in the ankles from the fluid that has pooled in the legs. Sometimes the legs feel heavy or achy, particularly after extended periods of standing. The veins tend to worsen over time without treatment.

What causes it

Genetic and hormonal factors play key roles in the occurrence of varicose veins. The condition tends to run in families and is four times more common in women than men.

Other possible causes include obesity, pregnancy, or frequent heavy lifting, all of which can create excessive pressure on the veins. Pregnancy also produces hormonal changes believed to weaken the veins in the legs. Varicose veins tend to affect people who spend a lot of time on their feet, who habitually cross their legs, or who get too little exercise. Also at risk are people with congestive heart failure (an inability of the heart to pump blood properly) or liver disease.

The herb gotu kola is an effective remedy for treating varicose veins.

Vitamin C/ Flavonoids	**Dosage:** 1,000 mg vitamin C and 500 mg flavonoids 3 times a day. **Comments:** Reduce vitamin C dose if diarrhea develops.
Vitamin E	**Dosage:** 400 IU twice a day. **Comments:** Check with your doctor if taking anticoagulant drugs.
Gotu kola	**Dosage:** 200 mg extract or 400-500 mg crude herb 3 times a day. **Comments:** Extract standardized to contain 10% asiaticosides.
Bilberry	**Dosage:** 80 mg 3 times a day. **Comments:** Standardized to contain 25% anthocyanosides.
Horse chestnut	**Dosage:** 500 mg each morning. **Comments:** Standardized to contain 16%-21% escin.
Butcher's broom	**Dosage:** 150 mg 3 times a day. **Comments:** Standardized to contain 9%-11% ruscogenin.

Note: Consider using supplements in blue first; those in black may also be beneficial. Some dosages may be supplied by supplements you are already taking—see page 39.

How supplements can help

If you have varicose veins, taking **vitamin C** with **flavonoids** (which help the body use vitamin C) and **vitamin E** can improve blood circulation and strengthen the walls of the veins and capillaries. The herb **gotu kola** can be added to these vitamins and is probably the most valuable botanical for this condition. Gotu kola enhances blood flow, increases the tone of the connective tissue surrounding the veins, and keeps the veins supple. **Bilberry** complements gotu kola; in fact, these two herbs are often sold in a single supplement. **Horse chestnut** can be used in place of gotu kola and bilberry. This herb appears to control inflammation and swelling and to reduce the accumulation of fluid. If you cannot find the standardized extract of horse chestnut, you can substitute the herb **butcher's broom**. It may take up to three months to see results. You can take the vitamins and herbs that work best for you indefinitely.

What else you can do

☑ Exercise, but avoid high-impact activities. Walk, bike, or swim rather than jog. If you lift weights, don't use very heavy ones.

☑ Elevate your legs whenever possible. This helps prevent the blood from pooling in the veins.

☑ Avoid prolonged standing or sitting and don't cross your legs.

☑ Don't wear tight clothing, including shoes, panty hose, or belts. These items can constrict veins in and around the legs and make it hard for blood to move upward as it should.

C·a·s·e H·i·s·t·o·r·y

GREAT LEGS OVER 40

More than most of her friends, Carol S. dreaded turning 40. This was the age when the varicose vein problem would begin—the one that plagued all the women in her family. She looked down at her own spidery blue veins and then nervously at the huge ropy veins of her mother and aunts, some of whom also had swollen legs, deep color changes, and open sores.

Then, one day, Carol decided to make "varicose vein prevention" her pet project. She began regular exercise, wore support stockings, changed her diet, avoided extended standing and leg crossing, and faithfully took gotu kola, bilberry, and other supplements she'd read about for "optimal vein health."

Now 45, Carol's varicose veins are virtually gone. When she looks in the mirror she can't believe her eyes. "No doubt about it," she says. "Simple changes gave my legs new life."

warts

They are the single most common skin complaint—and sooner or later, one in every ten people develops at least one. Though many warts disappear on their own, a variety of natural treatments can hasten healing for the millions of Americans who suffer from these unsightly blemishes.

SYMPTOMS

Warts may grow singly or in clusters; some may also itch or bleed, though most are painless.

- *Common wart: A flat or raised growth, usually just a bit darker than the skin, generally on the hands or fingers.*
- *Plantar wart: A flat or slightly raised bump on the bottom of the foot that can resemble a callus.*
- *Genital wart: Usually a reddish pink growth, with a small flowery head, that appears in the genital or anal area.*

When to Call Your Doctor

- If you have any unusual or worrisome skin growths.
- If a wart develops after age 45.
- If a wart is larger than pencil eraser size; bleeds, hurts, or interferes with daily tasks; or is located in the genital area.
- If a wart does not respond to self-care within 12 weeks.
- Reminder: If you have a medical condition, talk to your doctor before taking supplements.

What it is

Although warts may look serious, in most cases these small skin growths are harmless. There are many different kinds, including common warts, usually found on the fingers or hands, and plantar warts, which appear on the feet. Genital warts are considered the most serious because, unlike other types, they are highly contagious, and some types may increase the risk of skin, cervical, or penile cancers.

What causes it

Warts result when a human papilloma virus (there are dozens of different types) invades the top layer of skin, usually through a small cut or abrasion. Once an infection occurs, it may take from one to eight months—or sometimes many years—for a wart to appear. Low immunity may play a role in activating the wart virus and causing the growths to emerge.

How supplements can help

Because the development of warts is often linked to the health and potency of the immune system, supplements that strengthen immunity—including **vitamin A** and **vitamin C**—may also help eliminate the growths and, when taken long term, prevent recurrences.

In addition, try one of the following topical treatments: **vitamin E, garlic oil,** and **tea tree oil; goldenseal** and **pau d'arco** tinctures; or **aloe vera gel.** A powdered form of vitamin C, mixed with water, can also be used topically. All need to be applied to a skin compress, such as a piece of flannel or cotton gauze. Each is believed to contain virus-fighting

Mixed with a little water and applied to a compress, vitamin C in powder form may help warts disappear.

Supplement Recommendations

Vitamin A
Dosage: 50,000 IU twice a day for 10 days.
Comments: Women who are pregnant or considering pregnancy should not exceed 5,000 IU a day.

Vitamin C
Dosage: 1,000 mg 3 times a day.
Comments: Powdered vitamin C (½ tsp.) can also be mixed with a little water and applied as a skin compress twice daily.

Vitamin E
Dosage: Break open a capsule; add contents to a skin compress.
Comments: Apply at bedtime, remove in morning, until wart heals.

Garlic oil
Dosage: Moisten a skin compress with garlic oil.
Comments: Apply at bedtime, remove in morning, until wart heals.

Tea tree oil
Dosage: Put several drops on a skin compress.
Comments: Apply at bedtime, remove in morning, until wart heals.

Goldenseal
Dosage: Soak a skin compress with tincture.
Comments: Apply at bedtime, remove in morning, until wart heals.

Pau d'arco
Dosage: Soak a skin compress with tincture.
Comments: Apply at bedtime, remove in morning, until wart heals.

Aloe vera gel
Dosage: Put dab of gel on skin compress.
Comments: Use fresh aloe leaf or store-bought gel.

Note: Consider using supplements in **blue** first; those in **black** may also be beneficial. Some dosages may be supplied by supplements you are already taking—see page 39.

ingredients that may promote healing. If one doesn't seem to work, experiment with another. If skin irritation develops, dilute the preparation with a little water or vegetable oil, and rub a dab of petroleum jelly on the surrounding skin. Always dilute the preparations if you're applying them to the genitals, which may be especially sensitive. Change the compresses daily. Benefits should be noticed within three to four days. Continue topical treatment until the wart heals.

Other supplements that can be applied as skin compresses are castor oil (mix it with a little baking soda) and clove oil. You can try these remedies on most warts, even genital ones. But consult your doctor first, especially in the case of genital warts, which require close medical attention.

What else you can do

☑ Wear shower shoes at the gym or by the pool. Some plantar wart viruses are spread via locker room floors.

☑ Persistent warts may require prescription wart removers or freezing, burning, or laser treatments in a dermatologist's office.

FACTS & Tips

■ For stubborn warts, try soaking the affected area in very warm water for about 20 minutes before applying a topical treatment. Soaking may help the remedy penetrate the skin.

■ Over-the-counter wart remedies are sometimes effective, but be careful: They can contain harsh chemicals that are much more likely than natural supplements to irritate the skin.

■ If warts are on the face, legs, or other areas you shave, avoid straight razors, which can cause warts to spread, and try an electric shaver or depilatory instead. Cutting or scratching a wart can also result in bleeding, infection, and scarring.

LATEST FINDINGS

■ Can alcohol make you more susceptible to developing genital warts? Studies from the Fred Hutchinson Cancer Research Center in Seattle suggest it may. Researchers found that after adjusting for diet, sexual behavior, and other possible contributing factors, those who drank two to four alcoholic beverages a week doubled their risk of genital warts. Five or more drinks a week further increased risks.

■ Another recent study points to smoking as a possible risk factor for genital warts. Women who smoked were five times more likely to develop genital warts than nonsmokers.

yeast infection

At some point in life, most women experience the unpleasant burning and itching sensation of a vaginal yeast infection. If you're prone to this problem, you may find natural supplements useful to strengthen your overall defenses against yeast overgrowth.

SYMPTOMS

- *Intense genital itching.*
- *Inflammation and redness in the external genital area.*
- *White, curdlike, or thick vaginal discharge that may smell "yeasty" (similar to bread) or is odorless.*

When to Call Your Doctor

- If you experience any of above symptoms for the first time.
- If vaginal discharge has a strong, foul-smelling odor, or is tinged with blood.
- If symptoms don't disappear in five days despite treatment.
- If the yeast infection returns within two months.
- Reminder: If you have a medical condition, talk to your doctor before taking supplements.

What it is

The organism responsible for the majority of yeast infections, *Candida albicans,* is normally present in the body in small and harmless amounts. Under certain conditions, however, yeast multiplies rapidly and causes uncomfortable symptoms. Like most fungi, *Candida albicans* thrives in warm, moist areas, such as the vagina. Other species of *Candida* may also contribute to yeast infections.

What causes it

Anything that disturbs the normal balance of yeast and bacteria or the pH (acid/base) level in the vagina can create ideal conditions for yeast to grow uncontrolled. The normal vaginal environment can be upset by something as simple as the wearing of tight jeans or nylon underwear. The risk of yeast infections is also increased by hormonal changes during pregnancy, by the use of birth control pills or spermicides, or by diabetes.

In addition, a yeast infection is likely to develop when the immune system is weakened by illness, stress, or lack of sleep, or if it is severely compromised by HIV infection or chemotherapy. Taking certain antibiotics, such as ampicillin or tetracycline, commonly leads to yeast infections, because these drugs destroy not only the bacteria causing the illness, but also the "friendly" bacteria that keep yeast levels in check.

How supplements can help

Begin taking the supplements at the recommended dosages from the time you first notice symptoms until the infection is gone. Except for the suppositories, they all can be used in combination with prescription or over-the-counter yeast treatments. Strengthening your immune system with **vitamin C** and **echinacea** helps your body fight an acute yeast infection. The herb echinacea seems to stimulate white blood cells to destroy the yeast, and vitamin C may inhibit yeast growth. If you are susceptible to

Acidophilus supplements can supply friendly bacteria that help control the growth of yeast.

Supplement Recommendations	
Vitamin C	**Dosage:** 1,000 mg 3 times a day. **Comments:** Reduce dose if diarrhea develops.
Echinacea	**Dosage:** 200 mg 3 times a day. **Comments:** Use in a cycle of 3 weeks on, 1 week off, for recurrent infections; standardized to contain at least 3.5% echinacosides.
Acidophilus	**Dosage:** 1 pill twice a day orally or as a suppository. **Comments:** Get 1-2 billion live (viable) organisms per pill. Can insert oral pill into vagina; discontinue after 5 days.
Bifidus	**Dosage:** 1 pill twice a day. **Comments:** Use a supplement that contains 1-2 billion live (viable) organisms per pill.
FOS	**Dosage:** 2,000 mg twice a day. **Comments:** Use in combination with acidophilus and bifidus.
Tea tree oil	**Dosage:** Insert suppository into vagina every 12 hours for 5 days. **Comments:** Available in health-food stores.
Vitamin A/ Calendula	**Dosage:** Insert suppository into vagina every 12 hours for 5 days. **Comments:** Available in health-food stores.

Note: Consider using supplements in **blue** first; those in **black** may also be beneficial. Some dosages may be supplied by supplements you are already taking—see page 39.

FACTS & Tips

■ Men can get genital yeast infections too, especially if they are uncircumcised. The only sign may be an inflammation of the head of the penis, but often there are no symptoms. A man with a yeast infection may infect his partner, and should be treated.

■ In place of suppositories or capsules, make a douche from one of the following: 2 teaspoons each of powdered acidophilus and bifidus in a quart of warm water; lukewarm pau d'arco tea; or lukewarm goldenseal tea. Douche twice a day for up to seven days, using two cups of liquid each time.

■ Contrary to popular belief, a diet high in carbohydrates or sugar does not increase your risk of a yeast infection. Also, the yeast used to leaven bread is not the same type that causes yeast infections, so there's no benefit in a "yeast-free" diet.

yeast infections, take echinacea for three weeks, stop using it for a week, and then resume; use for six months along with vitamin C and acidophilus.

Boost your body's supply of friendly bacteria by taking supplements of **acidophilus** and **bifidus**; these are especially important if your infection is linked to antibiotic use. Also add **FOS** (fructo-oligosaccharides), because these indigestible carbohydrates feed the helpful bacteria and promote their growth.

If you would rather not use standard anti-yeast creams, try ready-made suppositories of either tea tree oil, or vitamin A and calendula. Clinical studies show that **tea tree oil** is an effective antifungal agent. **Vitamin A** supports the healthy maintenance of the mucous membranes that line the vagina; the herb **calendula** has anti-inflammatory and anti-fungal properties.

What else you can do

☑ Wear cotton underwear; stop wearing panty hose.

☑ Avoid deodorant tampons, feminine sprays, or commercial douches.

☑ Use a mild, nonperfumed soap to wash the vaginal area.

☑ Eat yogurt with live (active) cultures. Some studies show that having a cup a day reduces the incidence of yeast infections.

LATEST FINDINGS

■ Many women cannot correctly identify the symptoms of a yeast infection, according to a recent study. Nearly 90% of women who had never had a yeast infection and 65% of those who had were not able to accurately "diagnose" a yeast infection after reading medical descriptions of this and other gynecological problems. Many participants said they would use over-the-counter (OTC) yeast creams to treat more serious conditions (pelvic inflammatory disease and urinary tract infections), for which they are ineffective. Be sure to get a proper diagnosis before treating a vaginal infection on your own.

PART II

supplements

IN THIS SECTION of the book, you will find detailed profiles of more than 80 popular supplements, arranged alphabetically from acidophilus to zinc. Each entry is color-coded according to basic supplement type (for a general explanation of these basic types, see page 15). Look for:

- Vitamins
- Minerals
- Herbs
- Nutritional Supplements

Every profile describes what the supplement is, the forms it comes in, and the way it works to promote your health and prevent or relieve specific ailments. How much you need, appropriate dosages, and other guidelines for using the supplement are spelled out, along with possible side effects. For vitamins and minerals, leading food sources are also indicated.

Be sure to read the cautionary notes in the left-hand corner of each entry. To learn more about your particular disorder, refer to Part I, the "Ailments" section of this book. And always consult your doctor if you have a serious medical condition—or one that hasn't been properly diagnosed—before treating it with any supplement.

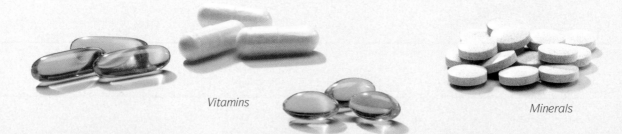

Vitamins

Minerals

About the recommendations

DOSAGE SUGGESTIONS are given in the supplement profiles that follow. These numbers are the total daily amount of a supplement that you'll need to treat a particular disorder. In practical terms, this means you may have to adjust these numbers to factor in the amount of these same supplements you may already be getting in your daily multivitamin or in individual supplements you're using for other health reasons.

For example, we suggest taking 400 IU of vitamin E a day for cancer prevention. If your daily multivitamin supplies 400 IU, you won't need to take any additional vitamin E to meet the recommendation. If you also suffer from angina (which calls for

800 IU of vitamin E) you'll have to take only 400 IU more to meet that requirement as well.

The dosages here are meant to be informative, but each person is different. If you have a serious medical condition, check with your doctor about your own case and the appropriate dose. Always read the label and never exceed the recommended dosage, even though you may be treating several ailments.

A final word: Though we've made every effort to include widely available dosages, the strengths of individual supplement products vary greatly. Many qualified people—health professionals, pharmacists, health-store staff—can help you determine an equivalent dose.

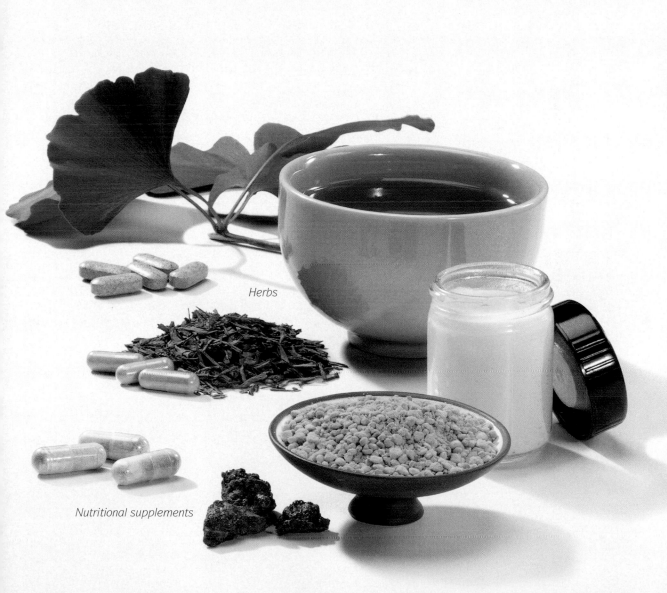

Herbs

Nutritional supplements

acidophilus

The "friendly" bacteria called acidophilus help create a healthy environment within the gastrointestinal tract. Taking acidophilus may combat digestive disorders, control vaginal yeast infections, and help the body resist diseases caused by "unfriendly" bacteria.

Lactobacillus acidophilus

COMMON USES

■ Treats chronic gastrointestinal tract disorders, such as irritable bowel syndrome, recurrent gas and bloating, and inflammatory bowel disease.

■ Controls vaginal yeast infections.

FORMS

■ Capsule
■ Tablet
■ Powder
■ Suppository
■ Douche
■ Liquid

CAUTION!

■ If you have a vaginal infection for the first time, see your doctor before treating it yourself. Acidophilus is useful against the yeast *Candida albicans,* but has little effect on other types of vaginal problems and may worsen their symptoms.

■ Reminder: If you have a medical condition, talk to your doctor before taking supplements.

What it is

Some 500 species of bacteria inhabit the digestive tract. Of these, the most beneficial are two strains of *Lactobacilli* bacteria: acidophilus and bifidus. Both are probiotics, meaning they help provide a proper balance of health-promoting bacteria in the intestine. They also manufacture natural antibiotics that kill dangerous microbes.

Yogurt, the traditional source of acidophilus, has been used as an elixir in folk medicine for hundreds, and very possibly thousands, of years. It can be difficult, however, to determine how much acidophilus is really in yogurt. When using supplements, read labels carefully: A therapeutic form should contain at least 1 billion organisms in each pill; smaller amounts may not be potent enough to have beneficial effects. Acidophilus is sometimes sold in combination with bifidus or with another ingredient that promotes the growth of friendly bacteria called FOS (fructo-oligosaccharides).

What it does

Acidophilus aids in restoring a normal balance of healthy bacteria in the gastrointestinal tract and vagina, which helps fight digestive disorders and control vaginal yeast infections. It may contain cancer-fighting agents, and may possibly lower serum cholesterol levels. Acidophilus also supplies certain vitamins, including B_{12}, K, thiamin, and folic acid.

⊡ **MAJOR BENEFITS:** Some studies show that when taken orally or inserted into the vagina as a suppository or douche, acidophilus may prevent or control vaginal yeast infections caused by *Candida albicans*. This property is particularly helpful if you're taking certain types of antibiotics that suppress acidophilus and allow yeast to flourish.

Indeed, acidophilus may be especially useful for anyone taking antibiotics to treat an infection. A healthy colon should contain about 85% *Lactobacilli* (including acidophilus and bifidus) and 14% coliform bacteria (including healthy types of *E. coli* and other bacterial strains). In many people—and particularly those on antibiotics—these counts can be upset, causing flatulence, diarrhea, constipation, and poor absorption of nutrients. Acidophilus creates an inhospitable environment for harmful types of *E. coli*, as well as for salmonella, streptococcus, and many other strains of bacteria that can be dangerous or even life-threatening.

✳ **ADDITIONAL BENEFITS:** Acidophilus can reduce the symptoms of inflammatory bowel disease, a chronic inflammation of the intestines. Along with a high-fiber diet, acidophilus contributes to overall colon health, which is necessary to help avert diverticulosis, a disorder in which the mucous lining of the colon bulges into the colon wall and creates small sacs (diverticula). Acidophilus may also relieve diarrhea triggered by irritable bowel syndrome and replenish beneficial intestinal microorganisms that diarrhea flushes out of the body.

Moreover, studies in animals suggest that acidophilus may be valuable in combating some cancers. When given to patients surgically treated for bladder cancer, acidophilus helped prevent the recurrence of single tumors. This result may have occurred because acidophilus prevents harmful bacteria from creating cancer-causing substances when the bacteria react with foods. Acidophilus may also lower blood cholesterol levels. Certain strains of these bacteria absorb cholesterol in the intestine before it reaches the arteries and does damage.

How to take it

📋 **DOSAGE:** *To make a vaginal douche:* Mix 2 teaspoons of acidophilus/bifidus powder in a quart of warm water; use twice a day for up to 10 days to restore normal bacterial growth. *To promote intestinal health:* Mix acidophilus/bifidus powder in water and drink; see label for exact dose. In capsule form, take one or two, each containing at least 1 billion live organisms, one to three times daily. For other forms, follow label directions.

◈ **GUIDELINES FOR USE:** Douching is best reserved for treating vaginal yeast infections, or for those times you are taking antibiotics. When using acidophilus orally, take it half an hour to an hour before eating. If you are on antibiotics, do not take them at the same time of day as acidophilus; continue the acidophilus even after you finish the antibiotics.

Possible side effects

Ingested in large quantities, acidophilus may cause diarrhea or other gastrointestinal complaints. Prolonged douching can irritate the vagina.

SHOPPING HINTS

■ Acidophilus products should say they contain "live cultures" or "active cultures." Be sure to check for an expiration date.

■ Whatever form you purchase, store it in a cool, dry place, such as the refrigerator. Heat can easily kill live acidophilus, as can freezing temperatures.

LATEST FINDINGS

■ A recent study showed that eating yogurt containing live acidophilus greatly reduced the recurrence of vaginal yeast infections. The women in the study ate 8 ounces of yogurt every day for six months. Researchers theorize that additional acidophilus bacteria grow in the vaginal canal, bolstering the normal *Lactobacilli* flora but leaving no room for the growth of yeast.

■ When used in a recent study of patients undergoing cancer radiation treatments, acidophilus prevented the diarrhea that is a typical side effect of this therapy. Patients drank a fermented milk product containing live acidophilus bacteria daily.

Did You Know?

Because high heat kills acidophilus cultures, some commercial yogurt manufacturers add active cultures after the entire pasteurization process has been completed.

aloe vera

Since the reign of Cleopatra, the cool, soothing gel from inside the leaf of the aloe vera plant has been gently applied to the skin to treat burns and minor wounds. This clear gel is also the basis of aloe vera juice, which can calm digestive complaints.

Aloe vera
A. barbadensis
A. vulgaris

COMMON USES

Applied topically
- *Heals minor burns (including sunburn), cuts and abrasions, insect bites and stings, welts, small skin ulcers, and frostbite.*
- *Relieves the itch of shingles (herpes zoster).*
- *May help clear up warts.*

Taken internally
- *Soothes ulcers, heartburn, and other digestive complaints.*

FORMS

- Cream/Ointment
- Fresh herb/Gel
- Liquid
- Capsule
- Softgel

CAUTION!

- Don't confuse aloe vera with the bitter yellow aloe latex, which is sold as a laxative and can cause severe cramping and diarrhea. Pregnant or breast-feeding women in particular should avoid aloe latex.
- Reminder: If you have a medical condition, talk to your doctor before taking supplements.

What it is

A succulent in the Lily family, aloe vera has fleshy leaves that provide a gel widely used as a topical treatment for skin problems—a practice dating back to at least 1500 B.C., when Egyptian healers described it in their treatises. The plant is native to the Cape of Good Hope and grows wild in much of Africa and Madagascar; commercial growers cultivate it in the Caribbean, the Mediterranean, Japan, and the United States.

What it does

Scientists aren't exactly sure how aloe vera works, but they have identified many of its active ingredients. Rich in anti-inflammatory substances, the gel contains a gummy material that acts as a soothing emollient, as well as bradykininase, a compound that helps treat pain and reduce swelling, and magnesium lactate, which quells itching. Aloe vera also dilates the tiny blood vessels known as capillaries, allowing more blood to get to an injury and thus speeding up the healing process. In addition, some studies show that it destroys, or at least inhibits, a number of bacteria, viruses, and fungi.

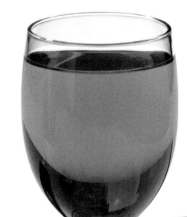

The fleshy, gel-filled leaf of the aloe vera plant is the source of healing pills and juice.

✳ MAJOR BENEFITS: Aloe vera gel is particularly helpful when applied to damaged skin. It aids in the healing of first-degree burns, sunburn, minor skin wounds, and even painful shingles by relieving pain and reducing itching. The gel also provides an airproof moisturizing barrier, so that wounds do not dry out. Furthermore, aloe vera's capillary-dilating properties increase blood circulation, speeding the regeneration of skin and relieving mild cases of frostbite. The gel's antiviral effects may promote the healing of warts as well.

Though effective against minor cuts and abrasions, aloe vera may not be a good choice for more serious, infected wounds. In a study of 21 women in a Los Angeles hospital whose cesarean-section wounds had become infected, applying aloe vera gel actually increased the length of time—from 53 to 83 days—it took for the wounds to heal.

✳ ADDITIONAL BENEFITS: Aloe vera gel is also used to make a juice that may be taken internally for inflammatory digestive disorders, including ulcers and heartburn. However, there's very little research on its internal use. In Japan, purified aloe vera compounds have been found to inhibit stomach secretions and lesions. In one study, aloe vera juice cured 17 of 18 patients with peptic ulcers, but, unfortunately, there was no comparison group taking a placebo. A U.S. commercial lab is currently conducting trials with an aloe-derived compound as a treatment for people with ulcerative colitis—a common type of inflammatory bowel disease.

Other studies are exploring aloe vera's effectiveness as a possible antiviral and immune-boosting agent for people with AIDS; as a treatment for leukemia and other types of cancer; and as a therapy to help those with diabetes manage the demands of their disease.

How to take it

⊘ DOSAGE: *For external use:* Liberally apply aloe vera gel or cream to the injured skin as needed or desired. *For internal use:* Take one-half to three-quarters of a cup of aloe vera juice three times a day; or take one or two capsules as directed on the label.

◉ GUIDELINES FOR USE: Topically, aloe vera gel can be applied repeatedly, especially in the case of burns. Just rub it on the affected area, let it dry, and reapply when needed. Fresh gel from a live leaf is the most potent—and economical—form of the herb. If you have an aloe vera plant, cut off several inches from a leaf, then slice the cutting lengthwise. Spread the gel found in the center onto the affected area. For internal use, take aloe vera juice between meals. Another form of aloe called aloe latex, a yellow extract from the inner leaf, is a powerful laxative and should be used only sparingly under a doctor's care.

Possible side effects

Topical aloe vera is very safe. In rare cases, some people get a mild, allergic skin reaction with itching or rash; simply discontinue use. Aloe vera juice, however, may contain small amounts of the laxative ingredient in aloe latex because of poor processing. If you experience cramping, diarrhea, or loose stools, stop taking the juice immediately and replace it with a new supply. Never take aloe vera juice if you are pregnant or breast-feeding.

SHOPPING HINTS

- When buying aloe products, be sure aloe vera is near the top of the ingredients list. Creams and ointments should contain at least 20% aloe vera. For internal use, look for juice that contains at least 98% aloe vera and no aloin or aloe-emodin.

- The International Aloe Science Council, a voluntary certification program, provides the "IASC-certified" seal to products that use certified raw ingredients and process them according to standard guidelines. Look for this seal, especially when you are purchasing aloe vera juice.

LATEST FINDINGS

- Add another potential use for aloe vera gel: treating the inflammatory skin condition psoriasis. A study of 60 people with long-standing psoriasis found that applying aloe to skin lesions three times a day for eight months led to significant improvement in 83% of the patients, versus only 6% in those who used a placebo.

Did You Know?

Aloe vera makes a soothing bath, which is especially helpful for sunburn. Just add a cup or two of the juice to a tub of lukewarm water.

alpha-lipoic acid

This relatively recent addition to the supplement scene has shown great promise in treating nerve damage in people with diabetes. It may also protect the liver and brain cells, prevent cataracts, and serve as a powerful general antioxidant.

What it is

In the 1950s scientists discovered that versatile alpha-lipoic acid (also known as thioctic acid or simply lipoic acid) worked with enzymes throughout the body to speed the processes involved in energy production. More recently, in the late 1980s, researchers found that alpha-lipoic acid can be a powerful antioxidant as well, neutralizing naturally occurring, highly reactive molecules called free radicals that can damage cells. Although the body manufactures it in minute amounts, alpha-lipoic acid is mainly present in foods such as spinach, meats (especially liver), and brewer's yeast. It's difficult, however, to obtain therapeutic amounts of this vitaminlike substance through diet alone. Instead, many experts recommend using supplements to get the full benefits of alpha-lipoic acid.

What it does

Alpha-lipoic acid affects nearly every cell in the body. It assists all of the B vitamins—including thiamin, riboflavin, pantothenic acid, and niacin—in converting carbohydrates, protein, and fats found in foods into energy the body can store and later use. Alpha-lipoic acid is a cell-protecting antioxidant that may help the body recycle other antioxidants, such as vitamins C and E, boosting their potency. Thanks to its unique chemical properties, alpha-lipoic acid is easily absorbed by most tissues in the body, including the brain, nerves, and liver, making it valuable for treating a wide range of ailments.

✪ **MAJOR BENEFITS:** One of alpha-lipoic acid's primary uses is to treat nerve damage, including diabetic neuropathy, a dangerous long-term complication of diabetes that causes pain and loss of feeling in the limbs. The nerve condition may be partly due to free-radical damage to nerve cells caused by runaway levels of sugar (glucose) in the blood. Alpha-lipoic acid may play a role in countering nerve damage through its antioxidant effects. In addition, it can help people with diabetes respond to insulin, the hormone that regulates glucose. In a study of 74 people with type 2 diabetes who were given 600 mg or more of alpha-lipoic acid daily,

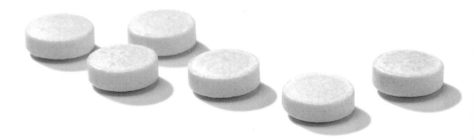

all benefited from lowered glucose levels. Studies in animals also show that alpha-lipoic acid increases blood flow to the nerves and enhances the conduction of nerve impulses. These effects may make alpha-lipoic acid suitable for the treatment of numbness, tingling, and other symptoms of nerve damage from any cause, not just diabetes.

Alpha-lipoic acid also assists the liver, protecting it against damage from free radicals and helping it clear toxins from the body. It is therefore sometimes used to treat hepatitis, cirrhosis, and other liver ailments, as well as in cases of poisoning—by lead or other heavy metals, or by hazardous industrial chemicals such as carbon tetrachloride.

✳ **ADDITIONAL BENEFITS:** Alpha-lipoic acid may have other potential uses, although more research is needed. Some compelling studies in animals show that it can prevent cataracts from forming. Additional animal experiments suggest that it may improve memory (making it potentially beneficial against Alzheimer's disease, for example) and protect brain cells against damage caused by an insufficient blood supply to the brain (the result of surgery or stroke, for example).

Some evidence indicates alpha-lipoic acid, through its antioxidant capacities, can suppress viral reproduction. In one study, alpha-lipoic acid supplements were shown to boost immune and liver function in a majority of patients infected with AIDS. It may also help in the fight against cancer, especially the forms of the disease thought to be related to free-radical damage. Finally, as part of a general high-potency antioxidant formula, alpha-lipoic acid may prove effective against disorders ranging from fibromyalgia to psoriasis, which may be aggravated, in part, by free-radical damage.

How to take it

🖊 **DOSAGE:** *To treat specific disorders:* Alpha-lipoic acid is usually taken in doses of 100 to 200 mg three times a day. *For general antioxidant support:* Lower doses of 50 to 150 mg a day may be used.

◐ **GUIDELINES FOR USE:** Alpha-lipoic acid can be taken with or without food. No major adverse effects have been reported.

Possible side effects

Alpha-lipoic acid appears to be very safe, and there have been no reports of serious side effects in people taking it. Occasionally, the supplement may produce mild gastrointestinal upset, and in rare cases, allergic skin rashes have occurred. If side effects appear, lower the dose or discontinue using the supplement.

LATEST FINDINGS

■ In a trial at multiple medical centers, 328 people with diabetic nerve damage were given 100 mg, 600 mg, or 1,200 mg of alpha-lipoic acid a day over a three-week period. Patients receiving 600 mg reported the most significant reduction in pain and numbness, compared with the other groups.

■ Alpha-lipoic acid may also benefit the 25% of diabetes sufferers who are at risk of sudden death from nerve-related heart damage. After four months of taking 800 mg of alpha-lipoic acid a day, these patients showed a notable improvement in their heart function tests.

■ A study of aged mice indicated that alpha-lipoic acid improved long-term memory, possibly by preventing free-radical damage to brain cells.

Did You Know?

Doctors have used an injectable form of alpha-lipoic acid to save the lives of people who mistakenly ate poisonous amanita mushrooms picked in the wild.

amino acids

The protein in food and in your body is a combination of chemical units called amino acids. A diet lacking even one amino acid can have a negative effect on your health. Supplements may be needed to help your body work more efficiently and to treat disease.

What it is

Every cell in the body needs and uses amino acids. Your body breaks down the protein from foods into its individual amino acids, which are then recombined to create the specific types of proteins the body requires. (Each cell, in fact, is programmed to produce exactly the right combination for its needs.) There are two types of amino acids: nonessential and essential. The body can manufacture nonessential amino acids, but must obtain essential amino acids from the foods you eat. Nonessential amino acids include alanine, arginine, asparagine, aspartic acid, cysteine, glutamic acid, glutamine, glycine, proline, serine, taurine, and tyrosine. Essential amino acids include histidine, isoleucine, leucine, lysine, methionine, phenylalanine, threonine, tryptophan, and valine.

What it does

Amino acids are needed to maintain and repair muscles, tendons, skin, ligaments, organs, glands, nails, and hair. They also aid in the production of hormones (such as insulin), neurotransmitters (message-carrying chemicals within the brain), various body fluids, and enzymes that trigger bodily functions. When even one amino acid is lacking, serious health problems will eventually occur.

Though the major cause of an amino acid deficiency is a poor diet (particularly one low in protein), amino acids may also be affected by infection, trauma, stress, medications, age, and chemical imbalances within the body. Nutritionally oriented doctors often give blood tests to determine whether a patient has a deficiency. Amino acid supplements can compensate for deficiencies and can also be taken therapeutically (even when patients aren't deficient) for a variety of health problems.

✪ **MAJOR BENEFITS:** Different amino acids (and their by-products) are very effective in the treatment of heart disease. Highly concentrated in the cells of the heart muscle, carnitine—a substance similar to an amino acid that the body produces from lysine—strengthens the heart, helps

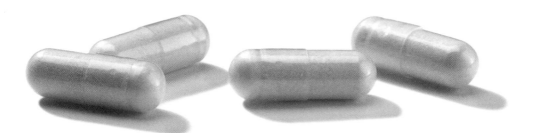

those with congestive heart failure, and can improve the chances of surviving a heart attack. Because it is also involved in fat metabolism, carnitine may help lower high levels of triglycerides (blood fats related to cholesterol). The nonessential amino acid arginine reduces the risk of heart attack and stroke by widening blood vessels and lowering blood pressure; it eases the symptoms and pains of angina as well. Taurine treats congestive heart failure and lowers high blood pressure by balancing the blood's sodium-to-potassium ratio and by regulating excessive activity of the central nervous system.

N-acetylcysteine (NAC), a by-product of the amino acid cysteine that's better absorbed than cysteine, stimulates the body's production of antioxidants and may be an antioxidant itself. As such, it aids in repairing cell damage and boosting the immune system. NAC also thins the mucus of chronic bronchitis and has been used to protect the liver in overdoses of acetaminophen (Tylenol). It may also be of value for disorders involving damage to brain or nerve cells, such as multiple sclerosis.

✳ **ADDITIONAL BENEFITS:** Concentrated in the cells of the digestive tract, glutamine can help heal ulcers and soothe irritable bowel syndrome and diverticulosis. By enhancing the production of certain brain chemicals, taurine may be a boon to people with epilepsy. It's also a key element in bile and may prevent gallstones. People with diabetes can also benefit from taurine because it facilitates the body's use of insulin.

Carnitine feeds the muscles by making it possible for them to burn fat for energy. Lysine is one of the most effective treatments for cold sores and is also useful for shingles and canker sores. (Arginine, on the other hand, can trigger cold sore or genital herpes outbreaks.)

How to take it

⊘ **DOSAGE:** For the recommended dosage of individual amino acids, see the appropriate ailment entry. When using any individual amino acid for longer than one month, take it with a mixed amino acid complex—a supplement that contains a variety of amino acids—to be sure you are receiving adequate, balanced amounts of all the amino acids.

◖ **GUIDELINES FOR USE:** Amino acid supplements are more effective when they don't have to compete with the amino acids in high-protein foods. Take the supplements at least an hour and a half before or after meals (first thing in the morning or at bedtime may be best).

Individual amino acid supplements should not be used for longer than three months, unless you are under the supervision of a doctor familiar with their use. Take mixed amino acid supplements on an empty stomach and also at a different time of day than you take the individual supplement.

Possible side effects

Amino acid supplements have no side effects as long as they are taken in the recommended amounts. High doses of certain amino acids, however, may be toxic and produce nausea, vomiting, or diarrhea.

SHOPPING HINTS

■ On supplement labels, amino acids are often prefaced by an L (L-carnitine, for example) or by a D. Buy the L forms: They most closely resemble the amino acids in the body. (One exception: D-L phenylalanine may be used for chronic pain.)

LATEST FINDINGS

■ Carnitine improved the symptoms of intermittent claudication (leg pain caused by the blockage of large arteries in legs) in 73% of people taking a specialized form of it, according to a study from Italy. Often people with this condition can't walk very far. L-carnitine in doses up to 2,000 mg a day increased the distance the participants could walk without pain.

■ Researchers at Stanford University found that arginine supplements may reduce the tendency for blood platelets to stick to each other and to artery walls, preventing clots that cause heart attacks and strokes. Arginine particularly benefits people with high cholesterol because they have stickier platelets than those with normal cholesterol.

astragalus

Astragalus membranaceus

For more than 2,000 years, astragalus has been an integral part of traditional medicine in China, where it is used to balance the life force, or *qi*. This herb is particularly valuable in fighting disease because of its powerful effect on the immune system.

COMMON USES

- *Enhances immunity.*
- *Helps fight respiratory infections.*
- *Bolsters the immune system in people undergoing cancer treatment.*

FORMS

- Tablet
- Capsule
- Tincture
- Dried herb/Tea

CAUTION!

- Pregnant women should consult with their doctor before using this herb.
- Reminder: If you have a medical condition, talk to your doctor before taking supplements.

What it is

Astragalus contains a variety of compounds that stimulate the body's immune system, and in China this native plant has long been used both to treat disease and to prevent it. Botanically, astragalus is related to licorice and the pea. And although its sweet-smelling pale yellow blossoms and delicate structure give the plant a frail appearance, it is actually a very hardy species. Medicinally, the herb's most important part is its root. The plant is harvested when it is four to seven years old; its flat, yellowish roots resemble wide popsicle sticks or tongue depressors. (The Chinese name for astragalus, *huang qi*, means "yellow leader," a testament both to its color and to its importance as a therapeutic herb.) Astragalus root is loaded with health-promoting substances, including polysaccharides, a class of carbohydrates that appear to be responsible for the herb's immune-boosting effects.

What it does

A tonic in the truest sense of the word, astragalus seems to enhance overall health by improving a person's resistance to disease, increasing stamina and vitality, and promoting general well-being. It also acts as an antioxidant, helping the body correct or prevent cell damage caused by free radicals. It may have antiviral and antibiotic properties as well. A distinct benefit of astragalus is that it can be safely used with conventional medicine and does not interfere with any standard treatment.

○ **PREVENTION:** This herb is particularly effective in fighting off colds, the flu, bronchitis, and sinus infections because it keeps viruses from gaining a foothold in the respiratory system. Like echinacea, astragalus can squash germs at the first sign of symptoms. And if an illness does develop, astragalus can shorten its duration and reduce its severity. People who frequently suffer from respiratory illnesses should consider using

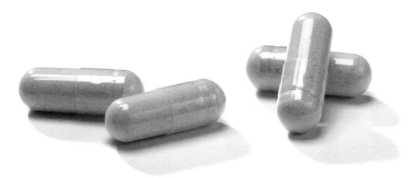

astragalus on a regular basis to prevent recurrences. It also appears to help minimize the health-damaging effects of excessive stress.

✴ **ADDITIONAL BENEFITS:** Astragalus is widely used in China to rebuild the immune system of people undergoing radiation or chemotherapy for cancer; in fact, this practice is gaining popularity in the West as well. The herb is especially valuable because it increases the body's production of T cells, macrophages, natural killer cells, interferon, and other immune cells. Astragalus may also protect bone marrow from the immune-suppressing effects of chemotherapy, radiation, toxins, and viruses. The herb, with its immune-stimulating action, might be a treatment possibility for people infected with HIV, the virus that causes AIDS.

In addition, astragalus widens blood vessels and increases blood flow, which makes it useful in controlling excessive perspiration (such as night sweats) and lowering blood pressure. Research has also shown that astragalus can have beneficial effects on the heart.

How to take it

🖉 **DOSAGE:** *For strengthening the immune system:* Take 200 mg of astragalus once or twice a day for three weeks, then alternate, in three-week stints, with echinacea, cat's claw, and pau d'arco. *For acute bronchitis:* Take 200 mg four times a day until the symptoms ease. Choose a product that contains a standardized extract of astragalus with 0.5% glucosides and 70% polysaccharides.

◈ **GUIDELINES FOR USE:** Astragalus can be taken at any time during the day, with or without meals.

Possible side effects

Remarkably, even after thousands of years of use in China, there are few (if any) negative reports about taking astragalus. The herb appears to have no side effects of any kind.

Astragalus root is dried for use in capsules.

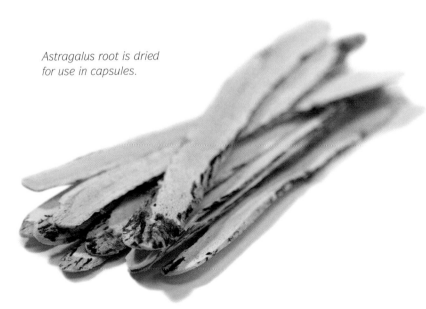

bee products

Although many intriguing claims are made for the healing powers of bee products, there is little evidence to support most of them. Yet bee pollen, royal jelly, and propolis are popular nutritional supplements and continue to be the subject of scientific studies.

COMMON USES

- *May help hay fever symptoms.*
- *Aids in healing skin abrasions.*

FORMS

- Tablet
- Capsule
- Softgel
- Liquid
- Powder
- Cream
- Lozenge
- Dried and fresh pollen

CAUTION!

- People with asthma or allergies to bee stings should be very careful when using bee products; they should avoid royal jelly entirely.
- Reminder: If you have a medical condition, talk to your doctor before taking supplements.

What it is

There are three types of bee products available in health-food stores: bee pollen, propolis, and royal jelly. The most familiar of these is bee pollen. After the bees gather pollen from plants, they compress it into pellets, which beekeepers then collect from the hives. (A second type of pollen, also sold as bee pollen, is collected directly from plants, not from bees at all.) Bee pollen contains protein, B vitamins, carbohydrates, and various enzymes. Propolis (also called bee glue) is a sticky resin that bees collect from the buds of pine trees and use to repair cracks in their hives. Then there's royal jelly, a milky-white substance produced by the salivary glands of worker bees as a food source for the queen bee. (The specialized nutritional content of royal jelly may account for the fertility, large size, and increased longevity of the queen.)

What it does

Bee products, especially bee pollen, have been touted as virtual cure-alls. Proponents assert that, among other things, these products slow aging, improve athletic performance, boost immunity, contribute to weight loss, fight bacteria, and alleviate the symptoms of allergies and hay fever. Although bee pollen shows some promise in treating allergies, and propolis may be effective as a salve for cuts and bruises, the scant research that has been conducted does not support the extravagant claims generally made for bee products.

✪ **MAJOR BENEFITS:** Bee pollen seems to help prevent the sneezing, runny nose, watery eyes, and other symptoms of seasonal pollen allergies. Some scientists believe that ingesting small amounts of pollen can desensitize an individual to its allergenic compounds, much as allergy shots do. Because your body produces antibodies when exposed to even

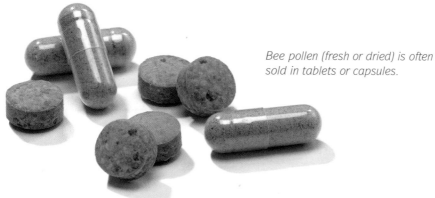

Bee pollen (fresh or dried) is often sold in tablets or capsules.

a tiny amount of pollen, your immune system then "remembers" it, preventing an extreme reaction that causes classic allergy symptoms. Testing of this theory is under way and until results are available, there appears to be no harm for most people in trying bee pollen. Various advocates maintain that to get the full anti-allergy benefit, you need to use bee pollen that comes from a local source, which will desensitize you to the specific pollens in your own environment.

✳ **ADDITIONAL BENEFITS:** Bee propolis may play some role as a skin softener or wound healer. Research has shown that though propolis contains antibacterial compounds, these are not as effective as standard antibiotics or over-the-counter antibiotic ointments in fighting infection.

Because royal jelly enhances the growth, fertility, and longevity of queen bees, many people think that it will do the same thing for humans. However, there's no evidence to support this view, and so there appears to be little reason to use royal jelly.

How to take it

🖉 **DOSAGE:** The amount of bee pollen needed to relieve allergy symptoms varies from person to person. In general, start with a few granules a day and increase the dose gradually until you're up to 1 to 3 rounded teaspoons a day.

◐ **GUIDELINES FOR USE:** Prior to hay fever season, start taking very small amounts of bee pollen each day—a few granules or a portion of a tablet. If you don't suffer any adverse reaction (see below), slowly increase your dosage until you experience relief from allergy symptoms. Have bee pollen supplements with plenty of water; you can also mix dried or fresh pollen with juice or sprinkle it over food.

Possible side effects

Because some individuals will have an allergic reaction to bee pollen, begin with a small amount so you can determine if it will have an adverse effect on you. Watch for hives, itchy throat, skin flushing, wheezing, or headache. Discontinue it immediately if any of these side effects occur.

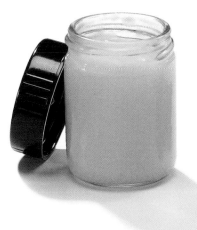
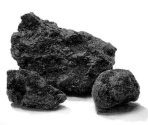
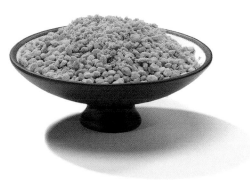

The three types of bee products on the market are royal jelly (left), propolis (center), and bee pollen (right).

beta-carotene

Once considered just a potent source of vitamin A, beta-carotene has gained prominence as a disease-fighting substance. Today, experts think that beta-carotene—along with the related nutrients called carotenoids—may protect against heart disease and cancer.

COMMON USES

- *Acts as a preventive for cancer and heart disease.*
- *May reverse some precancerous conditions.*
- *Has cell-protecting properties that may aid in the treatment of a wide variety of ailments from Alzheimer's to male infertility.*

FORMS

- Capsule
- Tablet
- Softgel
- Liquid

CAUTION!

- Consult your physician before using beta-carotene if you have a sluggish thyroid (hypothyroidism), kidney or liver disease, or an eating disorder.
- Many experts recommend that smokers, particularly those who consume large amounts of alcohol, avoid beta-carotene supplements.
- Reminder: If you have a medical condition, talk to your doctor before taking supplements.

What it is

Beta-carotene is part of a larger team of nutrients known as carotenoids, which are the yellow-orange pigments found in fruits and vegetables (see page 252). Because the body converts it to vitamin A, beta-carotene is sometimes called provitamin A. However, beta-carotene provides many additional benefits besides supplying the body with that vitamin.

What it does

An immune system booster and powerful antioxidant, beta-carotene neutralizes the free radicals that can damage cells and promote disease. By acting directly on cells, it combats—and may even reverse—some disorders. It appears to be most effective when combined with other carotenoids.

PREVENTION: Beta-carotene is a celebrated soldier in the war on heart disease. Results from a survey of more than 300 doctors enrolled in the Harvard University Physicians' Health Study revealed that taking 50 mg (85,000 IU) of beta-carotene a day cut the risk of heart attack, stroke, and all cardiovascular deaths in half. Other studies have shown that it can prevent LDL ("bad") cholesterol from damaging the heart and coronary vessels. High levels of beta-carotene may also offer protection against cancers of the lung, digestive tract, bladder, breast, and prostate.

MAJOR BENEFITS: Acting as an antioxidant, beta-carotene has reversed some precancerous conditions, particularly those affecting the skin, mucous membranes, lungs, mouth, throat, stomach, colon, prostate, cervix, and uterus. Further, it has been shown to inhibit the growth of abnormal cells, strengthen the immune system, fortify cell membranes, and increase communication among cells.

One hint of concern did arise, however, about beta-carotene's cancer-fighting benefits. In the early 1990s, landmark studies in Finland and the United States found that male smokers taking beta-carotene supplements had an increased risk of lung cancer. Though some found the studies flawed, many experts caution smokers to maintain adequate beta-carotene levels through natural food sources, not supplements.

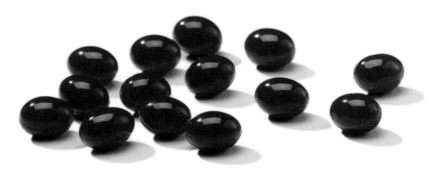

ADDITIONAL BENEFITS: As an antioxidant, beta-carotene may be helpful for a wide range of additional ailments, including Alzheimer's disease, chronic fatigue syndrome, male infertility, fibromyalgia, psoriasis, and a number of vision disorders.

How much you need

There is no RDA for beta-carotene, although about 10,000 IU meets the RDA for vitamin A. Higher doses are needed, however, to provide the full antioxidant and immune-boosting effects.

IF YOU GET TOO LITTLE: Signs of a beta-carotene deficiency are similar to those of inadequate vitamin A: poor night vision, dry skin, increased risk of infection, and the formation of precancerous cells. A deficiency may also increase your risk of cancer and heart disease. However, vitamin A deficiencies are rare: Even if you don't eat fruits and vegetables or take supplements, you can still meet your vitamin A needs with eggs, fortified milk, or other foods that supply it.

IF YOU GET TOO MUCH: It's almost impossible to get too much beta-carotene: The body discards what it doesn't process. If you ingest high levels—over 100,000 IU a day—your palms and soles may turn a harmless orange tone, which will disappear when you lower the dose.

How to take it

DOSAGE: Beta-carotene is probably most effective when combined with other carotenoids in a mixed carotenoid formula. Most people benefit from 25,000 IU (15 mg) of mixed carotenoids a day. Those at high risk for cancer can take up to 50,000 IU (30 mg) twice a day.

GUIDELINES FOR USE: Take supplements with meals. No adverse effects have been noted in pregnant or nursing women taking up to 50,000 IU a day.

Other sources

Carrots are a rich source of beta-carotene, as are other yellow, orange, and red fruits and vegetables, from sweet potatoes to cantaloupe. Green vegetables, such as broccoli, spinach, or lettuce, are also beneficial—the darker the green, the more beta-carotene they contain.

LATEST FINDINGS

■ Beta-carotene may help protect against many types of cancer—but in smokers, it may actually increase the risk of lung cancer. Recent studies show that this surprising effect seems strongest in men who smoke at least 20 cigarettes daily and increases further when alcohol intake is "above average." (Interestingly, former smokers do not appear to be at heightened risk.) One theory is that smokers generally have low vitamin C levels, and this imbalance causes beta-carotene to heighten, rather than decrease, free-radical formation.

Did You Know?

You'd have to eat more than a pound of fresh cantaloupe to get the beta-carotene in one 25,000 IU capsule.

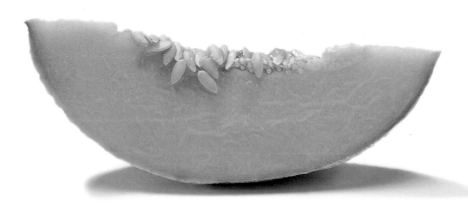

bilberry

Vaccinium myrtillus

During World War II, British RAF pilots noted the curious fact that their night vision improved after eating bilberry preserves. Their anecdotal reports sparked scientific research into this herb, which today is used to treat a wide range of visual disorders and other complaints.

What it is

Although the fruit of the bilberry bush has been enjoyed since prehistoric times, its first recorded medicinal use was in the sixteenth century. Historically, dried berry or leaf preparations were recommended for a variety of conditions, including scurvy (a disease caused by a vitamin C deficiency), urinary tract infections, and kidney stones.

A relative of the American blueberry, bilberry is a short, shrubby perennial that grows in the forests and wooded meadows of northern Europe. Bushes of these sweet blue-black berries are also found in western Asia and the Rocky Mountains of North America. The medically active components in the ripe fruit consist primarily of flavonoid compounds known as anthocyanosides. Accordingly, the modern medicinal form of bilberry is an extract containing a highly concentrated amount of these compounds.

What it does

Many of the medicinal qualities of bilberry derive from its major constituents, anthocyanosides, which are potent antioxidants. These compounds help counteract cell damage caused by unstable oxygen molecules called free radicals.

⭐ **MAJOR BENEFITS:** Bilberry extract is the leading herbal remedy for maintaining healthy vision and managing various eye disorders. In particular, bilberry helps the retina, the light-sensitive portion of the eye, adapt properly to both dark and light. It has been widely used to treat night blindness, as well as poor vision resulting from daytime glare.

Bilberries, available in capsule form, are now a popular herbal remedy for treating eye disorders.

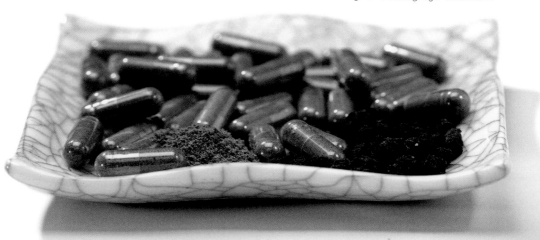

With its ability to strengthen tiny blood vessels (capillaries)—and, in turn, facilitate the delivery of oxygen-rich blood to the eyes—bilberry may also play a significant role in preventing and treating degenerative diseases of the retina (retinopathy). In one study, 31 patients were treated with bilberry extract daily for four weeks. Use of the extract fortified the capillaries and reduced hemorrhaging in the eyes, especially in cases of diabetes-related retinopathy.

In addition, bilberry is useful for preventing macular degeneration (a progressive disorder affecting the central part of the retina) and cataracts (loss of transparency of the eye's lens)—two leading causes of vision loss in older people. A study of 50 patients with age-related cataracts found that bilberry extract combined with vitamin E supplements inhibited cataract formation in almost all of the participants. Because it can strengthen collagen—the abundant protein that forms the "backbone" of healthy connective tissue—bilberry may also be valuable in preventing and treating glaucoma, a disease caused by excessive pressure within the eye.

✸ **ADDITIONAL BENEFITS:** Because the anthocyanosides in bilberry improve blood flow in capillaries, as well as in larger blood vessels, bilberry in standardized extract form may be worthwhile for people with poor circulation in their extremities. It's helpful for varicose veins and for the pain and burning of hemorrhoids, particularly during pregnancy, when these conditions can be quite troublesome. People who bruise easily may also benefit from bilberry's salutary effect on capillaries.

Although more study is needed, limited data indicate that bilberry may have other uses as well. One study showed that long-term use of bilberry extract improved the vision of normally nearsighted people—although how it produced this effect is unknown. Preliminary results in women show that bilberry helps treat menstrual cramps because anthocyanosides relax smooth muscle, including the uterus. And animal studies suggest that bilberry anthocyanosides may fight stomach ulcers.

How to take it

◯ **DOSAGE:** Normal dosages range from 40 to 160 mg of bilberry extract two or three times a day. The lower dose is generally recommended for long-term use, including prevention of macular degeneration; higher doses—up to 320 mg a day—may be needed by those with diabetes.

◉ **GUIDELINES FOR USE:** Bilberry can be taken with or without food. No adverse effects have been noted in pregnant or nursing women who use the herb. In addition, there are no known adverse interactions with prescription or over-the-counter drugs.

Possible side effects

At therapeutic doses, bilberry appears to be very safe and has no known side effects, even when taken long term.

biotin and pantothenic acid

It's surprising that these two B vitamins don't get more attention. They work together at the most basic level to produce enzymes that trigger many bodily functions, and they may assist in the treatment of various diseases.

COMMON USES

Biotin
- *Promotes healthy nails and hair.*
- *Helps the body use carbohydrates, fats, and protein.*
- *May improve blood sugar control in people with diabetes.*

Pantothenic acid
- *Promotes a healthy central nervous system.*
- *Helps the body use carbohydrates, fats, and protein.*
- *May improve chronic fatigue syndrome, migraines, heartburn, and allergies.*

FORMS
- Capsule
- Tablet
- Softgel
- Liquid

CAUTION!
- Reminder: If you have a medical condition, talk to your doctor before taking supplements.

What it is

The names of these two vitamins suggest their widespread presence in the body. Both words have Greek roots: *pantothenic* from *pantos,* which means "everywhere," and *biotin* from *bios,* which means "life." Because these vitamins are in many foods, deficiencies are virtually nonexistent. Biotin is also produced by intestinal bacteria, though this form may be difficult for the body to use. Multivitamins and B-complex vitamins usually include biotin and pantothenic acid (also called vitamin B_5) and both are also available as individual supplements. The main form of biotin is d-biotin. Pantothenic acid comes in two forms: pantethine and calcium pantothenate; the latter is suitable for most purposes and is less expensive than pantethine.

What it does

Both biotin and pantothenic acid are involved in the breakdown of carbohydrates, fats, and protein from foods and in the production of various enzymes. Biotin plays a special role in helping the body use glucose, its basic fuel, and it also promotes healthy nails and hair. The body needs pantothenic acid to maintain proper communication between the brain and nervous system and to produce certain stress hormones.

⭐ **MAJOR BENEFITS:** Biotin improves the quality of weak and brittle fingernails and may help slow hair loss, if it is due to a biotin deficiency. Research suggests the overproduction of stress hormones during long periods of emotional upset, depression, or anxiety increases the need for pantothenic acid, which is used to manufacture these hormones. Because stress is a factor in quitting smoking, migraines, and chronic fatigue, pantothenic acid may be useful for these conditions. In combination with the B vitamins choline and thiamin, pantothenic acid can be an effective heartburn remedy; it also helps reduce the nasal congestion of allergies.

❊ **ADDITIONAL BENEFITS:** In very high doses, biotin may help people with diabetes, increasing the body's response to insulin so blood sugar (glucose) levels stay low. In addition, it may protect against the nerve damage that sometimes occurs in diabetes (diabetic neuropathy).

Biotin (left) and pantothenic acid (right) are important B vitamins.

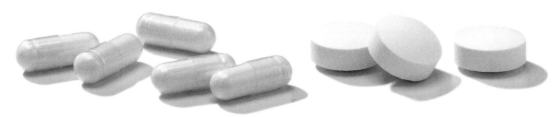

How much you need

There is no RDA for biotin or pantothenic acid, but experts recommend that you get 30 to 100 mcg of biotin and 4 to 7 mg of pantothenic acid a day. These amounts appear to be enough to maintain normal body functioning, but for the treatment of specific diseases or disorders, higher doses may be needed.

⊖ **IF YOU GET TOO LITTLE:** Deficiencies of biotin or pantothenic acid are virtually unknown in adults. Long-term use of antibiotics or antiseizure medications, however, can lead to less-than-optimal levels of biotin.

⊕ **IF YOU GET TOO MUCH:** There are no known serious adverse effects from high doses of biotin or pantothenic acid. Some people report diarrhea when taking doses of 10 grams a day or more of pantothenic acid.

How to take it

⊘ **DOSAGE:** *For hair and nails:* Take 1,000 to 1,200 mcg of biotin a day. *To aid in quitting smoking:* Take 500 mg of pantothenic acid twice a day. *During periods of stress:* Take 100 mg of pantothenic acid a day as part of a vitamin B complex. *For migraines:* Take 400 mg of pantothenic acid twice a day. *For chronic fatigue syndrome:* Take 500 mg of pantothenic acid twice a day. *For chronic heartburn:* Take 1,000 mg of pantothenic acid twice a day along with 500 mg of thiamin first thing in the morning and 500 mg choline three times a day. *For allergies:* Take 500 mg of pantothenic acid three times a day. *For diabetes:* Talk with your doctor about taking high doses of biotin to help or even prevent diabetic neuropathy.

◈ **GUIDELINES FOR USE:** Most people will get enough biotin and pantothenic acid from a multivitamin or a B-complex supplement. Individual supplements are necessary only to treat a specific disorder. In most cases, take individual supplements with meals.

Other sources

Biotin is found in liver, soy products, nuts, oatmeal, rice, barley, legumes, cauliflower, and whole wheat. Organ meats, fish, poultry, whole grains, yogurt, and legumes are the best sources of pantothenic acid.

black cohosh

Cimicifuga racemosa

Though baby boomers may claim black cohosh as the new "in" herb, its healing abilities were clearly recognized more than a century ago, when Native American and pioneer women singled out the root of this plant as one of the most useful natural medicines.

COMMON USES

- *Reduces menopausal symptoms, particularly hot flashes.*
- *Eases menstrual pain and other difficulties, such as PMS.*
- *Works as an anti-inflammatory; relieves muscle pain.*
- *Helps clear mucous membranes and relieve coughs.*

FORMS

- Capsule
- Tablet
- Tincture
- Dried herb/Tea

CAUTION!

- Never use black cohosh while pregnant or breast-feeding.
- This herb may interfere with hormonal medications (birth control pills or estrogen), so check with your doctor.
- Be careful if you're on a hypertension medication; black cohosh may intensify the drug's blood pressure-lowering effect.
- Reminder: If you have a medical condition, talk to your doctor before taking supplements.

What it is

Long used to treat "women's problems," black cohosh ("black" describes the dark color of the root; "cohosh" is derived from an Algonquian word for "rough") grows up to eight feet high and is distinguished by its tall stalks of fluffy white flowers. This member of the buttercup family is also known as bugbane, squawroot, rattle root, or *Cimicifuga racemosa,* its botanical name. However, its most common nickname, black snakeroot, describes its gnarled root, the part of the plant that is used medicinally. Contained in the root is a complex network of natural chemicals, some as powerful as the most modern pharmaceuticals.

What it does

Traditionally, black cohosh has long been prescribed to treat menstrual problems, pain after childbirth, nervous disorders, and joint pain. Today, the herb is recommended primarily for relief of the hot flashes that some women experience during menopause.

⭐ **MAJOR BENEFITS:** In Europe and increasingly in the United States, black cohosh is a popular remedy for hot flashes, vaginal dryness, and other menopausal symptoms. Scientific study has shown that black cohosh can reduce levels of LH (luteinizing hormone), which is produced by the brain's pituitary gland. The rise in LH that occurs during menopause is thought to be one cause of hot flashes.

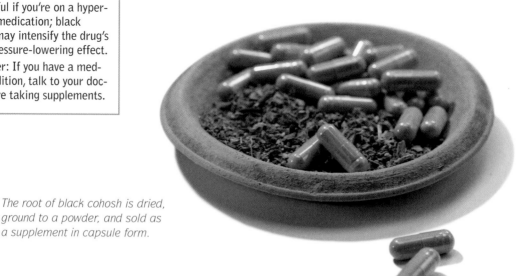

The root of black cohosh is dried, ground to a powder, and sold as a supplement in capsule form.

In addition, black cohosh contains phytoestrogens, plant compounds that have an effect similar to that of estrogen produced by the body. Phytoestrogens bind to hormone receptors in the breast, uterus, and elsewhere in the body, easing menopausal symptoms without increasing the risk of breast cancer, a possible side effect of hormone replacement therapy. In fact, some experts think phytoestrogens may even help prevent breast cancer by keeping the body's own estrogen from locking onto breast cells.

✱ **ADDITIONAL BENEFITS:** As a result of its antispasmodic properties, black cohosh can alleviate menstrual cramps by increasing blood flow to the uterus and reducing the intensity of uterine contractions. This action also makes it useful during labor and after childbirth. Because it evens out hormone levels, it may benefit women with premenstrual syndrome (PMS); however, chasteberry is probably better for this condition.

Although these effects are less frequently noted, black cohosh has demonstrated some mildly sedating and anti-inflammatory capabilities, which may be particularly valuable in treating muscle aches, as well as nerve-related pain such as sciatica or neuralgia. Because it has the ability to help clear mucus from the body, black cohosh has been recommended for coughs. This herb has been shown to be effective as a treatment for ringing in the ears (tinnitus).

How to take it

⬮ **DOSAGE:** Look for capsules or tablets containing extracts standardized to contain 2.5% of triterpenes, the active components in black cohosh. *For menopausal or PMS symptoms:* Take 40 mg of black cohosh twice a day. For PMS, begin treatment a week to 10 days before your period. *For menstrual cramps:* Take 40 mg three or four times a day as needed.

◆ **GUIDELINES FOR USE:** Black cohosh can be taken at any time of day, but to reduce the chance of stomach upset, you may prefer to use it with meals. Allow four to eight weeks to see its benefits. Many experts recommend a six-month limit on taking black cohosh, though recent studies show that longer use seems to be safe and free of significant side effects.

Possible side effects

Though it has virtually no toxic effects, black cohosh may cause stomach upset in certain people. One study suggested that it may induce slight weight gain and dizziness in some women. It may also lower blood pressure. A very high dose can cause nausea, vomiting, reduced pulse rate, heavy perspiration, and headache.

Did You Know?

Black cohosh was the main ingredient in one of the most popular folk medicines of all times—Lydia Pinkham's Vegetable Compound. Popular in the early 1900s, this "women's tonic" is still available today. Ironically, the current formula no longer contains any of this helpful native herb.

calcium

Renowned for preventing—or at least minimizing—the devastating effects of osteoporosis, calcium is now thought to lower high blood pressure and prevent colon cancer. Unfortunately, this important mineral is often seriously lacking in the modern American diet.

COMMON USES

- *Maintains bones and teeth.*
- *Helps prevent progressive bone loss and osteoporosis.*
- *Aids heart and muscle contraction, nerve impulses, and blood clotting.*
- *May help lower blood pressure in people with hypertension.*
- *Eases heartburn.*

FORMS

- Tablet
- Capsule
- Softgel
- Powder
- Liquid

What it is

Although it's the most abundant mineral in the body, most adults get just half the calcium they need each day. Eating enough calcium-rich foods may be difficult, but you can prevent a deficiency by taking supplements. A wide array of products line store shelves. The most common forms are calcium carbonate, calcium citrate, calcium citrate malate, calcium gluconate, calcium phosphate, and calcium lactate. A supplement's elemental (or pure) calcium depends on its accompanying compound. Calcium carbonate (useful in antacids to relieve heartburn) provides 40% elemental calcium, while calcium gluconate supplies 9%. The lower the calcium content, the more pills you need to meet recommended amounts.

What it does

The majority of the body's calcium is stored in the bones and teeth, where it provides strength and structure. The small amount circulating in the bloodstream helps move nutrients across cell membranes and plays a role in producing the hormones and enzymes that regulate digestion and metabolism. Calcium is also needed for normal communication among nerve cells, for blood clotting, for wound healing, and for muscle contraction. To have enough of this mineral available in the blood to perform vital functions, the body will steal it from the bones. Over time, too many calcium withdrawals leave bones porous and fragile. Only an adequate daily calcium intake will maintain healthy levels in the blood—and provide enough extra for the bones to absorb as a reserve.

PREVENTION: Getting enough calcium throughout life is a central factor in preventing osteoporosis, the bone-thinning disease that leads to a higher risk of hip and vertebrae fractures, spinal deformities, and loss of height. The body is best equipped to absorb calcium and build up bone mass before age 35, but it's never too late to increase your intake of it. Several studies show that even in people over age 65, taking calcium supplements and eating calcium-rich foods help maintain bone density and reduce the risk of fractures.

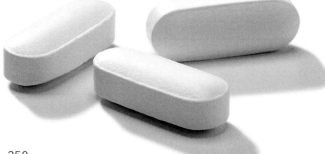

⊛ ADDITIONAL BENEFITS: By limiting the irritating effects of bile acids in the colon, calcium may reduce the incidence of colon cancer. Other research indicates that diets that include plenty of calcium—as well as fruits and vegetables—may actually help lower blood pressure as much as some prescription medications do.

How much you need

The National Academy of Sciences, which sets the Recommended Dietary Allowances (RDAs), has recently increased its recommendations for daily calcium intake to 1,000 mg for men and women ages 19 to 50, and to 1,200 mg for those ages 50 to 70.

⊖ IF YOU GET TOO LITTLE: A prolonged calcium deficiency can lead to bone abnormalities, such as osteoporosis. Muscle spasms can result from low levels of calcium in the blood.

⊕ IF YOU GET TOO MUCH: A daily calcium intake as high as 2,500 mg from a combination of food and supplements appears to be safe. However, taking calcium supplements may impair the body's absorption of the minerals zinc, iron, and magnesium. And very high doses of calcium from supplements might lead to kidney stones. Calcium carbonate may cause gas or constipation; if this is a problem, switch to calcium citrate.

How to take it

⊘ DOSAGE: Be sure to get the recommended amount of 1,000 to 1,200 mg of elemental calcium a day from foods, supplements, or both. It's often a good idea to also add supplemental magnesium when taking calcium.

◑ GUIDELINES FOR USE: To enhance absorption, divide your supplement dose so that you don't consume more than 600 mg of calcium at any one time, and be sure to take the supplements with food.

Other sources

The most familiar and plentiful sources of calcium are dairy products, such as milk, yogurt, or cheese. Choose low- or nonfat varieties: They're better for you and also contain slightly more calcium, ounce for ounce. Orange juice fortified with calcium malate, canned salmon and sardines (eaten with the soft bones), collard greens, arugula, broccoli, and almonds are good nondairy sources.

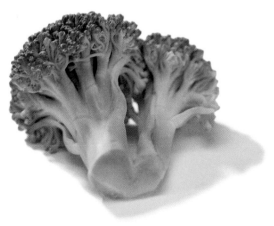

FACTS & Tips

■ Avoid calcium supplements made from dolomite, oyster shells, or bonemeal because these compounds may contain unacceptable levels of lead.

■ Calcium cannot be absorbed without vitamin D, which is made by the skin in response to sunlight. Because your body's ability to convert sunlight to vitamin D declines with age, your safest bet is to get 200 to 400 IU of vitamin D a day in your diet (fortified milk is the best source) or in supplement form. You can also buy calcium supplements with vitamin D.

■ Spinach is not a good source of calcium. It contains high levels of substances called oxalates, which lock up the calcium and limit the amount available to the body. The oxalates don't interfere with calcium absorption from other foods eaten at the same time, however.

SHOPPING HINTS

■ If you are over age 65, purchase calcium citrate. People over this age often lack sufficient stomach acid to absorb calcium carbonate.

Did You Know?

You'd have to eat nearly 80 florets of broccoli to get the 1,200 mg of calcium recommended daily.

carotenoids

The pigments that give some fruits and vegetables their rich red, orange, and yellow colors are called carotenoids. These natural compounds are also potent disease fighters. If your diet doesn't contain enough of them, supplements are a handy option.

COMMON USES

■ May lower the risk of certain types of cancers, including prostate and lung cancer.
■ May provide protection against heart disease.
■ Slow the development of macular degeneration.
■ Enhance immunity.

FORMS

■ Capsule
■ Tablet
■ Softgel

CAUTION!

■ Reminder: If you have a medical condition, talk to your doctor before taking supplements.

What it is

Although more than 600 carotenoid pigments have been identified in foods, it appears that only six of them are used in significant ways by the blood or tissues of the body. Besides beta-carotene (see page 242), which is probably the best-known carotenoid, these include alpha-carotene, lycopene, lutein, zeaxanthin, and cryptoxanthin.

Though carotenoids are found in various fruits and vegetables, the foods that represent the most concentrated sources may not be part of your daily fare. Alpha-carotene is found in carrots and pumpkin; lycopene is abundant in red fruits, such as watermelon, red grapefruit, guava, and especially processed tomatoes. Lutein and zeaxanthin are plentiful in dark green vegetables, pumpkin, and red peppers; and cryptoxanthin is present in mangoes, oranges, and peaches. To prevent certain diseases, supplements providing a mix of the six key carotenoids may be in order.

What it does

The primary benefit of carotenoids lies in their antioxidant potential. Antioxidants are compounds that protect the cells from damage by unstable oxygen molecules called free radicals. Though the carotenoids are similar, each acts on a specific type of body tissue. In addition, alpha-carotene and cryptoxanthin can be converted into vitamin A in the body, but not to the same extent as beta-carotene.

🛡 **PREVENTION:** Carotenoids may guard against certain types of cancer, apparently by limiting the abnormal growth of cells. Lycopene, for instance, appears to inhibit prostate cancer formation. Researchers at Harvard University found men who ate 10 or more servings a week of tomato-based foods—tomatoes are the richest dietary source of lycopene—cut their risk of prostate cancer by nearly 45%. Lycopene may also be effective against cancers of the stomach and digestive tract. Studies show that high intakes of alpha-carotene, lutein, and zeaxanthin decrease the risk of lung cancer, and that cryptoxanthin and alpha-carotene lower the risk of cervical cancer.

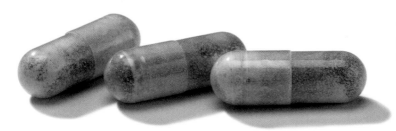

Though capsules for individual carotenoids such as lycopene (left) are available, it's best to take a mixed carotenoid supplement.

In addition, carotenoids may fight heart disease. In a survey of 1,300 elderly people, those who ate the greatest amount of carotenoid-rich foods had half the risk of developing heart disease and a 75% lower chance of heart attack than those who ate the least amount of these foods. This was true even after the researchers took other heart-disease risk factors—such as smoking and high cholesterol levels—into account. Scientists believe that all carotenoids, particularly alpha-carotene and lycopene, block the formation of LDL ("bad") cholesterol, which can lead to heart attacks and other cardiovascular problems.

✱ **ADDITIONAL BENEFITS:** The carotenoids lutein and zeaxanthin promote clear vision by absorbing the sun's harmful ultraviolet rays and neutralizing free radicals in the retina (the light-sensitive portion of the eye). This may help reduce the risk of macular degeneration, an age-related vision disorder that is the leading cause of blindness in older adults. Other carotenoids may prevent damage to the lens of the eye and so decrease the risk of cataracts.

Preliminary studies also indicate a link between low levels of carotenoids and menstrual disorders. And other studies show that, even after the onset of cancer, a diet high in carotenoids may improve the prognosis.

How to take it

⊘ **DOSAGE:** If you don't eat a wide variety of carotenoid-rich foods, take a supplement that contains mixed carotenoids—alpha-carotene, beta-carotene, lycopene, lutein, zeaxanthin, and cryptoxanthin—and supplies a minimum of 25,000 IU vitamin A activity each day. Higher doses of mixed carotenoids may be recommended for the prevention of specific disorders.

◆ **GUIDELINES FOR USE:** Take carotenoid supplements with foods that contain a bit of fat, which helps the body absorb the carotenoids more effectively. Some experts also believe that your body will absorb more of these nutrients if you divide the total daily amount of carotenoids you plan to take in half and have them at two different times during the day.

Possible side effects

Large doses of carotenoids (through food or supplements) can turn your skin orange, especially the palms of your hands and the soles of your feet. This effect is harmless and will gradually go away if you reduce your intake of them. Though there are no other known side effects associated with large amounts of mixed carotenoids, taking high doses of individual carotenoids may interfere with the workings of the other carotenoids.

F A C T S & Tips

■ Women who take oral contraceptives and postmenopausal women who use estrogen-based hormone replacement therapy have reduced levels of carotenoids in their blood. A mixed carotenoid supplement can be worthwhile for women in both groups.

■ Cooked tomatoes contain less water and consequently more lycopene than raw ones. And some experts think that the oil used in tomato sauce makes the lycopene more absorbable.

LATEST FINDINGS

■ In a major European study, lycopene was shown to help prevent heart attacks. Men who consumed large amounts of lycopene had only half the risk of a heart attack of men who consumed small amounts. Lycopene's protective effect was most beneficial to nonsmokers.

Did You Know?

Dark green vegetables contain carotenoids. The green chlorophyll masks the yellow-orange pigments that they contain.

cat's claw

Uncaria tomentosa
U. guianensis

Although Western researchers have studied cat's claw since the 1970s and European doctors have used it since the 1980s, popular interest in this herb has surged only recently. Studies suggest it may give the immune system a needed boost, which may benefit people with cancer.

COMMON USES

- *May enhance immunity, making it useful for sinusitis and other infections.*
- *Supports cancer treatment.*
- *May help relieve chronic pain.*
- *Reduces pain and inflammation from gout or arthritis.*

FORMS

- Tablet
- Capsule
- Softgel
- Tincture
- Dried herb/Tea

CAUTION!

- Never take cat's claw if you are pregnant, considering pregnancy, or breast-feeding. Its safety is not established in these situations, and it may bring on a spontaneous miscarriage.
- Reminder: If you have a medical condition, talk to your doctor before taking supplements.

What it is

In the Amazon basin, one woody tropical vine twining up trees in the rain forest features at the base of its leaves two curved thorns that resemble the claws of a cat. The herb derived from the inner bark or roots of this plant is known as cat's claw, or *uña de gato* (its Spanish name). Although there are dozens of related species, two specific ones, *Uncaria tomentosa* and *U. guianensis,* are harvested in the wild (primarily in Peru and Brazil) for medicinal purposes. Large pieces of their bark are a common sight in South American farmers' markets; native Indians have long made tea from the bark and used it to treat wounds, stomach ills, arthritis, cancer, and other ailments.

What it does

Modern scientific studies have identified several active ingredients in cat's claw that enhance the activity of the immune system and inhibit inflammation. Their presence may help explain why this herb traditionally has been employed to fight cancer, arthritis, dysentery, ulcers, and other infectious and inflammatory conditions.

⭐ **MAJOR BENEFITS:** In Germany and Austria, physicians prescribe cat's claw to stimulate the immune response in cancer patients, many of whom may be weakened by chemotherapy, radiation, or other conventional cancer treatments. Several compounds in the herb—some of which have been studied for decades—may account for its cancer-fighting and immune-boosting effects. In the 1970s, researchers reported that the inner bark and root contain compounds called procyanidolic oligomers (PCOs), which inhibit tumors in animals. In the 1980s, German scientists identified other compounds in cat's claw that enhance the immune system, in part by stimulating immune cells called phagocytes that engulf and

Once made into tablets, the woody, reddish brown bark of the cat's claw vine provides a natural way to enhance immunity.

devour viruses, bacteria, and other disease-causing microorganisms. Then, in 1993, an Italian study detected another class of compounds, called quinovic acid glycosides, that have multiple benefits. These act as antioxidants, ridding the body of cell-damaging molecules called free radicals. They also kill viruses, reduce inflammation, and inhibit the transformation of normal cells into cancerous ones.

In addition to its antitumor potential, cat's claw may be of value in combating stubborn infections such as sinusitis.

✳ **ADDITIONAL BENEFITS:** Traditionally the herb has been relied on to treat pain. Because of its anti-inflammatory properties, it may be effective in relieving joint pain caused by arthritis or gout. Additional studies are needed, however, to define the precise role that cat's claw plays in treating arthritis and other inflammatory complaints.

Some preliminary reports found that cat's claw, in conjunction with conventional AIDS drugs, may benefit people infected with HIV, because it seems to boost the immune response; further studies are necessary. Some experts caution against taking the herb for chronic conditions affecting the immune system, including tuberculosis, multiple sclerosis, and rheumatoid arthritis, because they believe it may overstimulate the immune system and make symptoms worse. Other doctors, however, recommend it for autoimmune disorders, including rheumatoid arthritis and lupus. More research must be undertaken.

How to take it

◐ **DOSAGE:** Take 250 mg of a standardized extract in pill form twice a day. Alternatively, consume 1 to 2 ml (20 to 40 drops) of the tincture twice a day. Pills containing the crude herb (the ground root or inner bark in a nonconcentrated form) are often available in 500 or 1,000 mg capsules. Have these twice daily (up to 2,000 mg a day). Cat's claw tea is sold in health-food stores; use 1 or 2 teaspoons of dried herb per cup of very hot water (follow package directions). You can drink up to three cups a day.

◐ **GUIDELINES FOR USE:** You can combine or rotate cat's claw with other immune-stimulating herbs, such as echinacea, goldenseal, reishi and maitake mushrooms, astragalus, or pau d'arco.

Pregnant or nursing women should avoid cat's claw. In Peru, cat's claw has been long valued as a contraceptive; in animals, it stimulates uterine contractions. This effect suggests the herb could induce a miscarriage.

Possible side effects

Although there have been few studies on the safety of this plant, there have been no reports that it is toxic at recommended doses. Taking higher doses, however, may cause diarrhea.

cayenne

Capsicum species

This fiery spice, made from dried hot peppers, is said to have originated in Cayenne, French Guiana. Ever since a physician sailing with Columbus first described these pungent fruits, cayenne's popularity as a painkiller, digestive aid—and food enhancer—has grown.

COMMON USES

Topical cream and ointment
- *Relieve arthritis pain.*
- *Reduce nerve pain of shingles (post-herpetic neuralgia), diabetes, surgery, or trigeminal neuralgia (tic douloureux).*

Tablet, capsule, and tincture
- *Alleviate indigestion.*

FORMS

- Cream/Ointment
- Tablet
- Capsule
- Softgel
- Tincture/Liquid
- Fresh or dried herb

CAUTION!

- Never apply cayenne cream to raw or open skin. And avoid your eyes and contact lenses: The burning can be intense.
- Reminder: If you have a medical condition, talk to your doctor before taking supplements.

What it is

Derived from several varieties of the *Capsicum* species, cayenne is a hot pepper famous for the fiery taste it brings to Cajun, Mexican, Indian, Asian, and other cuisines. It's a cousin of the bell peppers used in salads and the hot peppers that produce chili powder and hot sauces, but it's unrelated to common black table pepper. The main active ingredient in cayenne—and what gives the pepper its hotness—is capsaicin (pronounced cap-SAY-sin), an irritating, oily chemical that's also the prime component of pepper sprays sold for self-defense.

What it does

When applied to the skin, capsaicin is an effective painkiller. It causes the depletion of a component in nerve cells called substance P, which transmits pain impulses to the brain. When ingested in supplement form or in food, cayenne is believed to aid digestion.

⭐ **MAJOR BENEFITS:** Regular application to the skin of a cream or ointment containing capsaicin can be very effective for relieving the pain of arthritis. It also helps ease lingering post-shingles pain, as well as painful nerve damage from diabetes and from surgery (such as a mastectomy or an amputation).

Preliminary studies indicate cayenne cream may have other beneficial uses. It may reduce the itching of psoriasis (the itching sensation follows the same nerve pathways as pain). The cream has also shown promise in relieving the aches and pains of fibromyalgia and the coldness in the extremities caused by Raynaud's disease.

Hot cayenne peppers are the source of painkilling skin creams and digestion-aiding capsules.

✳ ADDITIONAL BENEFITS: Fresh peppers, tinctures, teas, tablets, and capsules are said to stimulate digestion and help relieve gas and ulcers by increasing blood circulation in the stomach and bowel and by promoting the secretion of digestive juices. Liquid forms mixed with water can be used as a gargle to soothe a sore throat. Special nasal preparations have been studied that may relieve congestion, fight colds, and alleviate the piercing pain of cluster headaches (try these only under a doctor's supervision). Claims that cayenne may reduce heart disease risk (by lowering blood cholesterol and triglyceride levels) or help prevent cancer (by providing vitamin C and other antioxidants) are unfounded.

How to take it

⊘ DOSAGE: *For external use:* Cayenne cream or ointment containing 0.025% to 0.075% capsaicin is most effective with regular, daily use; apply it thinly over the affected areas at least three or four times a day for pain, rubbing it in well. Pain may take several weeks to subside. *For internal use:* Follow the package instructions.

◉ GUIDELINES FOR USE: *For external use:* Because sensitivity to cayenne varies, test it first on a small, particularly painful area. If it works—which may take a week or more—and causes no lasting discomfort, you can enlarge the coverage area. To avoid getting cayenne in the eyes, wash your hands afterward with warm, soapy water or wear latex gloves during application and promptly discard them; you can also cover the area with a loose bandage. (If you're using capsaicin to relieve pain in the fingers or hands, wait 30 minutes before washing it off to allow the cream to penetrate the skin. In the meantime, avoid touching contact lenses and sensitive areas, such as your eyes and nose.) Store cayenne cream away from light and extreme heat or cold, and keep it out of the reach of children.

For internal use: Cayenne can be taken with or without food. No adverse effects have been reported in pregnant or breast-feeding women who use it internally or externally, but discontinue cayenne if a nursing baby becomes irritable.

Possible side effects

Cayenne cream or ointment frequently promotes warmth or a mildly unpleasant burning sensation that lasts half an hour or so during the first few days of topical application, but this effect usually disappears after several days of regular use.

Cayenne can also cause intense pain and burning—though no lasting damage—if it gets in your eyes (or other moist mucous membranes). If this occurs, flush the affected area with water or milk. To remove cayenne from the skin, wash with warm, soapy water. Vinegar may also work, but don't use it in or near your eyes.

Taken internally, cayenne may cause stomach pain or diarrhea. Capsaicin passing in the stool can also produce a burning sensation during bowel movements. Cayenne can sometimes trigger coughing, sneezing, tearing, or an irritated throat. These may be a result of using too much cream or inhaling the powder.

chamomile

Matricaria recutita

Sometimes called the world's most soothing plant, chamomile has traditionally been enjoyed as a tea to relax the nerves and ease digestive complaints. In concentrated form, this herb is increasingly found in pills and tinctures, and in skin formulas to treat sores and rashes.

COMMON USES

- *Promotes general relaxation and relieves anxiety.*
- *Alleviates insomnia.*
- *Heals mouth sores and treats gum disease.*
- *Soothes skin rashes and burns, including sunburn.*
- *Relieves red and irritated eyes.*
- *Eases menstrual cramps.*
- *Treats bowel inflammation, digestive upset, and heartburn.*

FORMS

- Capsule
- Dried herb/Tea
- Tincture
- Oil
- Cream/Ointment

CAUTION!

- Reminder: If you have a medical condition, talk to your doctor before taking supplements.

What it is

Chamomile is actually two herbs: German chamomile and Roman chamomile. The more popular one (and the one discussed in this book) is German—sometimes called Hungarian—chamomile. It comes from the dried daisylike flowers of the *Matricaria recutita* plant (its older botanical names are *Matricaria chamomilla* and *Chamomilla recutita).* The other type of chamomile, called Roman or English chamomile *(Chamaemelum nobile* or *Anthemis nobilis),* has properties similar to those of the German species; it is sold mainly in Europe.

This herb has long been used to prepare a gently soothing tea. Because of its pleasing, applelike aroma and flavor (the name "chamomile" is derived from the Greek *kamai melon,* which means "ground apple"), many people find the ritual of brewing and sipping the tea a relaxing experience. Concentrated chamomile extracts are also added to creams and lotions or packaged as pills or tinctures. The healing properties of the herb are related in part to its volatile oils, which contain a compound called apigenin as well as other therapeutic substances.

What it does

Chamomile is a great soother. Its anti-inflammatory, antispasmodic, and infection-fighting effects can benefit the whole body—inside and out. When taken internally, it calms digestive upsets, relieves cramping, and relaxes the nerves. It also works externally on the skin and the mucous membranes of the mouth and eyes, relieving rashes, sores, and inflammation.

★ **MAJOR BENEFITS:** When Peter Rabbit's mother put him to bed, she gave him a spoonful of chamomile tea. Scientists have confirmed her wisdom. Studies in animals have shown chamomile contains substances that act on the same parts of the brain and nervous system that anti-anxiety drugs affect, promoting relaxation and reducing stress.

Chamomile appears to have a mildly sedating effect, but more important, it also calms the body, making it easier for the person taking it to fall asleep naturally. In addition, the herb has a relaxing, anti-inflammatory effect on the smooth muscles that line the digestive tract: It helps ease a wide range of gastrointestinal complaints, including heartburn, diverticular disorders, and inflammatory bowel disease. In addition, its muscle-relaxing action may assist those suffering from menstrual cramps.

✳ **ADDITIONAL BENEFITS:** Used externally, chamomile helps soothe skin inflammation. It contains bacteria-fighting compounds that may speed the healing of infections as well. A dressing soaked in chamomile tea is often beneficial when applied to mild burns. For sunburn, chamomile oil can be added to a cool bath or mixed with almond oil and rubbed on sunburned areas. Chamomile creams, available ready-made in health-food stores, may relieve sunburn, as well as skin rashes such as eczema. The herb can also treat inflammation or infection of the eyes or mouth. Eyewashes made from the cooled tea may alleviate the redness or irritation of conjunctivitis and other eye inflammations; prepare a fresh batch of tea daily and store it in a sterile container. Used daily as a gargle or mouthwash, the tea can help heal mouth sores and prevent gum disease.

How to take it

⊘ **DOSAGE:** *To make a soothing cup of chamomile tea:* Pour a cup of very hot (not boiling) water over 2 teaspoons of dried flowers. Steep for five minutes and strain. Drink up to three cups a day or a cup at bedtime. The tea should be cooled thoroughly and kept sterile if you're using it on the skin or eyes. *For the skin:* Add a few drops of chamomile oil to half an ounce of almond oil (or another neutral oil) or buy a ready-made cream. Pills and tinctures are also available; follow package directions. A single pill, or up to 1 teaspoon of tincture, often has the therapeutic effects of a cup of tea.

◉ **GUIDELINES FOR USE:** Chamomile is gentle and can be used long term. It can be combined safely with prescription and over-the-counter drugs, as well as with other herbs and nutritional supplements. At recommended doses, the herb seems to be safe for children and pregnant and nursing women.

Possible side effects

Whether the herb is used internally or externally, side effects are extremely rare. Those taking higher-than-recommended doses of the herb have reported a few instances of nausea and vomiting. Though some red flags have been raised about possible allergic reactions, which cause bronchial tightness or skin rashes, these appear to be so rare that most people needn't worry about them.

FACTS & Tips

■ A chamomile bath can be relaxing—and provide relief for dry, irritated skin or sunburn. Add 10 drops of chamomile oil, or several cups of chamomile tea, to a cool bath and soak for half an hour or longer.

■ To treat burns, stick with chamomile creams or teas rather than greasy ointments. The latter contain oils that can trap the heat, slow healing, and increase the risk of infection. Creams, on the other hand, are made with a non-oily base.

SHOPPING HINTS

■ Pills and tinctures are formulated with concentrated extracts of chamomile. Buy standardized extracts that contain at least 1% apigenin, one of the herb's healing ingredients.

■ Check the labels of chamomile skin products carefully. Some feature the herb but contain only minuscule amounts. Buy creams or ointments that have at least 3% chamomile.

Did You Know?

Some people have successfully grown chamomile in their garden by simply tearing open a bag of chamomile tea and sprinkling its contents on the soil.

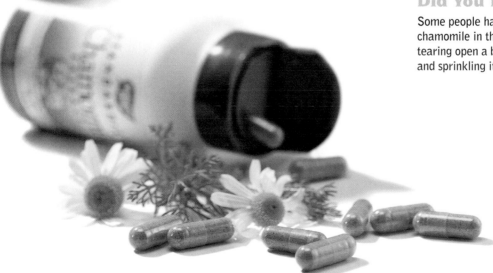

chasteberry

Vitex agnus-castus

Although chasteberry has been used since ancient times for menstrual complaints, European doctors first began prescribing it in the 1950s. Today, it has become the most commonly recommended herb in Europe to treat the symptoms of premenstrual syndrome (PMS).

COMMON USES

- *Alleviates symptoms of premenstrual syndrome (PMS).*
- *Regulates menstruation.*
- *Promotes fertility.*
- *Eases menopausal hot flashes.*

FORMS

- Tincture
- Tablet
- Capsule
- Dried herb/Tea

CAUTION!

- Chasteberry affects hormone production, so it should not be used by women taking hormonal medications, including birth control pills and estrogen, or by those who are pregnant.
- Reminder: If you have a medical condition, talk to your doctor before taking supplements.

What it is

Also called vitex, chaste tree berry, or monk's pepper, chasteberry is the fruit of the chaste tree. Actually a small shrub with violet flower spikes and long, slender leaves, the chaste tree is native to the Mediterranean region, but grows in subtropical climates throughout the world. Its red berries are harvested in the fall and then dried. They resemble peppercorns in shape, and the taste they impart to a therapeutic cup of tea is distinctively peppery.

What it does

The use of chasteberry for "female complaints" dates back to the time of Hippocrates. Although the herb does not actually contain hormones or hormonelike substances, it does spark the pituitary gland (located at the base of the brain) to send a signal to the ovaries to increase production of the female hormone progesterone. Chasteberry also inhibits the excessive production of prolactin, a hormone that primarily regulates breast-milk production but has other less-understood actions as well.

✪ **MAJOR BENEFITS:** Some scientists believe that women who routinely suffer from PMS produce too little progesterone in the last two weeks of their menstrual cycle. This deficiency causes an imbalance in the body's natural estrogen-progesterone ratio. Chasteberry helps restore hormonal equilibrium, relieving such PMS-related complaints as irritability, bloating, and depression. Studies in Germany indicate that the herb offers at least some relief for PMS symptoms in about 90% of women—and in one-third of them, the symptoms disappear. Chasteberry's prolactin-lowering action aids in reducing the breast pain and tenderness some women experience prior to menstruation, even if they have no other premenstrual symptoms.

The tiny dark red fruit of the chasteberry tree contains the herb's active ingredients.

ADDITIONAL BENEFITS: Because high levels of prolactin and low levels of progesterone in the body can inhibit monthly ovulation, chasteberry may be useful to those who are having trouble getting pregnant. The herb works best in women with mild or moderately low progesterone levels. When too much prolactin causes menstruation to stop (a condition called amenorrhea), the herb can help restore a normal monthly cycle.

Menopausal hot flashes are also the result of hormonal changes controlled by the pituitary gland, so women going through menopause may want to try chasteberry. Used either alone or in combination with other herbs such as dong quai or black cohosh, it can alleviate the periodic flushing and sweating that occur. Chasteberry is sometimes also recommended for menstrual-related acne.

How to take it

DOSAGE: Whether you are using chasteberry to treat PMS, breast tenderness, infertility, amenorrhea, or other menstrual disorders, the dose is the same. In tincture form, add ½ teaspoon twice a day to a glass of water. The equivalent dose for the powdered extract in tablet or capsule form is 225 mg, standardized to contain 0.5% agnuside (an active component in chasteberry). For menopausal hot flashes, take this same dosage (40 drops/225 mg) twice a day.

GUIDELINES FOR USE: Take chasteberry on an empty stomach to increase absorption; your first dose should always be taken in the morning. Even after just 10 days, a woman with PMS symptoms will probably notice at least some improvement during her next menstrual cycle. However, it may take three months of use to benefit from the full effect of this herb. Six months of treatment with chasteberry may be necessary to correct infertility or amenorrhea.

Possible side effects

Most people will not have any adverse side effects from taking chasteberry, but studies have shown that stomach irritation or an itchy rash can occur in a small percentage of women. Discontinue using it if you develop any rash. In addition, some women may experience an increased menstrual flow after taking this herb.

chromium

The second best-selling mineral supplement after calcium, chromium has been hyped as a fat burner, muscle builder, treatment for diabetes, and weapon against heart disease. Though this mineral is essential for growth and health, its more spectacular claims remain controversial.

COMMON USES

- *Essential for the breakdown of protein, fat, and carbohydrates.*
- *Helps the body maintain normal blood sugar (glucose) levels.*
- *May lower total blood cholesterol, LDL ("bad") cholesterol, and triglyceride levels.*
- *May enhance weight-loss efforts.*

FORMS

- Capsule
- Tablet
- Softgel
- Liquid

CAUTION!

- People with diabetes should consult their doctor before taking chromium. This mineral may alter the dosage for insulin or other diabetes medications.
- Reminder: If you have a medical condition, talk to your doctor before taking supplements.

What it is

Chromium is a trace mineral that comes in several chemical forms. Supplements usually contain chromium picolinate or chromium polynicotinate. Another type of chromium called chromium dinicotinic acid glutathione is found in brewer's yeast. Supplements may be worthwhile because many people today don't get enough chromium in their diet.

What it does

Chromium helps the body use insulin, a hormone that transfers blood sugar (glucose) to the cells, where it is burned as fuel. With enough chromium, the body uses insulin efficiently and maintains normal blood sugar levels. Chromium also aids the body in breaking down protein and fat.

PREVENTION: Getting sufficient chromium may prevent diabetes in people with insulin resistance. This disorder makes the body less sensitive to the effects of insulin, so the pancreas has to produce more and more of it to keep blood sugar (glucose) levels in check. When the pancreas can no longer keep up with the body's demand for extra insulin, type 2 diabetes develops. Chromium may help avert this progression by helping the body use insulin more effectively in the first place. Chromium also helps break down fats, so it may reduce LDL ("bad") and increase HDL ("good") cholesterol levels, reducing the risk of heart disease.

ADDITIONAL BENEFITS: Chromium may relieve headaches, irritability, and other symptoms of low blood sugar (hypoglycemia) by keeping blood sugar levels from dropping below normal. In people with diabetes, it may help control blood sugar levels. The mineral's most controversial claims relate to weight loss and muscle building. Though some studies indicate that large doses of chromium picolinate can aid in weight reduction or increase muscle mass, others have found no benefit. At best, the mineral may give you a slight edge in weight loss when combined with a sensible diet and regular exercise. But more research is needed to determine chromium's role in this regard.

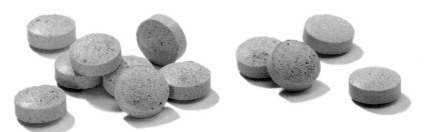

How much you need

No RDA has been established for chromium, but scientists believe that 50 to 200 mcg a day can prevent a deficiency. (But even on a healthy, varied diet, getting the high end of this recommendation would be difficult.)

⊖ **IF YOU GET TOO LITTLE:** A chromium deficiency can lead to inefficient use of glucose. In itself, a lack of chromium is probably not a cause of diabetes, but it can help precipitate the disease in those who are prone to it. In addition, anxiety, poor metabolism of amino acids, and high triglyceride and cholesterol levels may occur in individuals who don't get enough chromium.

⊕ **IF YOU GET TOO MUCH:** Chromium does not seem to have any adverse effects even at high doses, although there is some concern that megadoses can impair the absorption of iron and zinc. This can usually be corrected by getting extra iron or zinc through diet or supplements.

How to take it

▨ **DOSAGE:** Chromium supplements are generally available in 200 mcg doses. *For general good health:* Take 200 mcg a day. *As an aid to a weight-loss program:* Take 200 mcg twice a day. *To improve the effectiveness of insulin:* Use 200 mcg three times a day.

◉ **GUIDELINES FOR USE:** Take chromium in 200 mcg doses with food or a full glass of water to decrease stomach irritation. Chromium is better absorbed when combined with foods high in vitamin C (or taken with a vitamin C supplement). Calcium carbonate supplements or antacids can reduce chromium absorption.

Don't be confused by labels suggesting that one type of chromium—whether picolinate or polynicotinate—is absorbed better than any other. No reliable research supports these claims.

Other sources

Chromium is found in whole grains, whole grain breads and cereals, potatoes, prunes, peanut butter, nuts, seafood, and brewer's yeast. Low-fat diets tend to be higher in chromium than high-fat ones.

Did You Know?

Whole grain bread is a good source of chromium. Refined grains, found in white bread, contain little of this essential mineral.

coenzyme Q$_{10}$

Touted as a wonder supplement, coenzyme Q$_{10}$ is said to enhance stamina, help weight loss, combat cancer and AIDS, and even stave off aging. Although these claims may be extravagant, this nutrient does show promise for heart disease, weak gums, and other ailments.

COMMON USES

- *Improves the heart and circulation in those with congestive heart failure, a weakened heart muscle (cardiomyopathy), high blood pressure, heart rhythm disorders, chest pain (angina), or Raynaud's disease.*
- *Treats gum disease and maintains healthy gums and teeth.*
- *Protects the nerves and may help slow Alzheimer's or Parkinson's disease.*
- *May help prevent cancer and heart disease, and play a role in slowing down age-related degenerative changes.*
- *May improve the course of AIDS or cancer.*

FORMS

- Capsule
- Softgel
- Tablet
- Liquid

CAUTION!

- Pregnant or nursing women should be especially vigilant about checking with their doctor before using coenzyme Q$_{10}$; the nutrient has not been well studied in this group.
- Reminder: If you have a medical condition, talk to your doctor before taking supplements.

What it is

Coenzyme Q$_{10}$, a natural substance produced by the body, belongs to a family of compounds called quinones. When it was first isolated in 1957, scientists called it ubiquinone, because it is ubiquitous in nature. In fact, coenzyme Q$_{10}$ is found in all living creatures and is also concentrated in many foods, including nuts and oils. In the past decade, coenzyme Q$_{10}$ has become one of the most popular dietary supplements around the world. Proponents of the nutrient use it to maintain general good health, as well as to treat heart disease and a number of other serious conditions. Some clinicians believe it is so important for normal body functioning that it should be dubbed "vitamin Q."

What it does

The primary function of coenzyme Q$_{10}$ is as a catalyst for metabolism—the complex chain of chemical reactions during which food is broken down into packets of energy that the body can use. Acting in conjunction with enzymes (hence the name "coenzyme"), the compound speeds up the vital metabolic process, providing the energy that the cells need to digest food, heal wounds, maintain healthy muscles, and perform countless other bodily functions. Because of the nutrient's essential role in energy production, it's not surprising that it is found in every cell in the body. It is especially abundant in the energy-intensive cells of the heart, helping this organ beat more than 100,000 times each day. In addition, coenzyme Q$_{10}$ acts as an antioxidant, much like vitamins C and E, helping to neutralize the cell-damaging molecules known as free radicals.

PREVENTION: Coenzyme Q$_{10}$ may play a role in preventing cancer, heart attacks, and other diseases linked to free-radical damage. It's also used as a general energy enhancer and anti-aging supplement. Because

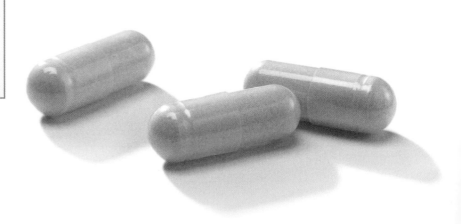

264

levels of the compound diminish with age (and with certain diseases), some doctors recommend daily supplementation beginning about age 40.

⊛ **MAJOR BENEFITS:** Coenzyme Q_{10} has generated much excitement as a possible therapy for heart disease, especially congestive heart failure or a weakened heart. In some studies, patients with a poorly functioning heart have been found to improve greatly after adding the supplement to their conventional drugs and therapies. Other studies have shown that people with cardiovascular disease have low levels of this substance in their heart. Further research suggests that coenzyme Q_{10} may help protect against blood clots, lower high blood pressure, diminish irregular heartbeats, treat mitral valve prolapse, lessen symptoms of Raynaud's disease (poor circulation in the extremities), and relieve chest pains (angina). If you have heart disease, talk with your doctor about taking this supplement. And remember: Coenzyme Q_{10} is intended as a complement to—and not as a replacement for—conventional medical treatments. Do not take this nutrient in place of heart drugs or other prescribed medications.

⊛ **ADDITIONAL BENEFITS:** A few small studies suggest that coenzyme Q_{10} may prolong survival in those with breast or prostate cancer, though results remain inconclusive. It also appears to aid healing and reduce pain and bleeding in those with gum disease, and speed recovery following oral surgery. The supplement shows some promise against Parkinson's and Alzheimer's diseases and fibromyalgia, and it may improve stamina in those with AIDS. Certain practitioners believe the nutrient helps stabilize blood sugar levels in people with diabetes. There are many other claims made for the supplement: that it slows aging, aids weight loss, enhances athletic performance, combats chronic fatigue syndrome, relieves multiple allergies, and boosts immunity. But more research is needed to determine the effectiveness of coenzyme Q_{10} for these and other conditions.

How to take it

⬗ **DOSAGE:** The general dosage is 50 mg twice a day. Higher dosages of 100 mg twice a day may be useful for heart or circulatory disorders, or for Alzheimer's disease and other specific complaints.

◈ **GUIDELINES FOR USE:** Take a supplement morning and evening, and ideally with food to enhance absorption. Coenzyme Q_{10} should be continued long term; it may require eight weeks or longer to notice results.

Possible side effects

Most research suggests that the supplement is harmless, even in large doses. In rare cases, it may cause upset stomach, diarrhea, nausea, or loss of appetite. But it appears to be very safe overall. Because coenzyme Q_{10} has not been extensively studied, however, check with your doctor before using it, especially if you are pregnant or nursing.

copper

Essential in preventing cardiovascular disease, maintaining good skin and hair color, and promoting fertility, copper is the least discussed but third most abundant trace mineral in the body. Even so, some experts believe that many people may be marginally deficient in this important nutrient.

What it is

Copper, the reddish brown malleable metal commonly used in cookware and plumbing, is also found in at least 15 proteins in the human body. This mineral is available in nutritional supplement form as copper aspartate, copper citrate, and copper picolinate. Although it can be obtained from a wide variety of foods, the typical American diet is low in copper, because the foods that are the best sources, such as oysters and liver, are not eaten frequently.

What it does

Copper is essential in the formation of collagen, a fundamental protein in bones, skin, and connective tissue. It also may help the body use its stored iron and play a role in maintaining immunity and fertility. Involved in the formation of melanin (a dark natural color found in the hair, skin, and eyes), copper promotes consistent pigmentation as well.

PREVENTION: Evidence suggests that copper can be a factor in preventing high blood pressure and heart rhythm disorders (arrhythmias). And some experts believe that it may protect tissues from damage by free radicals, helping to prevent cancer, heart disease, and other ailments. Getting enough copper may also help keep cholesterol levels low.

ADDITIONAL BENEFITS: Copper is necessary for the manufacture of many enzymes, especially superoxide dismutase (SOD), which appears to be one of the body's most potent antioxidants. It may also help stave off bone loss that can lead to osteoporosis.

How much you need

Although there is no daily RDA for copper, adults are advised to obtain 1.5 to 3 mg daily to keep the body functioning normally.

IF YOU GET TOO LITTLE: A true copper deficiency is rare. It usually occurs only in individuals with illnesses such as Crohn's disease or celiac

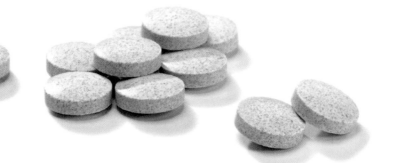

disease or in those with inherited conditions that inhibit copper absorption, such as albinism. Symptoms of deficiency are fatigue; heart rhythm disorders; brittle, discolored hair; high blood pressure; skeletal defects; and infertility.

But even a mild deficiency may have some adverse health effects. For example, a preliminary study involving 24 men found that a diet low in copper caused a significant increase in LDL ("bad") cholesterol and a decrease in HDL ("good") cholesterol. These changes in their cholesterol profile increased the participants' risk of heart disease.

⊕ **IF YOU GET TOO MUCH:** Just 10 mg of copper taken at one time can produce nausea, muscle pain, and stomachache. Severe copper toxicity from oral copper supplements has not been noted to date. However, some people who work with pesticides containing copper have suffered liver damage, coma, and even death.

How to take it

⊘ **DOSAGE:** Though there is no need to consume megadoses of copper, it is preferable to get amounts in the upper range of the recommended intake, 3 mg a day from food and supplements. If you take zinc supplements for longer than one month, add 2 mg of copper to your regimen. People who take antacids regularly may need extra copper as well.

◀ **GUIDELINES FOR USE:** It is advisable to take a supplement at the same time every day, preferably with a meal to decrease the chance of stomach irritation.

Other sources

Shellfish (oysters, lobsters, crabs) and organ meats (liver) are excellent sources of copper. However, if you're concerned about your cholesterol levels, there are many vegetarian foods rich in copper as well. These include legumes; whole grains, such as rye and wheat, and products made from them (bread, cereal, pasta); nuts and seeds; vegetables such as peas, artichokes, avocados, radishes, garlic, mushrooms, and potatoes; fruits such as tomatoes, bananas, and prunes; and soy products.

. . . .
SHOPPING HINTS

■ Individual copper supplements may be hard to find at the pharmacy or health-food store. Much more commonly this mineral is sold in combination with zinc. It's important to take extra copper when using zinc for longer than a month, because zinc interferes with the body's ability to absorb copper.

■ Ignore the label claims that one particular form of copper is better for you than another. There is no evidence that any one form (copper aspartate, copper citrate, or copper picolinate) is better absorbed than another or otherwise preferred by the body.
. . . .

LATEST FINDINGS

■ Copper may help prevent osteoporosis. In a recent study involving healthy women ages 45 to 56, those taking a daily 3 mg copper supplement showed no loss in mineral bone density, but women given a placebo showed a significant loss.

Did You Know?

You'd have to eat about **6 medium** avocados to get the **3 mg** of copper that you need to have each day.

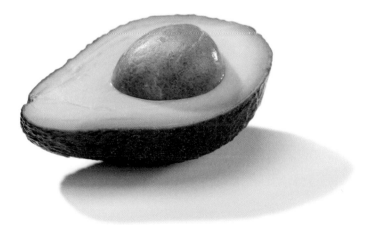

cranberry

Vaccinium macrocarpon

These tangy, ruby red berries, such an integral part of the American Thanksgiving tradition, have long been considered nature's cure for the urinary tract infections that frequently plague women of all ages. Modern science has now confirmed that this folk wisdom has real merit.

COMMON USES

- *Treats lower urinary tract infections (also called bladder infections or cystitis).*
- *May prevent recurrence of urinary tract infections.*
- *Helps deodorize urine.*

FORMS

- Capsule
- Tablet
- Softgel
- Liquid/Tincture
- Fresh or dried fruit
- Tea

CAUTION!

- Cranberry is not a substitute for antibiotics during an acute urinary tract infection (UTI). See your doctor if you don't feel better after 24 to 36 hours of using cranberry for a suspected UTI.
- See your doctor right away if symptoms include fever, chills, back pain, or blood in the urine, which may be signs of a kidney infection (upper UTI) requiring medical attention.
- Reminder: If you have a medical condition, talk to your doctor before taking supplements.

What it is

The cranberry, a native American plant closely related to the blueberry, has been used for centuries in both healing and cooking. The name is a shortened form of craneberry—the flowers of the low-growing shrub were thought to resemble the heads of the cranes that frequented the bogs where it grew. The berries are now widely cultivated throughout the United States, especially in Massachusetts and Washington. In early American medicine, cranberries were crushed and used as poultices for treating wounds and tumors, and also as a remedy for scurvy, a gum and bleeding disorder caused by a deficiency of vitamin C. In this century, medicinal interest in cranberry has focused on its important role in preventing and treating urinary tract infections (UTIs), which are caused by *E. coli* and other types of bacteria.

What it does

In the 1920s, it was discovered that people who consumed large amounts of cranberries produced a more acidic urine, and that the urine was purified in the process. During this purification process, a powerful substance

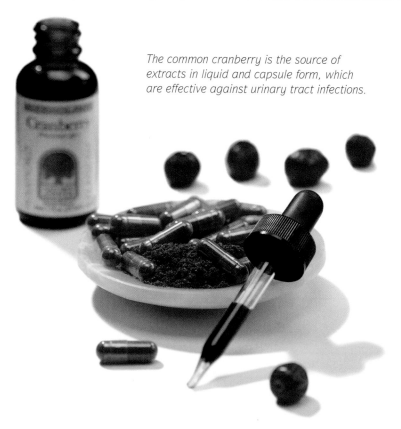

The common cranberry is the source of extracts in liquid and capsule form, which are effective against urinary tract infections.

called hippuric acid was created. It proved to have a strong antibiotic effect on the urinary tract. In fact, it discouraged and sometimes even eliminated harmful infection-causing bacteria.

More recent studies, however, indicate that cranberry's main infection-fighting capabilities may be due to a different property: Cranberry appears to inhibit the adhesion of harmful microorganisms to certain cells lining the urinary tract. This makes the environment a less hospitable place for *E. coli* and other bacteria to replicate, and thus reduces the likelihood of infection. Scientists have isolated two substances that produce this effect. One is fructose, a sugar that is found in many fruit juices. The other is a poorly understood compound present in cranberry and blueberry juices but absent from grapefruit, orange, guava, mango, and pineapple juices.

✪ **MAJOR BENEFITS:** Scientists have now confirmed the effectiveness of cranberry in preventing and treating UTIs. Several studies have shown that daily consumption of cranberry, either in juice or capsule form, dramatically reduces the recurrence of UTIs. Women are 10 times more likely to develop these infections than men—in fact, 25% to 35% of women ages 20 to 40 have had at least one. There's no reason, however, why men can't benefit from cranberry as well.

Cranberry also appears to shorten the course of urinary tract illness, helping to alleviate pain, burning, itching, and other symptoms. It's important to remember, though, that persistent UTIs should be treated promptly with antibiotics to prevent more serious complications. However, cranberry juice can be safely taken along with conventional drugs. It may even help hasten healing.

✱ **ADDITIONAL BENEFITS:** Because it helps deodorize urine, cranberry should be in the diet of anyone suffering from the embarrassing odors associated with incontinence. In addition, cranberry's high vitamin C content makes it a natural vitamin supplement.

How to take it

✐ **DOSAGE:** *To help treat urinary tract infections:* You should get about 800 mg of cranberry extract a day (two 400 mg pills). Or you can drink at least 16 ounces of undiluted juice a day or take it in tincture form (follow the package directions). *To prevent recurrences:* The dose can be cut in half to 400 mg of cranberry a day.

◆ **GUIDELINES FOR USE:** Cranberry can be taken with or without food. Drinking plenty of water or other fluids along with cranberry and throughout the day should speed recovery. Cranberry has no known interactions with antibiotics or other medications. But by acidifying the urine, cranberry may lessen the effect of another herb sometimes used for UTIs called uva ursi (also known as bearberry). Try one or the other.

Possible side effects

There are no known side effects from either the short-term or long-term use of cranberry. In addition, cranberry appears to be safe for pregnant and lactating women.

SHOPPING HINTS

■ For best medical effect, choose cranberry capsules or undiluted juice (which contains higher concentrations of the active ingredients) over presweetened juice. The processed commercial product (cranberry juice cocktail) is only one-third cranberry juice with added water and sweeteners to mask the berry's tart taste.

■ High-quality undiluted cranberry juice can be found at health-food stores. To make it more palatable, add sugar or other sweeteners to taste.

LATEST FINDINGS

■ A major study in the *Journal of the American Medical Association* looked at 153 elderly women (average age 78) who had no urinary tract symptoms. Half the women drank 300 ml (about a cup) of undiluted cranberry juice every day, and the other half received a placebo. After four to eight weeks, those who drank the cranberry juice were much less prone to urinary tract infections and had lower levels of potentially harmful bacteria in their urine.

■ Research confirms that cranberry is effective for younger as well older women. In a study in Utah, women ages 28 to 44 who took cranberry capsules (400 mg a day) for three months were only 40% as likely to have a urinary tract infection as the women who were given a placebo.

Did You Know?

You would have to eat 2 cups of fresh cranberries to get the equivalent of two 400 mg cranberry capsules.

dandelion

Taraxacum officinale

Known mostly as a persistent and prolific weed in the United States, dandelion is grown commercially in Europe. Its leaves and roots are a rich source of vitamins and minerals, and its active ingredients are particularly useful for treating digestive and liver problems.

COMMON USES

- Bolsters the liver; useful during cases of hepatitis (liver inflammation) and jaundice.
- Aids digestion by stimulating release of bile from the liver and gallbladder; may help prevent gallstones.
- Helps treat endometriosis.

FORMS

- Capsule
- Tablet
- Tincture
- Liquid
- Dried or fresh herb/Tea

What it is

Dandelion grows wild throughout much of the world and is cultivated in parts of Europe for medicinal uses. Closely related to chicory, this perennial plant can grow a foot high; its spatula-shaped leaves are shiny, hairless, and deeply toothed. The solitary yellow flower blooms for much of the growing season, opening at daybreak and closing at dusk and in wet weather (some cultures have used dandelions to signal the approach of rain). After the flower matures, the plant forms a puffball of seeds that are dispersed by the wind (or by playful children). Supplements usually contain the root (which is tapered and sweet tasting) or leaves, though the whole plant and flowers are also valued for their healing properties.

What it does

Folk healers have long prescribed dandelion for liver and digestive problems. Because its various active ingredients enhance the performance of the liver, this herb is useful for a wide range of disorders.

✪ **MAJOR BENEFITS:** Studies of dandelion's beneficial effects on the liver have shown that the herb increases the production and flow of bile (a digestive aid) from the liver and gallbladder, helping to treat such conditions as gallstones, jaundice, and hepatitis. It is thought that the plant's positive effect on various liver functions is probably related to its high content of the B vitamin choline.

Dandelion is sometimes mixed with other nutritional supplements that bolster liver function, including milk thistle, black radish, celandine, beet leaf, fringe tree bark, inositol, methionine, choline, or others. Such combinations are usually sold as liver or lipotropic ("fat-metabolizing") formulas in health-food stores.

Because it improves liver function, dandelion (in combination with other liver-strengthening nutrients) may be effective for relieving the pain and other symptoms of endometriosis. It also enhances the ability of the liver to remove excess estrogen from the body, thereby helping to restore a healthy balance of hormones in women who are afflicted with these disorders.

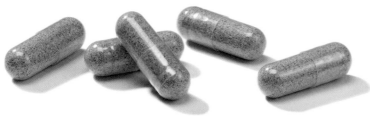

❋ ADDITIONAL BENEFITS: Dandelion root acts as a mild laxative, so a tea made from it may provide a gentle remedy for constipation. The herb may also enhance the body's ability to absorb iron from either food or supplements, which may help combat some cases of anemia. Some studies also indicate that dandelion may be of value in treating cancer. The Japanese have patented a freeze-dried extract of dandelion root to use against tumors; the Chinese are employing dandelion extracts in fighting breast cancer (a treatment supported by positive effects in animal studies). But additional studies need to be conducted in humans to determine the herb's true effectiveness against specific types of cancer.

As for other medical applications, studies have found that dandelion can lower blood sugar levels in animals, suggesting it may have some role to play in the treatment of diabetes. It may also have some diuretic effects, so it is sometimes given for water retention and bloating.

How to take it

⦿ DOSAGE: *To strengthen liver function in hepatitis, gallstones, and endometriosis:* Take 500 mg of a powdered solid dandelion root extract twice a day. This amount may also be found in some lipotropic (liver) combinations. Or take 1 or 2 teaspoons of a liquid dandelion extract three times a day. *For constipation:* Drink one cup of dandelion root tea three times a day. *For anemia:* Have 1 teaspoon of fresh dandelion juice or tincture each morning and evening with half a glass of water.

◉ GUIDELINES FOR USE: Drink fresh dandelion juice or liquid extract with water; take pills containing dandelion root extract with or without food. No adverse effects have been reported in pregnant or nursing women, though dandelion preparations may have diuretic effects, so this group of women may want to avoid the herb.

Possible side effects

Dandelion has no serious side effects. In large doses, it may cause a skin rash, upset stomach, or diarrhea. Stop using it if this happens, and discuss the reaction with your doctor.

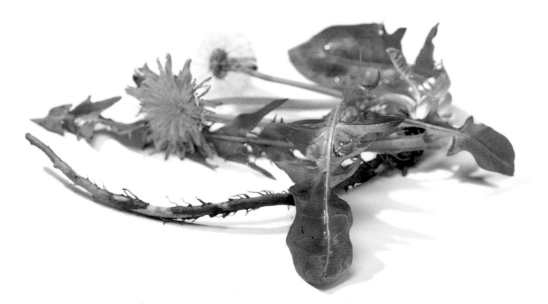

DHEA

Some advocates of DHEA call it the fountain of youth. Although the claim may be overblown, this hormone has shown promise in combating certain age-related diseases. More study is needed, however, to identify the exact effects of DHEA—as well as those who could benefit most from it.

What it is

Known as the "mother of hormones," DHEA (dehydroepiandrosterone) is needed by the body to produce many types of hormones including estrogen and testosterone. DHEA is secreted by the adrenal glands—located on top of the kidneys—as well as by the skin, brain, testicles, and ovaries. Although women make less DHEA than men, in both sexes DHEA production declines dramatically with age; levels are 80% lower at age 70 than at age 30. The significance of these falling DHEA levels, however, has not been determined.

What it does

There has been plenty of hype surrounding DHEA, so it is difficult to separate wishful thinking from sound scientific evidence. DHEA has been said to stimulate weight loss, increase libido, enhance memory, and prevent osteoporosis—but these claims are unsupported. Studies do indicate, however, that DHEA may improve general well-being in older people (although just how isn't clear), reduce the risk of heart disease, ease symptoms of the autoimmune disease lupus, help manage diabetes, and bolster immunity.

⭐ **MAJOR BENEFITS:** Having blood levels of DHEA on the high end of normal may lower the risk of heart disease for older men. In one study, men with naturally high DHEA levels had less body fat and higher HDL ("good") cholesterol levels than men with low DHEA levels. Those with high DHEA levels also did better on an exercise stress test, which measures the condition of the heart during physical exertion. These associations weren't seen in women, however. In fact, women taking DHEA seemed to have a slightly higher risk of heart disease. Other research suggests that DHEA may help "thin" the blood and so reduce the likelihood of blood clot formation and possible heart attack.

Some evidence of DHEA's immune-boosting action was noted in a study of older people who had received flu shots. Their immune response to the weakened flu virus in the injection was significantly increased after taking DHEA. Researchers are hopeful that DHEA can improve immune responses in people infected with HIV, the virus that causes AIDS.

✳ **ADDITIONAL BENEFITS:** A small study of postmenopausal women indicated that those taking DHEA had lower levels of triglycerides (a blood fat related to cholesterol) and were able to use insulin more efficiently than women not given DHEA. This finding suggests a possible role for the supplement in the treatment of diabetes.

DHEA has also been reported to have beneficial effects on patients with lupus, an autoimmune disease. It relieved some symptoms and reduced the amount of medication needed.

How to take it

▢ **DOSAGE:** DHEA supplements should be taken only to raise hormone levels to within a normal range—not to exceed those levels. Start with a low dose (5 mg for women; 10 mg for men) and slowly increase to achieve the desired effect. The maximum dose should not exceed 25 mg a day unless you are using it for a specific disorder, such as lupus or HIV. It's best to take DHEA in the morning. Healthy people under age 50 don't need the supplement at all.

◈ **GUIDELINES FOR USE:** Although DHEA is readily available in health-food stores and vitamin shops, it is more potent than many other nutrients or herbs. The long-term effects of DHEA supplementation are simply not known. Most experts believe you should take DHEA only under the supervision of a doctor, so try to find a physician familiar with the use of this nutritional supplement (see page 31).

Before taking DHEA, make sure your doctor checks for prostate cancer (men) or breast cancer (women), because such cancers are influenced by hormone levels in the body. Then, have a blood test to determine your current DHEA levels and use this supplement only if your blood level of this hormone is low. After three weeks, have another blood test to assess whether your dosage needs adjustment. Once obtained, a satisfactory blood level can often be maintained with as little as 5 to 10 mg of DHEA a week.

Possible side effects

When used to excess, DHEA supplements can cause acne, extremely oily skin, hair growth in women, deepening of the voice, and mood changes. In addition, one animal study demonstrated an association between liver cancer and excessively high doses of DHEA.

SHOPPING HINTS

■ The labels on wild yam products sometimes claim that the herb contains substances that are converted to DHEA or other hormones once within the body. In fact, this conversion can be achieved only in a laboratory, not by the human body.

LATEST FINDINGS

■ Although there's no evidence that DHEA will lengthen your life, it may enhance your quality of life. In a recent study, older men and women taking DHEA reported increased feelings of well-being, improved sleep, more energy, and a greater ability to handle stress. More than 80% of the women and 67% of the men had a positive response to DHEA, compared with less than 10% of the people taking a placebo.

dong quai

An ingredient in many herbal "women's supplements," dong quai, or angelica, is a traditional tonic used in Asia to aid the female reproductive system. Its popularity is second only to ginseng's in China and Japan, but Western experts continue to debate the effectiveness of this herb.

Angelica sinensis
A. acutiloba

What it is

Although dong quai grows wild in Asia, it's also widely cultivated for medicinal purposes in China (the *Angelica sinensis* variety) and in Japan (*A. acutiloba*), where many women take it daily to maintain overall good health. The most widely available therapeutic form is derived from the root of *A. sinensis,* a plant with hollow stems that grows up to eight feet tall and has clusters of white flowers. When it's in bloom, angelica resembles Queen Anne's lace, its botanical relative. Other names for dong quai include dang gui, tang kuie, and Chinese angelica.

What it does

Generally, dong quai is believed to keep the uterus healthy and to regulate the menstrual cycle. It may also widen blood vessels and increase blood flow to various organs. Even among herbal experts, however, questions linger about its benefits. One reason dong quai has been difficult to assess is that it is often taken in combination with other herbs.

✪ **MAJOR BENEFITS:** Traditionally, dong quai has been used for menstrual and menopausal difficulties. Claims for the herb include balancing the menstrual cycle, correcting abnormal bleeding patterns, alleviating symptoms of premenstrual syndrome (PMS), easing menstrual cramps, reducing menopausal hot flashes, and improving the vaginal dryness associated with menopause.

There are two theories about how dong quai may help relieve these problems. Some herbalists believe it contains plant estrogens (phytoestrogens), which are weaker than estrogens produced by the body but which still chemically bind with estrogen receptors in human cells. Because of this, phytoestrogens may minimize the potential negative effects of a woman's own estrogen, which include an increased risk of breast cancer. Phytoestrogens also may prevent hot flashes by compensating for the decline in estrogen levels that occurs after menopause.

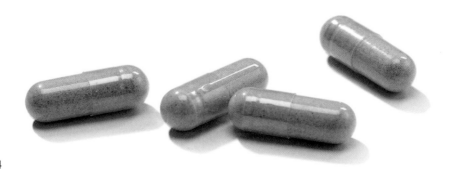

Other experts attribute the effectiveness of dong quai to its abundance of coumarins. This group of natural chemicals dilates blood vessels, increases blood flow to the uterus and other organs, and stimulates the central nervous system. Coumarins also appear to reduce inflammation and muscle spasms, which may account for dong quai's ability to reduce the severity of menstrual cramps.

✳ **ADDITIONAL BENEFITS:** Although dong quai is not typically used to lower blood pressure, it does have this effect because it dilates blood vessels, making it easier for the heart to pump blood through the body. The herb is also rich in vitamin B_{12}, and so may help build red blood cells.

How to take it

📄 **DOSAGE:** *For PMS, menstrual irregularities, menstrual cramps, or hot flashes:* Be sure to get 600 mg of dong quai daily. (Available too from 30 drops (1.5 ml) of tincture three times a day.) In either pill or liquid form, extracts should be standardized to contain 0.8% to 1.1% ligustilide. You can also use a single preparation in which dong quai is combined with such menstrual-regulating herbs as chasteberry, licorice, and Siberian ginseng.

◆ **GUIDELINES FOR USE:** For symptoms of PMS, use dong quai on the days you're not menstruating. If you also get menstrual cramps, continue using dong quai until menstruation stops. For cramps without PMS, begin taking dong quai the day before your period is due. For hot flashes, use it daily. Continue the herb for two months before deciding if it works.

Possible side effects

Dong quai may have a mild laxative effect and may promote heavy menstrual bleeding. Protect yourself from the sun when using dong quai, because its root contains compounds called psoralens that can make some people more sensitive to sunlight and cause a severe sunburn.

SHOPPING HINTS

■ If you want to try dong quai for menstrual cramps or menopausal symptoms, make sure to purchase Chinese or Japanese angelica *(Angelica sinensis* or *A. acutiloba).* Traditionally, the American and European angelicas *(A. archangelica* or *A. atropurpurea)* have both been widely used for respiratory ailments and stomach upset, but they have shown no real effect for gynecological problems.

LATEST FINDINGS

■ A recent study found dong quai was no better than a placebo as a remedy for hot flashes and other menopausal problems, such as vaginal dryness. Both dong quai and the placebo reduced the frequency of hot flashes by 25% to 30%. But this study tested the effect of dong quai alone. In Asia, it is traditionally used in combination with other herbs.

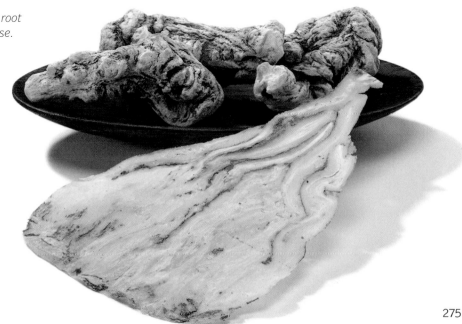

Dong quai's naturally gnarled root is flattened out for medicinal use.

echinacea

Long used by Native Americans, midwestern settlers, and earlier generations of doctors, this herb fell out of favor with the advent of modern antibiotics. But echinacea is regaining popularity as a safe and powerful immune-system booster to fight colds, flu, and other infections.

Echinacea angustifolia
E. purpurea
E. pallida

COMMON USES

- *Reduces the body's susceptibility to colds and flu.*
- *Limits the duration and severity of infections.*
- *Helps fight recurrent respiratory, middle ear, urinary tract, and vaginal yeast infections.*
- *Speeds the healing of skin wounds and inflammations.*

FORMS

- Capsule
- Tablet
- Softgel
- Lozenge
- Tincture
- Liquid
- Dried herb/Tea

CAUTION!

- If you're taking antibiotics or other drugs for an infection, use echinacea as an addition to, not as a replacement for, those medications.
- Echinacea can overstimulate the immune system and may worsen symptoms of lupus, multiple sclerosis, rheumatoid arthritis, or other autoimmune disorders. It may also be counterproductive in progressive infections such as tuberculosis.
- Reminder: If you have a medical condition, talk to your doctor before taking supplements.

What it is

Also known as the purple, or prairie, coneflower, echinacea (pronounced ek-in-NAY-sha) is a wildflower with daisylike purple blossoms native to the grasslands of the central United States. For centuries, the Plains tribes used the plant to heal wounds and to counteract the toxins of snakebites. The herb also became popular with European-American pioneers and their physicians, who considered it an all-purpose infection fighter.

Of the nine echinacea species, three *(Echinacea angustifolia, E. pallida, and E. purpurea)* are used medicinally. They appear in literally hundreds of commercial preparations, which utilize different parts of the plant (flowers, leaves, stems, or roots) and come in a variety of forms. Echinacea contains many active ingredients thought to strengthen the immune system, and in recent years, it has become one of the most popular herbal remedies in the world.

What it does

A natural antibiotic and infection fighter, echinacea helps to kill bacteria, viruses, fungi, and other disease-causing microbes. It acts by stimulating various immune-system cells that are key weapons against infection. In addition, the herb boosts the cells' production of an innate virus-fighting substance called interferon. Because these effects are relatively short-lived, however, the herb is best administered at frequent intervals—as often as every couple of hours during acute infections.

PREVENTION: Echinacea can help prevent the two most common viral ailments—colds and flu. It is most effective when taken at the first hint of illness. In one study of people who were susceptible to colds, those who used the herb for eight weeks were 35% less likely to come down with a cold than those given a placebo. Furthermore, they caught colds less often—40 days elapsed between infections, versus 25 days for the placebo group. Studies confirm that echinacea is also useful if you're already suffering from the aches, pains, congestion, or fever of colds or flu. Overall, symptoms are less severe and subside sooner.

ADDITIONAL BENEFITS: Echinacea may be of value for recurrent ailments, including vaginal yeast, urinary tract, and middle ear infections. It is also sometimes used to treat strep throat, staph infections, herpes infections (including genital herpes, cold sores, and shingles), bronchitis, and sinus infections. Moreover, the herb is being studied as a possible treatment for chronic fatigue syndrome and AIDS. And it may prove effective against some types of cancer, particularly in patients whose immune systems are depressed by radiation treatments or chemotherapy.

Echinacea can be applied to the skin as well. Its juice promotes the healing of all kinds of wounds, boils, abscesses, eczema, burns, canker or cold sores, and bedsores. To treat a sore throat or tonsillitis, the tincture can be diluted and used as a gargle.

How to take it

🖊 **DOSAGE:** Because echinacea comes in many different forms, check the product's label for the proper dosage. *For colds and flu:* A high dose is needed—up to 200 mg five a times a day. In one major study, patients with the flu who were given 900 mg of echinacea a day did better than those who received either a lower dosage of 450 mg a day or a placebo. *For other infections:* The recommended dose is 200 mg three or four times a day. *For long-term use as a general immune booster:* To derive the most benefits, especially for those prone to chronic infections, alternate echinacea every three weeks with other immune-enhancing herbs, including goldenseal, astragalus, pau d'arco, and medicinal mushrooms. Echinacea teas, often blended with other herbs, are available as well.

🔷 **GUIDELINES FOR USE:** Echinacea should be used no longer than eight weeks, followed by a one-week interval before you resume taking it. Some studies suggest that with continuous use, the herb's immunity-boosting effects diminish. Starting and stopping echinacea, or rotating it with other herbs, may maximize its effectiveness. You can take it with or without food.

Possible side effects

At recommended doses, echinacea has no known side effects, and no adverse reactions have been reported in pregnant or nursing women. However, people who are allergic to flowers in the daisy family may also be allergic to this herb. If you develop a skin rash or have trouble breathing, call your doctor right away.

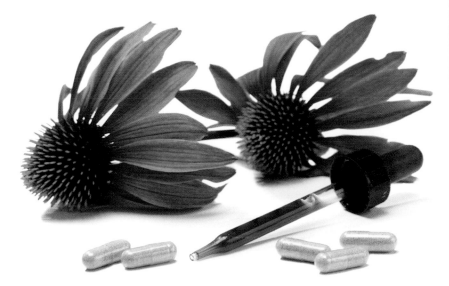

SHOPPING HINTS

■ Buying echinacea can be confusing because it comes in so many different forms. Experts often recommend a liquid—either the fresh-pressed juice (standardized to contain 2.4% beta-1, 2-fructofuranosides) or an alcohol-based tincture (containing a 5:1 concentration of the herb). Those who dislike the bitter taste of the liquids can take standardized extracts in pill form. Look for pills containing at least 3.5% echinacosides.

■ Some commercial preparations combine echinacea with another immune-enhancing herb called goldenseal, but the combination can be very pricey. For many ailments, just plain echinacea works fine, so you can skip the more costly mixture.

LATEST FINDINGS

■ Scientists are investigating whether echinacea may also be helpful against cancer. In a recent study in Germany, a small group of patients with advanced colon cancer received echinacea along with standard chemotherapy. The herb appeared to prolong survival in these patients, presumably by boosting the immune system's ability to fight cancer cells. Additional research is needed to define the possible role of this herb in combating colon and other forms of cancer.

Did You Know?

Echinacea contains a substance that makes the lips and tongue tingle when taken in liquid form. If you use a liquid preparation, look for this effect—it's often a good indication that you've bought a high-quality product.

ephedra

Sometimes called the world's oldest medicine, this herb has been used in China to treat colds and asthma since 3000 B.C. It's still considered an effective remedy for bronchial disorders, but concerns about safety have made ephedra controversial in recent years.

Ephedra sinica
E. intermedia
E. equisetina

COMMON USES

- *Eases congestion and labored breathing that are caused by allergies or asthma.*
- *Relieves pressure and congestion in sinus infections (sinusitis).*
- *May aid weight loss.*

FORMS

- Capsule
- Tablet
- Tincture
- Dried herb/Tea

CAUTION!

- Ephedra can cause blood pressure to soar. Check with your doctor if you have high blood pressure, heart disease, or heart rhythm disorders or take MAO inhibitors for depression.
- Ephedra can elevate blood sugar. People with diabetes should use it with caution.
- Talk to your doctor if you have thyroid disease, difficulty urinating from prostate problems, or are pregnant or breast-feeding.
- Reminder: If you have a medical problem, talk to your doctor before taking supplements.

What it is

Also known by its Chinese name *Ma huang*, ephedra is made from the dried stems of *Ephedra sinica*, a shrub native to desert regions of Asia. However, preparations from species such as *E. intermedia* or *E. equisetina* may also be effective. A synthetic version of ephedra's active ingredients is widely used in both prescription and over-the-counter drugs, including hundreds of cold, allergy, asthma, weight-loss, and energy-boosting formulas. Unfortunately, the herb has been abused in recent years, when some people began taking very high doses as a recreational stimulant—leading to heart attacks, strokes, and at least 28 deaths. As a result, the FDA considered banning the supplement in 1996. Though a ban was not imposed, the FDA has since proposed that all ephedra preparations carry a warning label.

What it does

Ephedra's primary active ingredients, the chemicals ephedrine and pseudo-ephedrine, have two major effects: They stimulate the central nervous system and they open the airways. Ephedra's stimulant effect is stronger than that of caffeine, but less potent than that of amphetamines or that of the natural adrenal hormone epinephrine (adrenaline), which prepares the body for stressful situations (the "fight-or-flight" response).

Ephedra makes the heart beat faster, increases blood pressure, speeds up the metabolism, and acts as a diuretic. But throughout its long history its main use has been as a bronchodilator, to treat the bronchial and nasal congestion of asthma, allergies, colds, and sinus infections. In the 1920s, U.S. drug companies began extracting active ingredients from the herb and using it in asthma and cold medicines—a practice that many companies still follow today.

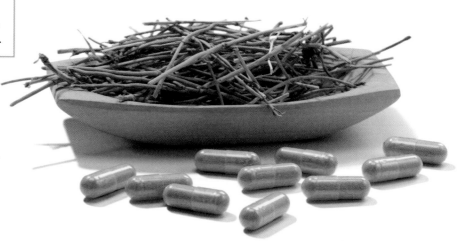

The dried stems of ephedra are made into capsules that have many therapeutic benefits.

* **MAJOR BENEFITS:** Ephedra dilates the small airways in the lungs (the bronchioles), which helps relieve congestion and coughing due to seasonal allergies or to mild asthma. It also plays a role in alleviating respiratory symptoms caused by colds, flu, and sinus infections.

* **ADDITIONAL BENEFITS:** Some weight-loss supplements claim that ephedra, usually in combination with St. John's wort, is an "herbal fen-phen," a natural alternative to the antiobesity prescription drugs fenfluramine (now banned for possibly causing heart disease) and phentermine. Though ephedra may make the body burn calories quickly and suppress appetite, studies of this herb as a weight-loss aid have been contradictory. For those in otherwise good health, it may be safe and effective in recommended doses.

More controversial is the claim that ephedra enhances athletic performance by boosting energy. Not only is there no scientific basis for this theory, but it has had tragic consequences: A number of athletes have become seriously ill—and several have died—after taking large doses of products containing ephedra. The herb is currently listed as a banned substance by the U.S. Olympic Committee.

How to take it

* **DOSAGE:** Check your bottle's label to see how much ephedrine is contained in each dose of ephedra. Most standardized extracts supply about 5.5% to 6.5% ephedrine (also known as "ephedra alkaloids"). Begin with a low daily dose, such as 100 mg of ephedra (about 6 mg of ephedrine). If side effects aren't a problem, increase the dose, but don't exceed 130 mg of ephedra (about 8 mg of ephedrine) three times a day.

To make a tea, pour 1 cup of very hot water over 1 teaspoon of dried ephedra (along with other herbs if desired) and steep for 10 to 15 minutes; drink one or two cups a day. Or take ¼ to 1 teaspoon ephedra tincture (up to 8 mg of ephedrine) in a glass of water up to three times daily.

* **GUIDELINES FOR USE:** Check with your doctor before using ephedra, especially if you have heart disease, diabetes, or other medical problems, or if your symptoms do not improve. Never exceed the recommended dose. This herb can be taken long term for certain conditions, such as chronic asthma, but try to use it only as needed—up to seven days at a time—to minimize the chance of side effects. Ephedra may be safely combined with many other herbs, including St. John's wort. But avoid taking it with caffeine, which can cause excessive stimulation. If it promotes insomnia, omit your evening dose.

Possible side effects

The higher the dose and the longer you take ephedra, the greater the incidence of such common side effects as nervousness, insomnia, heart palpitations, and paleness. Less often there may be dizziness, tingling, nausea and vomiting, loss of appetite, muscle cramps, headache, and difficult or painful urination. Extremely serious side effects include high blood pressure, stroke, seizures, and with very high doses, hallucinations and psychosis.

evening primrose oil

Native Americans and the early settlers valued the evening primrose plant for its healing powers. Today, research focuses on the therapeutic effect of the oil from its seeds, which contain a special fat called gamma-linolenic acid (GLA).

Oenothera biennis

COMMON USES

- *Eases rheumatoid arthritis pain.*
- *Can minimize symptoms of diabetic nerve damage.*
- *Relieves eczema symptoms.*
- *Helps treat premenstrual syndrome, endometriosis, and menstrual cramps.*
- *Lessens inflammation of acne, rosacea, and muscle strains.*

FORMS

- Capsule
- Softgel
- Oil

CAUTION!

- Reminder: If you have a medical condition, talk to your doctor before taking supplements.

What it is

Called evening primrose because its light yellow flowers open at dusk, this wildflower grows in North America and Europe. The plant and its root have long been used for medicinal purposes—to treat bruises, hemorrhoids, sore throat, and stomachaches. But the use of its seed oil, which contains gamma-linolenic acid (GLA), is relatively recent. GLA is an essential fatty acid that the body converts to hormonelike compounds called prostaglandins, which regulate a number of bodily functions.

Although the body can make GLA from other types of fat you consume, there is no one food that has appreciable amounts of GLA. Evening primrose oil provides a concentrated source: 7% to 10% of its fatty acids are in the form of GLA. There are, however, other sources of GLA. Borage seed oil and black currant seed oil contain higher amounts of GLA—20% to 26% for borage; 14% to 19% for black currant—than evening primrose oil, but they also have a higher percentage of other fatty acids that may interfere with GLA absorption. Most of the studies investigating the effects of GLA have used evening primrose oil, and for this reason it is the preferred source of GLA. Still, borage oil may be a good substitute: It is less expensive than evening primrose oil, and a lower dose is required to produce a therapeutic effect.

What it does

The body produces several types of prostaglandins: Some promote inflammation, others control it. The GLA in evening primrose oil is directly converted to important anti-inflammatory prostaglandins, which accounts for most of the supplement's therapeutic effects. In addition, GLA is an important component of cell membranes.

Although evening primrose oil comes in liquid form, softgels may be a more convenient way to take it.

PREVENTION: In people with diabetes, the GLA in evening primrose oil has been shown to help prevent nerve damage (neuropathy), a common complication of the disease. In a study of people with mild diabetic neuropathy, one year of treatment with evening primrose oil reduced numbness and tingling, loss of sensation, and other symptoms of the disorder better than a placebo did, suggesting that evening primrose may be of value in reversing neuropathy.

ADDITIONAL BENEFITS: One of the leading uses for evening primrose oil is to treat eczema, an allergic skin condition that may develop if the body has trouble converting fats from food into GLA. Studies of people with eczema indicate that taking evening primrose oil for three to four months can help alleviate itching and reduce the need for topical steroid creams and drugs with unpleasant side effects.

Because of its GLA content, evening primrose oil can be effective for menstrual disorders, such as PMS, menstrual cramps, and endometriosis. In particular, the oil blocks the inflammatory prostaglandins that cause menstrual cramps. It also appears to ease the breast tenderness that some women experience just before their periods and may play a role in reversing infertility in some women.

Rheumatoid arthritis is characterized by joint pain and swelling, and studies have found that these symptoms improve with the supplementation of evening primrose oil or another source of GLA. Conditions that involve inflammation, such as rosacea, acne, and muscle strain, can also benefit from evening primrose oil.

How to take it

DOSAGE: The recommended therapeutic dose for evening primrose oil is generally 1,000 mg three times a day. This supplies 240 mg of GLA a day. To get an equivalent amount of GLA from other sources, you would need to take 1,000 mg of borage oil or 1,500 mg of black currant oil each day. Evening primrose oil or borage oil can also be applied topically to the fingers to ease the symptoms of Raynaud's disease.

GUIDELINES FOR USE: Take evening primrose oil or other sources of GLA with meals to enhance absorption.

Possible side effects

In studies, about 2% of the participants using evening primrose oil experienced bloating or abdominal upset. However, consuming it with food may lessen this effect.

LATEST FINDINGS

■ In a study of 60 people with eczema, GLA—the essential fatty acid in evening primrose oil that accounts for its therapeutic benefits—was found to be superior to a placebo in reducing the itching and oozing of the condition. Those in the GLA group took 274 mg twice a day (an amount found in approximately seven 1,000 mg evening primrose capsules) for 12 weeks. Examinations by a dermatologist every four weeks confirmed the gradual improvement of symptoms reported by these patients.

■ A study from the University of Massachusetts Medical Center showed that very high doses of GLA in the form of borage oil (2.4 grams of GLA a day) reduced damage to joint tissue in people with rheumatoid arthritis. As a result, they had less joint pain and swelling.

feverfew

Tanacetum parthenium

Despite its name, feverfew is not a fever reducer but a migraine preventive. Though for centuries this herb was relied on for headaches, stomach problems, and menstrual irregularities, feverfew virtually disappeared from use until reports calling it a migraine cure began appearing in the late 1970s.

COMMON USES

- ■ *Helps prevent or reduce the intensity of migraines.*
- ■ *May ease menstrual complaints.*

FORMS

- ■ Capsule
- ■ Tablet
- ■ Tincture
- ■ Dried herb/Tea

CAUTION!

- ■ Pregnant women should avoid feverfew because it may cause contractions of the uterus. Women who are breast-feeding should also not use the herb.
- ■ Because feverfew may inhibit blood clotting, check with your doctor before using it if you are taking anticoagulant drugs.
- ■ Reminder: If you have a medical condition, talk to your doctor before taking supplements.

What it is

Recently celebrated for its effect on migraines, feverfew (also known as featherfew or febrifuge) is a member of the flower family that includes daisies and sunflowers. With its bright yellow and white blossoms and feathery yellow-green leaves, this herb resembles chamomile and is often mistaken for it. The leaves are used medicinally, and although the flowers have no health benefits, they do emit a strong aroma. In the Middle Ages, the plant was believed to purify the air and prevent malaria and other life-threatening diseases. Although feverfew probably can't kill germs in the atmosphere, the odor apparently is quite offensive to bees and bugs, and so feverfew planted in your garden can act as a natural insect repellent.

What it does

The active compound in feverfew (a chemical called parthenolide) seems to block substances in the body that widen and constrict blood vessels and cause inflammation.

🛡 **PREVENTION:** Though the exact cause of migraines is unknown, some experts think these headaches occur when blood vessels in the head constrict and then rapidly dilate. Such a dramatic change can trigger the release of chemicals stored in platelets (the small blood cells involved in blood clotting) that cause pain and inflammation. Researchers speculate that feverfew prevents the sudden dilation of blood vessels, and so inhibits the release of those chemicals. Though this action makes feverfew a good migraine preventive, the herb cannot relieve a migraine once it occurs.

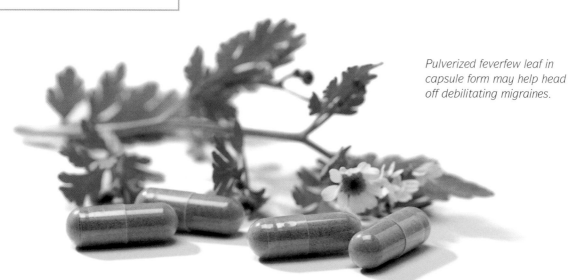

Pulverized feverfew leaf in capsule form may help head off debilitating migraines.

Word of mouth among people with chronic migraines led to widespread use of feverfew beginning in the 1970s. To determine the herb's effectiveness, British researchers recruited migraine sufferers who had already been using feverfew regularly. The researchers then divided them into two sections: One continued to take feverfew, and the other was given a placebo. Those on the placebo pills soon experienced more frequent, and more intense headaches, but those in the feverfew group had no increase in migraine occurrences. Another study showed that feverfew reduced the number of migraines by 24% and that even when the headaches did occur, they were much less severe. The results of these and other studies have led health authorities in Canada and other countries to approve the use of feverfew for migraine prevention.

✳ **ADDITIONAL BENEFITS:** Feverfew has long been used for menstrual complaints. The herb inhibits the production of prostaglandins, hormone-like substances that can cause pain and inflammation. Because menstrual cramps result from an excess of prostaglandins produced by the lining of the uterus, feverfew may still be suitable for this problem.

The anti-inflammatory action of the herb also led to its use as a treatment for the inflamed, sore joints that occur in rheumatoid arthritis (RA). However, a study of RA patients found no additional benefit from taking feverfew in conjunction with medications that are commonly prescribed for this condition. No studies have been done on how the herb might work alone, or in combination with other herbal treatments for RA.

How to take it

◑ **DOSAGE:** For migraines, a dose of 250 mg a day of a feverfew product standardized to contain at least 0.4% parthenolide is typical.

◈ **GUIDELINES FOR USE:** The experience of the migraine sufferers in the British study cited above underscores the importance of taking feverfew daily for an extended time, because stopping the herb may lead to a resumption of headaches.

Possible side effects

Few side effects have been noted, even when feverfew is used long term. There have been reports of sores and inflammation of the mucous membranes of the mouth, but this reaction seems to be limited to people who chew the fresh leaves (a common practice before feverfew supplements became available). Some people experience stomach upset from both the fresh leaves and supplements. Skin contact with the plant can cause a rash; anyone who develops a rash after touching feverfew should not use the product internally.

C·a·s·e H·i·s·t·o·r·y

A MIGRAINE PREVENTIVE

For a while, Nick L. considered the pricey new migraine medications nothing short of wonder drugs because of their amazing ability to stop the dizzying pain of his headaches. But what he really wanted was something that could prevent a migraine from starting. His doctor offered other drugs, but their side effects were troublesome. "Sure, the beta-blockers headed off my migraines," Nick remembers, "but my sex life vanished too." He tried several types, but the result was always the same.

During a trip to London, he saw a shop sign: "Migraine Sufferers—We have feverfew in stock." Though he was skeptical of herbal therapies, he bought a bottle, which sat unopened in his medicine chest for six months.

Then he read an article affirming the safety and effectiveness of feverfew. He decided to give it a try and took two capsules with his daily vitamin. "From that point on, it was a migraine-free year," he says. "My first since childhood."

fish oils

Scientists noticed a curiously low incidence of heart disease among Greenland Eskimos despite their high-fat diet. The reason? They were eating fish rich in omega-3 fatty acids. Later studies confirmed the cardioprotective effect of fish oils while uncovering other benefits as well.

What it is

The fat in fish has a form of polyunsaturated fatty acids called omega-3s. These differ from the polyunsaturated fatty acids found in vegetable oils (called omega-6s), and they have different effects on the body. (Fish don't manufacture such fats but get them from the plankton they eat—the colder the water, the more omega-3s the plankton contains.) The two most potent forms of omega-3s, eicosapentaenoic acid (EPA) and docosahexanoic acid (DHA), are found in abundance in cold-water fish such as salmon, trout, mackerel, and tuna (including the canned variety). The sources of a third type of omega-3, alpha-linolenic acid (ALA), are certain vegetable oils (such as flaxseed oil) and leafy greens (such as purslane). However, ALA doesn't affect the body in the same way that EPA and DHA do.

What it does

Omega-3s play a key role in a range of vital body processes, from blood pressure and blood clotting to inflammation and immunity. They may be useful for preventing or treating many diseases and disorders.

PREVENTION: Fish oils appear to reduce the risk of heart disease. They do this in several ways. Most importantly, the presence of omega-3s makes platelets in the blood less likely to clump together and form the clots that lead to heart attacks. Next, omega-3s can reduce triglycerides (blood fats related to cholesterol) and may lower blood pressure. In addition, recent research has shown that omega-3s strengthen the heart's electrical system, preventing heart-rhythm abnormalities. However, the strongest evidence for the cardiovascular benefits of fish oils comes from studies in which the participants ate fish rather than taking fish oil supplements.

Within the artery walls, omega-3s inhibit inflammation, which is a factor in plaque buildup. As a result, therapeutic doses of fish oils are one of the few successful ways to prevent the reblockage of arteries that commonly occurs after angioplasty, a procedure in which a small balloon is guided through an artery to a blockage and then is inflated to compress plaque, widen the vessel, and improve blood flow to the heart. This effect on blood vessels makes fish oils helpful for Raynaud's disease as well.

ADDITIONAL BENEFITS: Omega-3s are also effective general anti-inflammatories, useful for joint problems, lupus, and psoriasis. Studies indicate that people with rheumatoid arthritis experience less joint swelling and stiffness, and may even be able to manage on lower doses of anti-inflammatory drugs, when they take fish oil supplements. In a yearlong study of people with Crohn's disease (a painful type of inflammatory bowel disease), 69% of those taking enteric-coated fish oil supplements (about 3 grams of fish oils a day) stayed symptom-free, compared with just 28% of those receiving a placebo. Fish oils may also help ease menstrual cramps. In addition, omega-3s may play a role in mental health. Some experts believe there's a correlation between the increasing incidence of depression in the United States and the declining consumption of fish. And a preliminary study suggested that omega-3 fatty acids may reduce the severity of schizophrenia by about 25%.

How to take it

⊘ **DOSAGE:** *For heart disease, Raynaud's disease, lupus, and psoriasis:* Take 3,000 mg of fish oils a day. *For rheumatoid arthritis:* Take 6,000 mg a day. *For inflammatory bowel disease:* Take 5,000 mg a day.

◉ **GUIDELINES FOR USE:** Fish oil supplements are not necessary for heart disease prevention or treatment if you eat fish at least twice a week. However, supplements are recommended for rheumatoid arthritis and other inflammatory conditions. Take capsules with meals. Supplements may be easier to tolerate if you take them in divided doses; for example, 1,000 mg three times a day, instead of 3,000 mg in one sitting.

Possible side effects

Fish oil capsules may cause belching, flatulence, bloating, nausea, and diarrhea. Very high doses may result in a slightly fishy body odor. There's some concern high doses can lead to internal bleeding. But a study of people with heart disease who took 8,000 mg of fish oil supplements in addition to aspirin (an anticoagulant) found no increase in internal bleeding.

Some studies found high doses of fish oils worsen blood sugar control in people with diabetes; others have shown no effect. To be safe, people with diabetes should not take more than 2,000 mg of fish oil supplements a day without the advice of their doctor.

Individuals with high fasting triglycerides should be careful if they also have high LDL ("bad") cholesterol: Therapeutic doses of fish oils can increase LDL. Garlic supplements, however, may be the remedy. One study found garlic reversed the fish oils' LDL-raising effect. For rheumatoid arthritis and other inflammatory conditions, eating fish is probably not sufficient, and fish oil supplements are recommended.

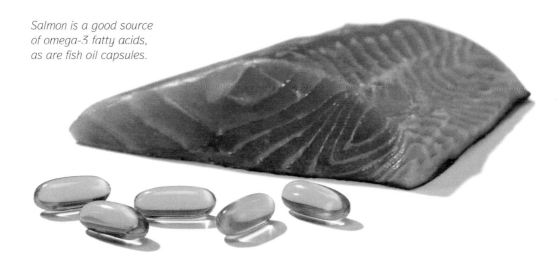

Salmon is a good source of omega-3 fatty acids, as are fish oil capsules.

5-HTP

Americans suffering from depression, insomnia, migraines, or obesity have a new supplement to consider: 5-HTP. Unlike its close chemical cousin, the amino acid tryptophan, which was recalled for safety concerns, 5-HTP appears to be safe—and it may be even more effective.

What it is

The nutrient 5-HTP, short for 5-hydroxytryptophan, is a derivative of the amino acid tryptophan, which is found in such high-protein foods as beef, chicken, fish, and dairy products. The body makes 5-HTP from the tryptophan present in our diets. It's also in the seeds of an African plant called *Griffonia simplicifolia,* which is the source of the 5-HTP supplements sold in health-food stores.

The focus of much recent interest, 5-HTP acts on the brain, helping to elevate mood, promote sleep and weight loss, and relieve migraines, among other uses. Unlike many other supplements (and drugs) that contain substances with molecules too large to pass from the bloodstream into the brain, 5-HTP is small enough to enter the brain. Once there, it is converted into a vital nervous system chemical, or neurotransmitter, called serotonin. Although it affects many parts of the body, serotonin's most important actions take place in the brain, where it influences everything from mood to appetite to sleep.

Because it is closely related to the amino acid tryptophan, 5-HTP remains somewhat controversial. In 1989 the FDA banned tryptophan supplements—which were often sold as L-tryptophan and used for many of the same purposes as 5-HTP—after reports of a fatal illness among those taking it. The illness was later found to be caused by contamination of the supplement during the manufacturing process, not by the tryptophan itself. In 1994 5-HTP began to be sold in the United States as an over-the-counter alternative to tryptophan. 5-HTP is not made in the same way as tryptophan, and so it avoids the contamination problems of its predecessor. Even though safety concerns have been raised, many experts believe the supplement is safe and effective.

What it does

In recent years 5-HTP has been studied as a treatment for such mood disorders as depression, anxiety, and panic attacks because it can boost levels of serotonin in the brain. Scientists are also investigating whether it

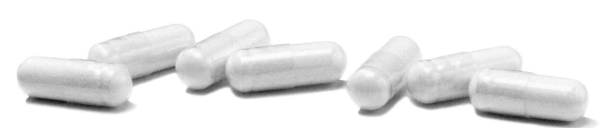

may work for a diverse array of additional complaints linked to low serotonin levels, including migraines, fibromyalgia, obesity, eating disorders, PMS, and even violent behavior. Although additional research is needed to determine its effectiveness against many of these conditions, preliminary studies suggest it may be very beneficial for some.

✴ **MAJOR BENEFITS:** For decades, European doctors have been prescribing 5-HTP for the treatment of depression and insomnia. In some cases, it may be more effective, lift depression quicker, and produce fewer side effects than standard antidepressant drugs. In one study, more than half of the patients who suffered from long-standing depression and were resistant to all other antidepressants felt better after taking 5-HTP. The nutrient has also been shown to promote sleep, and to improve the quality of sleep, by increasing the amount of time people spend in two key sleep stages: deep sleep and REM sleep (the dreaming stage). After dreaming longer, those on 5-HTP awaken feeling more rested and refreshed.

✴ **ADDITIONAL BENEFITS:** Individuals trying to lose weight or suffering from migraines may benefit from 5-HTP. In one study, overweight women who took the supplement ate fewer calories, lost more weight, and were more likely to feel full while on a diet than those given a placebo. It may also be useful in relieving severe headaches, including migraines, reducing not only their frequency, but also their intensity and duration.

The supplement may also work to increase pain tolerance in those with fibromyalgia, a chronic condition marked by aches and fatigue, in part by helping to relieve any underlying depression. In a recent Italian study of 200 fibromyalgia sufferers, those who took 5-HTP along with conventional antidepressants had less pain than those receiving either 5-HTP or the drugs alone. If you're taking antidepressants, don't try 5-HTP without consulting your doctor first: Adverse reactions can occur.

How to take it

⊘ **DOSAGE:** The recommended dosage for depression and most other ailments is 50 to 100 mg three times a day. *For migraines:* Take up to 100 mg three times a day if necessary. *For insomnia:* Take a single 100 mg dose half an hour before bedtime. When using 5-HTP, it is a good idea to begin with a low dose (such as 50 mg) and gradually increase it if needed.

◆ **GUIDELINES FOR USE:** To assure rapid absorption, take 5-HTP on an empty stomach. For weight control, take the supplement 30 minutes before meals. Don't use 5-HTP for more than three months without consulting your doctor. Some doctors combine it with the mood-enhancing herb St. John's wort. But you should not take it with that herb, with the St. John's wort/ephedra combination recommended for weight control, or with conventional antidepressants without checking with your doctor first.

Possible side effects

The generally mild side effects include nausea, constipation, gas, drowsiness, and a reduced sex drive. Nausea usually diminishes within a few days.

SHOPPING HINTS

■ Even though a product is billed as 5-HTP, it may include additional herbs or nutrients that you do not need. Carefully check the ingredient list on the label to make sure you know what you're getting.

■ Because 5-HTP is typically sold in 50 mg and 100 mg strengths, you can use the smaller dose to increase your dosage more gradually, minimizing your risk of suffering side effects.

LATEST FINDINGS

■ Though recent reports of adverse reactions in a few people taking 5-HTP have raised safety concerns, additional study is needed to determine whether these rare reactions are linked to possible contaminants in the supplement. Many experts have found 5-HTP to be safe and effective in large numbers of people.

■ In one recent study, 20 obese patients took either 5-HTP or a placebo for 12 weeks. During the first six weeks, they ate anything they wanted. Over the last six weeks, they restricted their daily diet to 1,200 calories. Those on 5-HTP lost 12 pounds, compared with barely two pounds for the placebo group.

flavonoids

What do citrus fruits, grape seed extract, red wine, pine bark extract, and onions have in common? The answer is they're all good sources of flavonoids, the plant pigments that help fight a host of disorders, from cataracts and cancer to hay fever and menopausal hot flashes.

What it is

More than 4,000 flavonoids (or bioflavonoids, as they are sometimes called on supplement labels) have been identified, and scientists suspect that there may be many more still to be discovered in nature. Flavonoids give color to fruits, vegetables, and herbs and are found in legumes, grains, and nuts as well. They are also potent antioxidants—some are even more powerful than vitamin C or vitamin E in preventing cell damage caused by unstable oxygen molecules (free radicals). So far only a few flavonoids have been investigated for their healing potential.

One of these, quercetin (found in onions and apples), also serves as a building block for other flavonoids. Rutin and hesperidin are the most active of the so-called citrus flavonoids, which, as the name suggests, are present in oranges, grapefruits, tangerines, and other citrus fruits.

Other flavonoids include PCOs (or procyanidolic oligomers; also called proanthocyanidins), anthocyanosides, polyphenols, and genistein. PCOs are plentiful in pine bark and grape seed extracts and in red wine. Anthocyanosides are found in the herb bilberry. Green tea is the primary source of polyphenols, especially EGCG (epigallocatechin-gallate), which experts believe is possibly the most effective cancer-fighting compound yet discovered. Genistein, found in soy products, has antioxidant properties and can also mimic the effects of estrogen. (For more information, see the entries on these individual supplements as well.)

What it does

The disease-fighting potential of flavonoids stems from their ability to reduce inflammation, prevent the release of histamine (which causes allergy symptoms such as congestion), fight free radicals, boost immunity, strengthen blood vessels, and increase blood flow, among other actions.

🛡 **PREVENTION:** The flavonoids quercetin and PCOs may protect against heart disease and other circulatory disorders because they inhibit bodily changes that can lead to blocked arteries; they also help strengthen blood

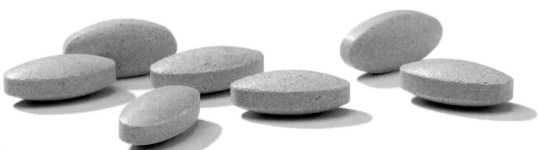

vessels in a variety of ways. Studies from Finland and the Netherlands found that people who get plenty of flavonoids, particularly quercetin, have a reduced risk of developing heart disease or having a stroke. In one study, a diet high in flavonoids appeared to cut the chances of dying from heart disease by 50% in women and 23% in men. Another study reported a 75% drop in stroke risk for men who had the highest intake of flavonoids, compared with those who had the lowest.

Polyphenols and quercetin have shown promise as anticancer compounds. Studies found lower rates of stomach, pancreatic, lung, and possibly breast cancer in people with a high intake of these flavonoids. In addition, soy-based genistein may help fight breast cancer and minimize hot flashes by interacting with estrogen receptors in the body. Quercetin also aids the body in using blood sugar and so may be valuable in preventing diabetes. Furthermore, it inhibits the buildup of sorbitol (a type of sugar) in the lens of the eye, a cause of cataracts.

✳ **ADDITIONAL BENEFITS:** Quercetin may help relieve hay fever, sinusitis, and asthma because it can block allergic reactions to pollen and reduce inflammation in the airways and lungs. This anti-inflammatory action also makes it useful for bug bites, eczema, and related skin conditions, as well as for inflammatory disorders of the joints and muscles, such as rheumatoid arthritis, gout, and fibromyalgia. Because they strengthen blood vessels, PCOs and citrus flavonoids are helpful in repairing varicose veins and hemorrhoids. Rutin and hesperidin play a role in preventing bruising.

How to take it

📗 **DOSAGE:** *For general health benefits:* Buy a flavonoid mixture that contains several types (such as quercetin, rutin, and hesperidin) and follow the dosage instructions on the label. *For allergies, asthma, gout, and insect bites:* Take 500 mg quercetin two or three times a day.

◑ **GUIDELINES FOR USE:** Grape seed extract and green tea are excellent sources of flavonoids and exert an antioxidant effect as well. It's usually best to combine flavonoids with vitamin C to enhance their protective properties. Quercetin should be taken 20 minutes before meals; other flavonoids can be taken at any time of the day.

Possible side effects

There are no known toxicities, adverse reactions, or other side effects from flavonoids.

Did You Know?

Eating an apple a day has always been associated with good health, and a recent study suggests that quercetin may be the magic ingredient. Lung cancer risk fell by 58% in people who ate the most apples (a major source of quercetin) compared with those who ate the fewest apples.

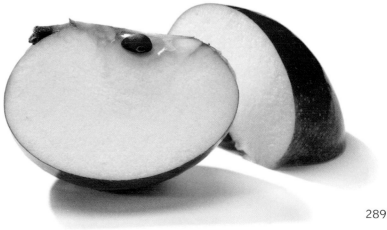

flaxseed oil

A rich source of healing oil, flaxseed has been cultivated for more than 7,000 years. Among the oil's most important uses are the prevention and treatment of cancer, heart disease, and a variety of inflammatory disorders and hormone-related problems.

Linum usitatissimum

COMMON USES

■ *Helps protect against cancer, heart disease, cataracts, and gallstones.*

■ *Reduces inflammation associated with gout and lupus.*

■ *Promotes healthy skin, hair, and nails; benefits acne, eczema, psoriasis, rosacea, and sunburn.*

■ *May be useful for infertility, impotence, menstrual cramps, and endometriosis.*

■ *Aids in treating nerve disorders.*

■ *Relieves constipation, gallstones, and diverticular disorders.*

FORMS

■ Capsule
■ Softgel
■ Oil
■ Powder

CAUTION!

■ Some people are allergic to flaxseed. If you experience difficulty breathing after taking the supplement, seek immediate medical attention.

■ Always take ground flaxseed with plenty of water (a large glass per tablespoon) to prevent it from swelling up and blocking your throat or digestive tract.

■ Reminder: If you have a medical condition, talk to your doctor before taking supplements.

What it is

It began as a fiber for weaving—and it remains the basis of natural linen fabric. However, the medicinal properties of flaxseed quickly became legendary. A slender annual that grows up to three feet high and bears blue flowers from February through September, the flax plant was first grown in Europe, then later brought to North America, where it continues to thrive. Both the oil from the flaxseeds (also known as linseeds) and the seeds themselves are used for therapeutic purposes.

What it does

Flaxseeds are a potent source of essential fatty acids (EFAs)—fats and oils critical for health, which the body cannot make on its own. One EFA, alpha-linolenic acid, is known as an omega-3 fatty acid. Found in fish and flaxseeds, omega-3s have been acclaimed in recent years for protecting against heart disease and for treating many other ailments. Flaxseeds also contain omega-6 fatty acids (in the form of linoleic acid)—the same healthy fats present in many vegetable oils. In addition, flaxseeds provide substances called lignans, which appear to have beneficial effects on various hormones and may help fight cancer, bacteria, viruses, and fungi. Ounce for ounce, flaxseeds boast up to 800 times the lignans in most other foods.

⭐ **MAJOR BENEFITS:** EFAs work throughout the body to protect cell membranes—the outer coverings that are gatekeepers for all cells, admitting healthy nutrients and barring damaging substances. That function explains why flaxseed oil has such far-reaching effects.

The brown seeds of the flax plant can be pressed to make an oil, which is also sold in capsule form.

Flaxseed oil works to lower cholesterol, thereby protecting against heart disease. It may provide benefits as well against angina and high blood pressure. A recent five-year study at Simmons College in Boston indicated that it may be useful in preventing a second heart attack. As an anti-inflammatory, it improves the treatment of such conditions as lupus and gout. As a digestive aid, it can help prevent or even dissolve gallstones. Flaxseed oil also boosts the health of hair and nails and speeds healing of skin lesions, so it is effective for everything from acne to sunburn. In addition, it may facilitate the transmission of nerve impulses, making it potentially useful for numbness and tingling, as well as for chronic brain and nerve ailments such as Parkinson's or Alzheimer's disease or nerve damage from diabetes. It may even help fight fatigue.

Crushed flaxseeds are an excellent natural source of fiber. They add bulk to stools, and their oil lubricates the stools, making flaxseeds useful for the relief of constipation and diverticular complaints.

✴ **ADDITIONAL BENEFITS:** Flaxseed oil seems to have cancer-fighting properties, though further studies are needed. It may reduce the risk of breast, colon, prostate, and possibly skin cancers, and studies at the University of Toronto found it may help treat women with both early and advanced breast cancer too.

Because flaxseeds contain plant-based estrogens (phytoestrogens) that mimic the female sex hormone estrogen, the oil can have beneficial effects on the menstrual cycle, balancing the ratio of estrogen to progesterone. It helps improve uterine function and can therefore treat fertility problems. As an anti-inflammatory, flaxseed oil can reduce menstrual cramps or the pain of fibrocystic breasts.

This oil can promote well-being in men as well. It has shown some promise against male infertility and prostate problems. In some studies, flaxseeds were also found to possess antibacterial, antifungal, and antiviral properties, which may partly explain why flaxseed oil is effective against ailments such as cold sores and shingles.

How to take it

⊘ **DOSAGE:** Liquid flaxseed oil is the easiest way to get a therapeutic amount, which ranges from 1 teaspoon to 1 tablespoon once or twice a day. To get 1 tablespoon of the oil in capsule form, you'll need to swallow about 14 capsules, each containing 1,000 mg of oil. For flaxseed fiber, mix 1 or 2 tablespoons of ground flaxseeds with a glass of water and drink it up to three times a day; the treatment may take a day or so to act.

◐ **GUIDELINES FOR USE:** Take flaxseed oil with food, which enhances absorption by the body. You can also mix it into juice, yogurt, cottage cheese, or other foods and drinks.

Possible side effects

Flaxseed oil appears to be very safe. Those using the ground seeds may experience some flatulence initially, but this should soon disappear.

folic acid

Getting enough of this B vitamin could prevent 50,000 deaths a year from cardiovascular disease. It could also reduce by nearly half the number of babies born with common birth defects and possibly prevent many cancers. Yet nine out of ten American adults take in too little folic acid.

COMMON USES

- *Protects against birth defects.*
- *Reduces heart disease and stroke risk.*
- *Lowers risk for several cancers.*

FORMS

- Tablet
- Capsule
- Powder
- Liquid

CAUTION!

- Folic acid supplements, even at normal doses, may mask a type of anemia caused by a vitamin B_{12} deficiency. Unchecked, this anemia can cause irreversible nerve damage and dementia. If you take folic acid supplements, be sure to take extra vitamin B_{12} as well.
- Reminder: If you have a medical or psychiatric condition, talk to your doctor before taking supplements.

What it is

This water-soluble B vitamin, also called folacin or folate, was first identified in the 1940s when it was extracted from spinach. Because the body can't store it very long, you need to replenish your supply daily. Cooking, or even long storage, can destroy up to half the folic acid in foods, so supplements may be the best way to get enough of this vital nutrient.

What it does

In the body, folic acid is utilized thousands of times a day to make blood cells, heal wounds, build muscle—in fact, it's necessary for every function that requires cell division. Folic acid is critical to DNA and RNA formation and assures that cells duplicate normally. It is especially important in fetal development and helps produce key chemicals for the brain and nervous system.

⬛ PREVENTION: Adequate folic acid at conception and for the first three months of pregnancy greatly reduces the risk of serious birth defects, including spina bifida. This B vitamin also appears to regulate the body's production and use of homocysteine, an amino acid-like substance that at high levels may damage the lining of blood vessels, making them more susceptible to plaque buildup. This makes folic acid an important weapon against heart disease. In addition, it may be useful in warding off certain cancers, including those of the lungs, cervix, colon, and rectum.

✳ ADDITIONAL BENEFITS: Folic acid may help depression. Because high levels of homocysteine may contribute to this condition, some experts think folic acid (which is often deficient in people who are depressed) may be of value because it reduces homocysteine levels. Studies also show that taking folic acid improves the effectiveness of antidepressants

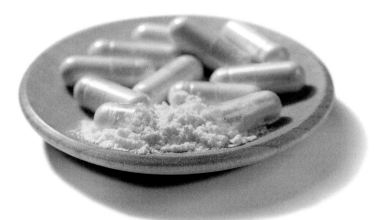

in people with low folic acid levels. Folic acid supplements have been useful in treating gout and irritable bowel syndrome as well. Because high homocysteine levels may be a factor in osteoporosis, folic acid may even help keep bones strong.

How much you need

The current adult RDA for folic acid is 400 mcg a day. Supplements are important for older people, who may not get enough of this vitamin in food.

⊟ **IF YOU GET TOO LITTLE:** Though relatively rare, a severe folic acid deficiency can cause a form of anemia (megaloblastic anemia), a sore red tongue, chronic diarrhea, and poor growth (in children). Alcoholics and people who are on certain medications (for cancer or epilepsy) or who have malabsorption diseases (Crohn's, celiac sprue) are susceptible to severe deficiency. Much more common is a low level of folic acid, which causes no symptoms but raises the risk of heart disease or birth defects.

⊞ **IF YOU GET TOO MUCH:** Very large doses—5,000 to 10,000 mcg—offer no benefit and may be dangerous for people with hormone-related cancers, such as those of the breast or prostate. High doses may also cause seizures in those with epilepsy. The National Academy of Sciences suggests an upper daily limit for folic acid of 1,000 mcg for adults.

How to take it

▱ **DOSAGE:** *For overall good health and the prevention of heart disease:* Take a dose of 400 to 800 mcg of folic acid a day. *For women who might become pregnant:* Take a total of 800 mcg a day. (Adequate folic acid stores are important because the vitamin plays a role in a baby's development from conception.) *For people with depression:* Take 400 mcg a day, as part of a vitamin B-complex supplement.

◉ **GUIDELINES FOR USE:** Folic acid can be taken at any time of the day, with or without food. When taking individual folic acid supplements for any reason, combine it with an additional 1,000 mcg of vitamin B_{12} to prevent a B_{12} deficiency.

Other sources

Excellent food sources of folic acid include green vegetables, beans, whole grains, and orange juice. Some refined grain products are now fortified with folic acid.

SHOPPING HINTS

■ Buy a folic acid supplement that also contains vitamin B_{12} (too much of one can mask a deficiency in the other). A combination supplement may be less expensive than buying each vitamin separately.

LATEST FINDINGS

■ For prevention of disease, the best way to get enough folic acid may be through supplements. In a small study, people taking 400 mcg of folic acid a day in pills or in specially fortified foods increased their folic acid level. But those who just ate foods naturally rich in folic acid showed no increase. Scientists speculate that the folic acid found naturally in foods may not be absorbed well enough to have a therapeutic effect.

■ A preliminary study from Oxford University hints that folic acid may play a role in preventing Alzheimer's disease. People with the disease tended to have lower blood levels of folic acid and vitamin B_{12} than healthy people of the same age.

Did You Know?

You'd need to eat 24 spears of asparagus a day to get the 400 mcg of folic acid recommended for good health.

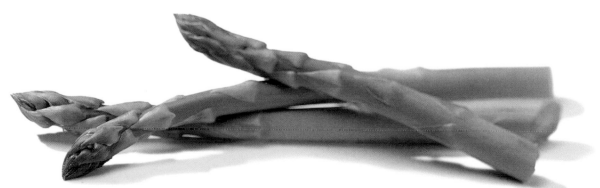

garlic

Allium sativum

There was a time when people who wanted to keep their friends wouldn't eat garlic-laced foods and suffer the resulting bad breath. Today, aging baby boomers are more likely to follow the lead of the ancient Egyptians, who worshiped this pungent and potent herb for its medicinal and culinary powers.

COMMON USES

- *May lower cholesterol levels.*
- *Reduces blood clotting.*
- *Fights infections.*
- *Acts to boost immunity.*
- *May prevent some cancers.*
- *May produce a slight drop in blood pressure.*
- *Combats fungal infections.*

FORMS

- Tablet
- Capsule
- Softgel
- Liquid
- Oil
- Powder
- Fresh herb

CAUTION!

- Consult your doctor if you're taking medications to prevent blood clots (anticoagulants or aspirin) or to reduce high blood pressure (antihypertensives). Garlic may intensify the effects of these drugs.
- Reminder: If you have a medical condition, talk to your doctor before taking supplements.

What it is

For thousands of years, garlic has been valued for its therapeutic potential. Egyptian pyramid builders took it for strength and endurance; Louis Pasteur investigated its antibacterial properties; and physicians in the two world wars used it to treat battle wounds. Garlic is related to the onion, scallion, and other plants in the genus *Allium*. The entire plant is odoriferous, but the strongest aroma is concentrated in the bulb, the site of garlic's healing powers and flavor.

Most of garlic's health benefits derive from the more than 100 sulfur compounds it contains. When the bulb is crushed or chewed, alliin, one of the sulfur compounds, becomes allicin, the chemical responsible for garlic's odor and health effects. In turn, some of the allicin is rapidly broken down into other sulfur compounds, such as ajoene, which can also have medicinal properties. Cooking garlic inhibits the formation of allicin and eliminates some of the other therapeutic chemicals.

What it does

Traditionally, garlic has been employed to treat everything from leprosy and parasites to hemorrhoids. Today, researchers are focusing on its potential to reduce the risk of heart disease and cancer.

PREVENTION: The liberal use of garlic in Italy and Spain may partly explain why these countries have such a low incidence of hardening of the arteries (atherosclerosis). Several studies suggest that garlic can prevent heart disease in various ways. For example, garlic makes platelets (the cells involved in blood clotting) less likely to clump and stick to artery walls, lessening the chance of a heart attack. There's evidence that the herb dissolves clot-forming proteins, which can affect plaque development. Garlic also lowers blood pressure slightly, mainly because of its ability to widen blood vessels and help blood circulate more freely.

Recent studies examined garlic's effect on cholesterol. Though the results are not clear-cut, most nutritionally oriented doctors think that

Garlic supplements come in many forms, including capsules (left) and enteric-coated softgels (right).

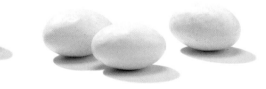

garlic, perhaps in combination with other cholesterol-lowering supplements, is worth a try. The herb may interfere with the metabolism of cholesterol in the liver; as a result, less cholesterol is released into the blood.

✳ **ADDITIONAL BENEFITS:** Garlic may have anticancer properties. It has been found to be particularly effective in preventing digestive cancers and possibly even breast and prostate cancers. Researchers aren't sure how garlic produces these benefits. Several mechanisms may be involved. First, there's the herb's ability to increase the level of enzymes that can detoxify cancer triggers. Then, it blocks the formation of nitrites linked to stomach cancer, and it's proficient at stimulating the immune system. Garlic's antioxidant properties are important as well.

Garlic is often effective against infectious organisms—viruses, bacteria, and fungi—because allicin can block the enzymes that give the organisms their ability to invade and damage tissues. The herb has also been shown to inhibit the fungi responsible for athlete's foot and swimmer's ear.

How to take it

⊘ **DOSAGE:** Look for supplements that supply 4,000 mcg of allicin potential per pill, approximately the same amount of allicin potential found in one clove of fresh garlic. *For general health or to help high cholesterol:* Take a 400 to 600 mg garlic supplement each day. *For colds and flu:* Take a 400 to 600 mg garlic supplement four times a day. *For topical benefits:* Apply garlic oil two or three times a day. Some skin conditions, including warts and insect bites, may respond to garlic oil or a crushed raw garlic clove applied directly to the affected area.

◐ **GUIDELINES FOR USE:** Garlic can be taken indefinitely. However, if you are using the herb for cholesterol problems, have your levels checked in three months to see if they have changed; if you've derived no benefits, talk to your doctor about other remedies.

Possible side effects

Some people develop heartburn, intestinal gas, and diarrhea when taking high doses of garlic. Using enteric-coated supplements may reduce such side effects. Skin rashes have also been reported.

SHOPPING HINTS

- Most experts believe supplements made from garlic powder are the most effective.
- Enteric-coating prevents garlic breath and allows the supplement to pass through the stomach undigested, which assures the formation of allicin.
- Deodorized garlic preparations appear to have the same benefits as regular supplements.

LATEST FINDINGS

- In a recent laboratory study, researchers found that garlic extract was powerful enough to neutralize *Helicobacter pylori*, the bacterium that causes ulcers. The next step is to see whether garlic will do the same in the body.
- Garlic may prevent stiffening of the aorta—the artery that carries blood from the heart to the rest of the body—which occurs naturally with age. In one study, some 200 people took either garlic supplements or a placebo daily for two years. At the end of the study, the aortas of the 70-year-olds in the garlic group were as supple as those of the 55-year-olds who didn't take the supplement. A flexible aorta may help reduce age-related organ damage.

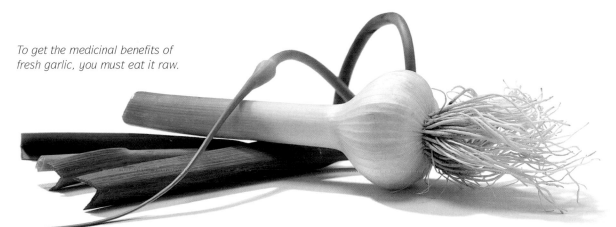

To get the medicinal benefits of fresh garlic, you must eat it raw.

ginger

Zingiber officinale

From ancient India and China to Greece and Rome, ginger was revered as a medicinal and as a culinary spice. Medieval Europeans traced this herb to the Garden of Eden, and it has long been valued by traditional healers. In modern homes and hospitals, it's used to quell nausea and much more.

COMMON USES

- *Alleviates nausea and dizziness.*
- *May relieve pain and inflammation of arthritis.*
- *Eases muscle aches.*
- *Relieves allergies.*
- *Reduces flatulence.*

FORMS

- Capsule
- Tablet
- Softgel
- Oil
- Tincture
- Liquid
- Fresh or dried root/Tea
- Crystallized, candied herb

CAUTION!

- Ginger may relieve morning sickness during the first two months of pregnancy (up to 250 mg four times a day). But longer use or higher doses should be taken only under a doctor's supervision.
- Chemotherapy patients should not take ginger on an empty stomach because it can irritate the stomach lining.
- Reminder: If you have a medical condition, talk to your doctor before taking supplements.

What it is

Renowned for its stomach-settling properties, ginger is native to parts of India and China, as well as Jamaica and other tropical areas. This warm-climate perennial is closely related to turmeric and marjoram, and its roots are used for culinary and therapeutic purposes. As a spice, ginger adds a hot and lemony flavor to foods as disparate as roast pork and gingersnap cookies. Medicinally, it continues to play a major role in traditional healing.

What it does

For thousands of years, all around the globe, this pungent spice has been popular as a treatment for digestive problems, ranging from mild indigestion and flatulence to nausea and vomiting. It's also been helpful for relieving colds and arthritis. Modern research into ginger's active ingredients confirms the effectiveness of many of these ancient remedies.

✪ **MAJOR BENEFITS:** What can you do with a seasick sailor? The answer is: Try ginger. In a Danish study, 40 naval cadets took 1 gram of powdered ginger a day; they were much less likely to break out in a cold sweat and vomit (classic symptoms of the seasick) than 39 others who took a placebo.

Because ginger works primarily in the digestive tract, boosting digestive fluids and neutralizing acids, it may be a good medical alternative to antinausea drugs that can affect the central nervous system and cause grogginess. Studies of women undergoing exploratory surgery (laparoscopy) or major gynecological surgery show that taking 1 gram of ginger before an operation can significantly reduce postoperative nausea and vomiting, a common side effect of surgery medications and anesthesia. Ginger also appears to counter the nausea created by chemotherapy, though it's best to take it with food to minimize any stomach irritation.

Ginger's antinausea effects make it useful for reducing dizziness, a common problem in older patients, as well as for treating morning sickness. For years, ginger has been a staple of folk medicine, primarily as a digestive aid to counter stomach upset. Ginger supplements (or fresh pulp mixed with lime juice) are also a fine remedy for flatulence.

✪ **ADDITIONAL BENEFITS:** Ginger's anti-inflammatory and pain-relieving properties may help relieve the muscle aches and chronic pain associated with arthritis and other conditions. In a study of seven women with rheumatoid arthritis (an autoimmune disease characterized by severe inflammation), just 5 to 50 grams of fresh ginger or capsules containing up to 1 gram of powdered ginger lessened joint pain and inflammation. Its anti-inflammatory properties suggest that ginger may ease bronchial constriction due to allergies or colds.

How to take it

⊘ **DOSAGE:** *To prevent motion sickness, dizziness, and nausea; reduce flatulence; and relieve chronic pain or rheumatoid arthritis:* Take ginger up to three times a day, or every four hours as needed. The usual dose is 100 to 200 mg of the standardized extract in pill form; 1 or 2 grams of fresh powdered ginger; or a ½-inch slice of fresh ginger root. Other preparations, including ginger tea (available in tea bags, or use ½ teaspoon of grated ginger root per cup of very hot water) or natural ginger ale (containing real ginger), can be used several times a day for similar purposes and for arthritis and pain relief. On trips, try crystallized ginger candy: A 1-inch square, about ¼-inch thick, contains approximately 500 mg of ginger. *For aching muscles:* Rub several drops of ginger oil, mixed with ½ ounce of almond oil or another neutral oil, on the sore areas. *For allergy relief:* Drink up to four cups of ginger tea a day as needed to reduce symptoms.

◈ **GUIDELINES FOR USE:** Take ginger capsules with fluid. If you're trying to prevent motion sickness, have ginger three to four hours before your departure, and then every four hours as needed, up to four times a day. For postoperative nausea, begin taking ginger the day before your operation, under your doctor's supervision.

Possible side effects

Ginger is very safe for a broad range of complaints, whether it's taken in a concentrated capsule form, eaten fresh, or sipped as a tea or ginger ale. Occasional heartburn seems to be the only documented side effect.

Whether eaten fresh or taken in capsules, ginger is a potent remedy for nausea and dizziness.

ginkgo biloba

Ginkgo biloba

This popular herbal medicine, derived from one of the oldest species of tree on earth, is widely marketed as a memory booster. Ginkgo biloba does help with age-related memory loss, but whether it's a "smart pill" meant for everyone remains to be seen.

COMMON USES

- *Slows the progression of Alzheimer's symptoms; sharpens memory and concentration, particularly in older people.*
- *Lessens depression and anxiety in some older people.*
- *Alleviates coldness in the extremities (Raynaud's disease) and painful leg cramps (intermittent claudication).*
- *Helps headaches, ringing in the ears (tinnitus), and dizziness.*
- *May restore erections in men with impotence.*

FORMS

- Tablet
- Capsule
- Softgel
- Tincture
- Powder
- Liquid

CAUTION!

- Don't use unprocessed ginkgo leaves in any form, including teas; they contain potent chemicals (allergens) that can trigger allergic reactions. Stick with standardized extracts (GBE): The allergens are removed during processing.
- Reminder: If you have a medical or psychiatric condition, talk to your doctor before taking supplements.

What it is

The medicinal form of the herb is extracted from the fan-shaped leaves of the ancient ginkgo biloba tree, a species that has survived in China for more than 200 million years. (The leaves are double- or bi-lobed; hence the name "biloba.") A concentrated form of the herb, ginkgo biloba extract (GBE), is used to make the supplement. Commonly called ginkgo, GBE is obtained by drying and milling the leaves and then extracting the active ingredients in a mixture of acetone and water.

What it does

Ginkgo may have beneficial effects on both the circulatory and the central nervous systems. It increases blood flow to the brain and to the arms and legs by regulating the tone and elasticity of blood vessels, from the largest arteries to the tiniest capillaries. It also acts like aspirin by helping to reduce the "stickiness" of the blood, thereby lowering the risk of blood clots. Ginkgo appears to have antioxidant properties as well, mopping up the damaging compounds known as free radicals and aiding in the maintenance of healthy blood cells. And some researchers report that it enhances the nervous system by promoting the delivery of additional oxygen and blood sugar (glucose) to nerve cells.

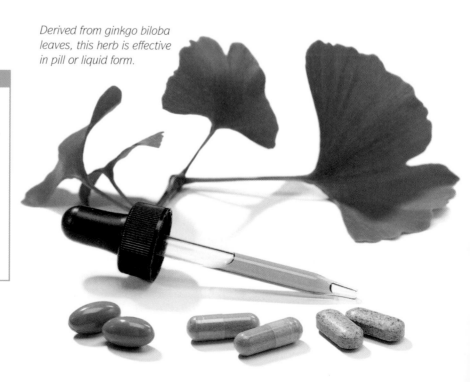

Derived from ginkgo biloba leaves, this herb is effective in pill or liquid form.

PREVENTION: Interest now centers on ginkgo's possible role as a preventive for age-related memory loss. Unfortunately, there's little scientific evidence ginkgo will make most people better able to focus or remember. So far, it is those already suffering from diminished blood flow to the brain—not healthy volunteers—who have benefited most from taking the herb. Current research is trying to determine whether ginkgo's ability to help prevent blood clots may stave off heart attacks or strokes.

MAJOR BENEFITS: The fact that ginkgo aids blood flow to the brain—thus increasing oxygen—is of particular relevance to older people, whose arteries may have narrowed with cholesterol buildup or other conditions. Diminished blood flow has been linked to Alzheimer's and memory loss, as well as to anxiety, headaches, depression, confusion, ringing in the ears, and dizziness. All may be helped by ginkgo.

ADDITIONAL BENEFITS: Ginkgo also promotes blood flow to the arms and legs, making it useful for reducing the pain, cramping, and weakness caused by narrowed arteries in the leg, a disorder called intermittent claudication. There are indications that the herb may improve circulation to the extremities in those with Raynaud's disease, or help victims of scleroderma, an uncommon autoimmune disorder.

In addition, by increasing blood flow to the nerve-rich fibers of the eyes and ears, some studies suggest ginkgo may be of value in treating macular degeneration or diabetes-related eye disease (both leading causes of blindness), as well as some types of hearing loss. Ongoing studies are assessing the possible effectiveness of ginkgo in speeding up recovery from certain strokes and head injuries, as well as in treating other conditions that may be related to circulatory or nervous system impairment, including impotence, multiple sclerosis, and nerve damage tied to diabetes. Traditional Chinese healers have long used ginkgo for asthma, because the herb appears to alleviate wheezing and other respiratory complaints.

How to take it

DOSAGE: Use supplements that contain ginkgo biloba extract, or GBE, the concentrated form of the herb. *As a general memory booster and for poor circulation:* Take 120 mg of GBE daily, divided into two or three doses. *For Alzheimer's disease, depression, ringing in the ears, dizziness, impotence, or other conditions caused by insufficient blood flow to the brain:* Take up to 240 mg a day.

GUIDELINES FOR USE: It commonly takes four to six weeks, and in some cases up to 12 weeks, to notice the herb's effects. Generally, it is considered safe for long-term use in recommended dosages. You can take ginkgo with or without food. No adverse effects have been reported in pregnant or lactating women who take the herb.

Possible side effects

In rare cases, ginkgo may cause irritability, restlessness, diarrhea, nausea, or vomiting, though these effects are usually mild and transient. People starting the herb may also notice a headache during the first day or two of use. If side effects are bothersome, discontinue it or reduce the dosage.

LATEST FINDINGS

■ A yearlong study, published in the *Journal of the American Medical Association,* evaluated 202 patients with dementia, most of whom also had Alzheimer's disease. Patients who took 120 mg of ginkgo biloba extract a day were more likely to stabilize or improve their mental and social functions, compared with those given a placebo. The effects were modest and of limited duration.

Did You Know?

Ginkgo trees have two "sexes"—male and female. The nuts from the female tree have long been valued in China and Japan as a culinary delicacy with healing properties.

ginseng (panax)

Panax ginseng

A wildly popular herb in the United States and Europe, ginseng is added to everything from fruit juices to vitamin supplements. Though most of these actually contain little ginseng, quality ginseng does exert a variety of protective effects on the body.

COMMON USES

- *Combats the physical effects of stress.*
- *May treat impotence and infertility in men.*
- *Boosts energy.*

FORMS

- Tablet
- Capsule
- Softgel
- Powder
- Tincture
- Dried herb/Tea

CAUTION!

- Don't take Panax ginseng if you have uncontrolled high blood pressure or a heart rhythm irregularity.
- Don't use Panax ginseng if you are pregnant.
- Don't use Panax ginseng if you take MAO inhibitor drugs.
- Reminder: If you have a medical condition, talk to your doctor before taking supplements.

What it is

Panax ginseng (also called Asian, Chinese, or Korean ginseng) has been used in Chinese medicine for thousands of years to enhance both longevity and the quality of life. *Panax ginseng* is the most widely available and extensively studied form of this herb. Another species, *Panax quinquefolius* or American ginseng, is grown mainly in the Midwest and exported to China.

The medicinal part of the plant is its slow-growing root, which is harvested after four to six years, when its overall ginsenoside content—the main active ingredient in ginseng—is at its peak. There are 13 different ginsenosides in all. Panax ginseng also contains panaxans, substances that can lower blood sugar, and polysaccharides, complex sugar molecules that enhance the immune system. "White" ginseng is simply the dried root; "red" ginseng has been steamed and dried.

What it does

The primary health benefits of Panax ginseng derive from its immune-stimulating and antioxidant properties, as well as from its ability to protect the body against the adverse effects of stress.

PREVENTION: Ginseng may help the body combat a variety of illnesses. It stimulates the production of specialized immune cells called "killer T cells," which destroy harmful viruses and bacteria.

Studies have also indicated that the herb may inhibit the growth of certain cancer cells. A large Korean study found that the risk of developing cancer in people who took ginseng was half that of subjects who did not take it. Although ginseng powders and tinctures were shown to have cancer-preventive effects, eating fresh ginseng root or drinking ginseng juice or tea did not lower cancer risk.

ADDITIONAL BENEFITS: Ginseng may benefit people who are feeling fatigued and overstressed and those recovering from a long illness. The herb has been shown to balance the release of stress hormones in the

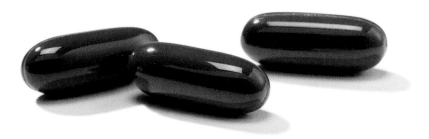

body and support the organs that produce these hormones, namely the pituitary gland and hypothalamus in the brain and the adrenal glands, located on top of the kidneys. Ginseng may also enhance the production of endorphins, "feel-good" chemicals produced by the brain.

Many long-distance runners and body-builders take ginseng to heighten physical endurance. Herbalists believe that ginseng can delay fatigue by enabling the exercising muscles to use energy more efficiently. Some research, however, contradicts this hypothesis.

Though the way it works is not clear, ginseng may be helpful for impotence. Some of its active ingredients appear to affect smooth muscle tissue and improve erectile function. Men with fertility problems may benefit from ginseng as well because animal studies indicate it increases testosterone levels and sperm production.

How to take it

⏻ **Dosage:** Select a product that is standardized to contain at least 7% ginsenosides. *For general health and combating fatigue:* Take 100 to 250 mg Panax ginseng once or twice a day. *To support the body in times of stress or during recovery from an illness:* Take 100 to 250 mg twice a day. *For male impotence and infertility:* Take 100 to 250 mg twice a day.

◉ **Guidelines for use:** Start at the lower end of the dosage range and increase your intake gradually. Some experts recommend that you stop taking ginseng for a week every two or three weeks and then resume your regular dose. In some cases, ginseng may be rotated with other immune-stimulating herbs, such as astragalus or Siberian ginseng.

Possible side effects

At the doses recommended here, ginseng is unlikely to cause any side effects. There have been reports that higher doses cause nervousness, insomnia, headache, and stomach upset; if you have any of these problems, reduce your dose. The combination of ginseng and caffeine may intensify these reactions, so cut back on or avoid caffeine. Some women report increased menstrual bleeding or breast tenderness with high doses of ginseng. If this occurs, reduce your dose or stop using it.

Did You Know?

The name "ginseng" is derived from the ancient Chinese word *jen shen* (meaning "man root") because the ginseng root (below) often resembles the shape of the human body.

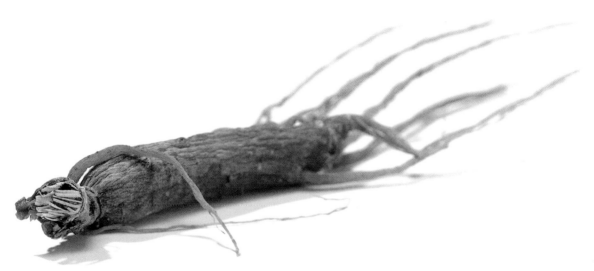

glucosamine

This promising arthritis fighter helps build cartilage—which provides cushioning at the tips of the bones—and protects and strengthens the joints as it relieves pain and stiffness. Although your body produces some glucosamine, a supplement is more effective.

COMMON USES

- *Relieves pain, stiffness, and swelling of the knees, fingers, and other joints due to osteo-arthritis or rheumatoid arthritis.*
- *Helps reduce arthritic back and neck pain.*
- *May speed the healing of sprains and strengthen joints, preventing future injury.*

FORMS

- Capsule
- Tablet

CAUTION!

- Reminder: If you have a medical condition, talk to your doctor before taking supplements.

What it is

Scientists have long known that the body manufactures a small amount of glucosamine (pronounced glue-KOSE-a-mean), a fairly simple molecule that contains the sugar glucose. It's found in relatively high concentrations in the joints and connective tissues, where the body uses it to form the larger molecules necessary for cartilage repair and maintenance. In recent years, glucosamine has become available as a nutritional supplement. Various forms are sold, including glucosamine sulfate and N-acetyl-glucosamine (NAG). Glucosamine sulfate is the preferred form for arthritis: It is readily used by the body (90% to 98% is absorbed through the intestine) and appears to be very effective for this condition.

What it does

Though some experts hail glucosamine as an arthritis cure, no one supplement can claim that title. It does, however, provide significant relief from pain and inflammation for about half of arthritis sufferers—especially those with the common age-related form known as osteoarthritis. It can also help people with rheumatoid arthritis and other types of joint injuries, and it offers additional benefits as well.

⭐ **MAJOR BENEFITS:** Approved for the treatment of arthritis in some 70 countries around the world, glucosamine can ease pain and inflammation, increase range of motion, and help repair aging and damaged joints in the knees, hips, spine, and hands. Recent studies show that it may be even more effective for relieving pain and inflammation than nonsteroidal anti-inflammatory drugs (NSAIDs), such as aspirin and ibuprofen, commonly taken by arthritis sufferers—without their harmful side effects. What's more, while NSAIDs mask arthritis pain, they do little to combat the progression of the disease—and may even make it worse by impairing the body's ability to build cartilage. In contrast, glucosamine helps make cartilage and may repair damaged joints. Though it can't do much for people with advanced arthritis, when cartilage has completely worn away, it may benefit the millions of people with mild to moderately severe symptoms.

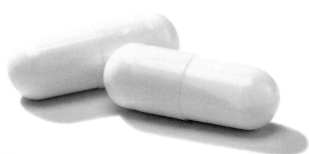

ADDITIONAL BENEFITS: As a general joint strengthener, glucosamine may be useful for the prevention of arthritis and all forms of age-related degenerative joint disease. It may also speed healing of acute joint injuries, such as a sprained ankle or finger.

In addition to aiding joints and connective tissues, glucosamine promotes a healthy lining in the digestive tract and may be beneficial in treating ailments such as irritable bowel syndrome. It is included in various "intestinal health" preparations sold in health-food stores, usually in the form of N-acetyl-glucosamine (NAG), which tends to act specifically on the intestinal lining.

How to take it

DOSAGE: The usual dosage for arthritis and other conditions is 500 mg glucosamine sulfate three times a day, or 1,500 mg daily. This amount has been shown to be safe for all individuals and effective for most. People weighing more than 200 pounds or taking diuretics may need higher daily doses (about 900 mg per 100 pounds of body weight); talk to your doctor about an appropriate dosage.

GUIDELINES FOR USE: Glucosamine is typically taken long term and appears to be very safe. It may not bring relief as quickly as pain relievers or anti-inflammatories (it usually works in two to eight weeks), but its benefits are far greater and longer-lasting when it's used over a period of time. Take glucosamine with meals to minimize the chance of digestive upset.

Glucosamine's anti-arthritis effects may be enhanced by using it along with another supplement, such as chondroitin sulfate (a related cartilage-building compound), niacinamide (a form of the B vitamin niacin), or S-adenosylmethionine (SAM), a form of the amino acid methionine. Other supplements that are sometimes taken along with glucosamine for the relief of arthritis include boswellia, a tree extract from India; sea cucumber, an ancient Chinese remedy; and the topical pain reliever cayenne cream. No adverse reactions have been reported when glucosamine is used with other supplements or with prescription or over-the-counter medications.

Possible side effects

Because it is a natural substance produced in the body, glucosamine is virtually free of side effects, though no long-term studies have been done. Gastrointestinal effects, such as heartburn or nausea, occur rarely in those who take glucosamine supplements.

goldenseal

The Cherokee, Iroquois, and other American tribes valued goldenseal as a remedy for everything from insect bites and bloating to eye infections and stomachaches. Today, the herb is officially recognized as a medicine in eleven countries, though not in the United States.

Hydrastis canadensis

COMMON USES

- *Promotes healing of canker sores and cold sores.*
- *Helps destroy the virus that causes warts.*
- *Bolsters the immune system.*
- *Calms a nauseated stomach.*
- *May help urinary tract infections.*
- *Treats eye infections.*

FORMS

- Capsule
- Softgel
- Tincture
- Liquid
- Dried herb/Tea
- Ointment/Cream

CAUTION!

- Goldenseal should not be used by pregnant women or people with heart disease, high blood pressure, diabetes, or glaucoma.
- Reminder: If you have a medical condition, talk to your doctor before taking supplements.

What it is

The dried root of this perennial herb has long been used to soothe inflamed or infected mucous membranes. Today, it is appreciated for its ability to help the body fight infection. The plant was first called goldenseal in the nineteenth century, deriving its name from the rich yellow of the root and the small cuplike scars found there. These scars, which appear on the previous year's root growth, resemble the wax seals formerly used to close envelopes—hence the name "goldenseal." Related to the buttercup, goldenseal is native to North America and once grew wild from Vermont to Arkansas. As interest in its medicinal properties grew, however, the plant was extensively harvested. Currently, most of the goldenseal on the market is commercially cultivated in Oregon and Washington.

The key medicinal compounds in goldenseal are the alkaloids berberine and hydrastine. Berberine is also responsible for the root's rich yellow color—so vibrant, in fact, that Native Americans and early settlers utilized goldenseal as a dye as well as a medicinal herb. Because the alkaloids have a bitter taste, goldenseal tea often includes other herbs or is mixed with a sweetener such as honey.

What it does

The primary benefit of goldenseal is its overall effect on immunity. Not only does it increase the immune system's production of germ-fighting compounds, it can combat both bacteria and viruses directly.

PREVENTION: Taking goldenseal at the first sign of a cold or the flu may prevent the illness from developing fully—or at least greatly minimize the symptoms—by enhancing the activity of virus-fighting white blood cells.

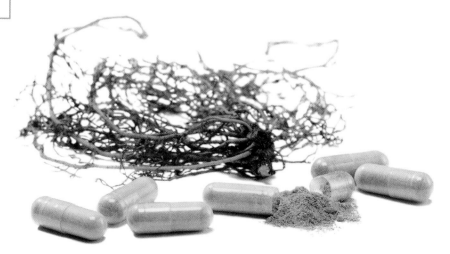

The root of the goldenseal plant is dried and then ground to a powder for use in supplements.

✳ ADDITIONAL BENEFITS: Goldenseal fights bacteria, making it useful for mild urinary tract infections (if you begin taking it early enough) and sinus infections. It may also help soothe nausea and vomiting, by stimulating digestive secretions and working to destroy the bacteria that may be causing the symptoms.

As one of several herbs that stimulate the immune system—others include echinacea, pau d'arco, and astragalus—goldenseal may play a role in relieving the symptoms of chronic fatigue syndrome, a disabling disorder that may be partially caused by a weakened immune system. It also helps to fight cold sores and shingles (both caused by the herpes virus). Use it for no more than a week or two at a time.

Applied topically, goldenseal tincture is beneficial for canker sores and warts. The tincture promotes the healing of the sores and directly fights the human papilloma virus that causes warts. Once cooled and strained, goldenseal tea can be used as an eyewash to relieve eye infections such as conjunctivitis. Be sure to prepare a fresh batch daily and store it in a sterile container, so the tea won't get contaminated.

How to take it

⬤ DOSAGE: *For colds, flu, and other respiratory infections:* As soon as you begin to feel sick, take 125 mg of goldenseal (in combination with 200 mg of echinacea) five times a day for five days. *For urinary tract infections:* Drink several cups of goldenseal tea a day. *For nausea and vomiting:* Take 125 mg every four hours as needed. *For chronic fatigue syndrome:* Use 125 mg twice a day in rotation with other immune-stimulating herbs. *For cold sores:* Take 125 mg of goldenseal with 200 mg echinacea four times a day. *For shingles:* Take 125 mg of goldenseal with 200 mg echinacea four times a day. *For canker sores and warts:* Apply goldenseal tincture directly to the sores three times a day. *For eye infections:* Use 1 teaspoon dried herb per pint of hot water. Steep, finely strain, cool, and apply as an eyewash three times a day; make a new solution every day.

◒ GUIDELINES FOR USE: Take goldenseal supplements with meals. Unlike echinacea and other herbs that stimulate the immune system, goldenseal should be used only when you feel that you're coming down with a cold, the flu, or some other illness, and just for the duration of the illness. The single exception is when you're taking goldenseal in rotation with other herbs to strengthen the immune system.

Possible side effects

When taken at recommended doses and for suggested lengths of time, goldenseal is safe to use and has few side effects. Very high doses may irritate the mucous membranes of the mouth and cause diarrhea, nausea, and respiratory problems.

C·a·s·e H·i·s·t·o·r·y

GO FOR THE GOLD

Alexa K. always reacted badly to antibiotics. Although she knew she needed them for her sinus infections, the side effects—dizziness, nausea, diarrhea—often made the drugs worse than the illness.

When an herbalist told her to try goldenseal extract, her doctor was skeptical. "Look," he said, "try the goldenseal, but keep my prescription handy. If you don't feel better, you can always get it filled."

Alexa took the goldenseal and, in a few days, her sinus infection was gone—without a single side effect. Now goldenseal is a part of her sinus first-aid kit. At the first sign of an infection, she starts taking it, along with the immune stimulator echinacea.

Though antibiotics are sometimes necessary, in the last few years Alexa has often been able to avoid them. "Those miserable side effects are history!" she happily reports.

gotu kola

Centella asiatica

This herb is a favorite food of elephants, notoriously long-lived animals, which has led many people to associate it with longevity. Though scientific research hasn't shown that it can extend your life, studies have found that gotu kola provides other important health benefits.

COMMON USES

- *Treats burns and wounds.*
- *Builds connective tissue.*
- *Strengthens veins.*
- *Improves memory.*

FORMS

- Capsule
- Tablet
- Tincture
- Powder
- Dried herb/Tea

What it is

The medicinal use of gotu kola has its roots in India, where the herb continues to be part of the ancient healing tradition called Ayurveda. Word of its therapeutic benefits for skin disorders gradually spread throughout Asia and Europe. In fact, gotu kola has been prescribed in France since the 1880s to treat burns and other wounds.

A red-flowered plant that thrives in hot, swampy areas, gotu kola grows naturally in India, Sri Lanka, Madagascar, middle and southern Africa, Australia, China, and the southern United States. The appearance of this slender, creeping perennial changes depending on whether it's growing in water (broad, fan-shaped leaves) or on dry land (small, thin leaves). The plant's leaf is most commonly used medicinally.

What it does

Whether taken internally or applied externally as a compress, gotu kola has many beneficial effects. The herb's workhorse substances are chemicals called triterpenes (especially asiaticoside), which appear to enhance the formation of collagen in bones, cartilage, and connective tissue. In addition, they promote healthy blood vessels and help produce neurotransmitters, the chemical messengers in the brain.

✪ **MAJOR BENEFITS:** Gotu kola's singular effect on connective tissue—promoting its healthy development and inhibiting the formation of hardened areas—makes it potentially important for treating many skin conditions. It can be therapeutic for burns, keloids (overgrown scar tissue), and wounds (including surgical incisions and skin ulcers). Gotu kola also seems to strengthen cells in the walls of blood vessels, improving blood flow and making it valuable for the treatment of varicose veins. Research results are often impressive. In more than a dozen studies observing gotu kola's effect on veins (which are surrounded by supportive connective-tissue sheaths), about 80% of patients with varicose veins and similar problems showed substantial improvement. Other studies indicate that applying gotu kola topically to psoriasis lesions may aid healing as well.

✪ **ADDITIONAL BENEFITS:** Gotu kola has been used to increase mental acuity for thousands of years. Current research supports a role for this herb in boosting memory, improving learning capabilities, and possibly reversing some of the memory loss associated with Alzheimer's disease. In one study, 30 developmentally disabled children were found to have significantly better concentration and attention levels after taking gotu kola for 12 weeks than they did at the start of the study. Preliminary findings reveal that animals given gotu kola for two weeks were able to learn and retain new behaviors much better than animals not on the herb.

How to take it

⦿ **DOSAGE:** *To treat varicose veins:* Take 200 mg of the standardized extract three times a day. *For burns:* Use 200 mg twice a day until they heal. *To improve memory or possibly slow the progress of Alzheimer's disease:* Take 200 mg three times a day. You can substitute 400 to 500 mg of the crude herb for each 200 mg dose of the standardized extract.

◈ **GUIDELINES FOR USE:** In most cases, gotu kola is taken internally as a tablet or capsule, with or without meals. However, gotu kola tea or tincture can also be applied externally to the skin for psoriasis, burns, wounds, incisions, or scars. You can use both the oral and topical preparations of the herb over the same period of time.

To apply gotu kola topically, soak a compress in tea or in tincture and apply it directly to problem areas. Start with a relatively weak solution and increase the strength as needed. To brew gotu kola tea, steep 1 or 2 teaspoons of dried leaf in a cup of very hot water for 10 to 15 minutes. You can also make a paste to apply to patches of skin affected by psoriasis: Break open capsules and mix 2 teaspoons of dried gotu kola powder in a small amount of water.

Possible side effects

Taking gotu kola orally or using a topical preparation generally does not cause problems. Skin rash (dermatitis), sensitivity to sunlight, and headaches are rare side effects. If you experience these symptoms, reduce the dosage or stop using the herb.

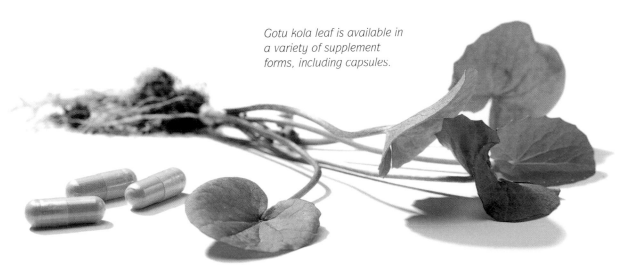

Gotu kola leaf is available in a variety of supplement forms, including capsules.

grape seed extract

With antioxidant properties many times more powerful than vitamin C or vitamin E, grape seed extract is a heart-smart and cancer-smart botanical. It also has the power to improve vascular health and increase your well-being in myriad ways.

What it is

This extract from the tiny seeds of red grapes is a flavonoid and one of Europe's leading natural treatments. Plant substances with potent antioxidant potential, flavonoids protect the cells from damage by unstable oxygen molecules called free radicals. Grape seed extract contains procyanidolic oligomers (PCOs), also called proanthocyanidins. Once called pycnogenols (pik-NODGE-en-alls), PCOs are believed to play an important role in preventing heart disease and cancer. "Pycnogenol" with a capital P is the trademark for a specific PCO derived from maritime pine bark; it can be used in place of grape seed extract, but it is more expensive, and many practitioners don't believe it's worth the extra cost.

What it does

Grape seed extract exerts a powerful, positive influence on blood vessels. Not coincidentally, the active substances in this extract, PCOs, are key ingredients in one of the drugs most frequently prescribed for blood vessel (vascular) disorders in western Europe.

Because it is both oil- and water-soluble, grape seed extract can penetrate all types of cell membranes, delivering antioxidant protection throughout the body. Moreover, it is one of the few substances that can cross the blood-brain barrier, which means it may protect brain cells from free-radical damage.

MAJOR BENEFITS: With its powerful ability to enhance the health of blood vessels, grape seed extract may both reduce the risk of heart attack and stroke and also strengthen fragile or weak capillaries and increase blood flow, particularly to the extremities. For this reason, many experts find it a beneficial supplement for almost any type of vascular insufficiency, as well as for conditions that are associated with poor vascular

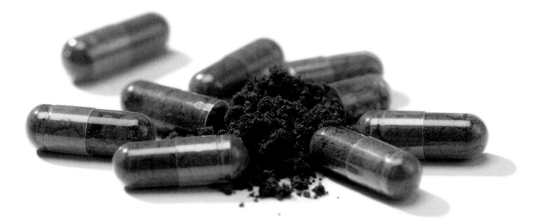

function, including diabetes, varicose veins, some cases of impotence, numbness and tingling in the arms and legs, and even painful leg cramps.

Because it can have an impact on even the tiniest blood vessels, grape seed extract also benefits circulation in the eye. It is frequently recommended as a supplement to combat macular degeneration and cataracts, two of the most common causes of blindness in older people. And if you use computers on a regular basis, grape seed extract may also be for you. At least one study showed that 300 mg daily for just 60 days reduced eyestrain associated with computer monitor work and improved contrast vision.

Many experts now endorse grape seed extract for its cancer-fighting properties. Working as antioxidants, PCOs correct damage to the genetic material of cells that could possibly cause tumors to form.

✳ **ADDITIONAL BENEFITS:** Helping to preserve and reinforce the collagen in the skin, grape seed extract is often used in the treatment of connective tissue disorders, such as rheumatoid arthritis. In Europe, it is often included in cosmetic creams to improve skin elasticity.

For allergy sufferers, grape seed extract offers relief; it inhibits the release of symptom-causing compounds such as histamine, which, in turn, helps control a variety of allergic reactions, from hives to hay fever. Grape seed also blocks the release of prostaglandins, chemicals involved in allergic reactions and in pain and inflammation, particularly that of the menstrual disorder called endometriosis.

How to take it

◍ **DOSAGE:** *For antioxidant protection:* Take 100 mg daily. *For therapeutic benefits:* Doses are usually 200 mg daily. Choose supplements standardized to contain 92% to 95% proanthocyanidins, or PCOs.

◈ **GUIDELINES FOR USE:** After 24 hours, only about 28% of grape seed extract's active components remain in the body. So it's important to take supplements at the same time every day, particularly when they are used to combat disease.

Possible side effects

No side effects from taking grape seed extract have been reported, and no toxic reactions have been noted.

FACTS
& Tips

■ Grape seed oil (not to be confused with grape seed extract) may offer health benefits too. A preliminary study at the University Health Science Center in Syracuse, New York, found that adding about 2 tablespoons of grape seed oil to the daily diet increased HDL ("good") cholesterol by 14% and reduced triglycerides by 15% in just four weeks. Use it in place of other oils in salads or cooking.

LATEST FINDINGS

■ A preliminary study from the University of Arizona at Tucson suggests that pine bark extract, which contains the same active ingredients as grape seed extract, may be as effective an anticoagulant as aspirin, and so may help lower the risk of heart attack and stroke. Researchers asked 38 smokers—who are more likely to develop the type of blood clots that cause heart attacks—to take either pine bark extract or aspirin. Blood tests revealed that both remedies were equally effective, but pine bark did not have aspirin's side effects—such as stomach irritation and increased risk for internal bleeding.

green tea

Camellia sinensis

According to legend, around 2700 B.C. a Chinese emperor sat under a tea shrub, and a few leaves fell into his cup of hot water. Presto! Green tea was born. Now, modern research has found that this type of tea contains one of the most promising anticancer compounds ever discovered.

COMMON USES

- *May help prevent cancer.*
- *Protects against heart disease.*
- *Inhibits tooth decay.*
- *Promotes longevity.*

FORMS

- Capsule
- Tablet
- Liquid
- Powder
- Tea

What it is

The traditional process that yields green tea is simple: The leaves from the tea plant are first steamed, then rolled and dried. The steaming kills enzymes that would otherwise ferment the leaves. With other types of tea, the leaves are allowed to ferment either partially (for oolong tea) or fully (for black tea). The lack of fermentation, however, gives green tea its unique flavor and, more important, preserves virtually all of the naturally present polyphenols (strong antioxidants that can protect against cell damage). Other substances in green tea that also may be beneficial are fluoride, catechins, and tannins.

What it does

Green tea possesses compounds that may provide powerful protection against several cancers and, possibly, heart disease. Studies indicate that it also fights infection and promotes longevity.

PREVENTION: The rate of certain types of cancer is lower among people who drink green tea. In one large-scale study, researchers found that Chinese men and women who drank green tea as seldom as once a week for six months had lower rates of rectal, pancreatic, and possibly colon cancer than those who rarely or never drank it. In women, the risk of rectal and pancreatic cancer was nearly cut in half. Preliminary research suggests that green tea may also fight breast, stomach, and skin cancer.

Studies investigating how green tea might guard against cancer have pointed to the potency of its main antioxidant, a polyphenol dubbed EGCG (for epigallocatechin-gallate). Some scientists believe EGCG may be one of the most effective anticancer compounds ever discovered, protecting cells from damage and strengthening the body's own production of antioxidant enzymes. According to a study from Ohio's Case Western Reserve University, EGCG seems to signal cancer cells to stop reproducing by stimulating a natural process of programmed cell death called apoptosis. Remarkably, EGCG does not harm healthy cells. In addition, research at the Medical College of Ohio indicates that EGCG inhibits the production of urokinase, an enzyme that cancer cells need in order to grow. In animals, blocking urokinase shrinks tumors, and sometimes causes cancer to go into complete remission.

ADDITIONAL BENEFITS: The antioxidant effect of green tea's polyphenols may also help protect the heart. In test-tube studies, these compounds appeared to suppress the damage to LDL cholesterol, thought to be an initial step in the buildup of plaque in the arteries. A Japanese study of 1,371 men linked daily green tea consumption to the prevention of heart disease. In addition, green tea contains fluoride, which may help protect against tooth decay, and provides an overall antibacterial effect.

How to take it

⊘ **DOSAGE:** You can get the benefits of green tea either by taking green tea capsules or tablets, or by drinking several cups of the brew each day. Your aim should be to get 240 to 320 mg of polyphenols.

When using supplements, buy those standardized to contain at least 50% polyphenols. At this concentration, two 250 mg supplements would provide 250 mg of polyphenols. Studies show that four cups of freshly brewed green tea also supply a recommended amount of polyphenols.

◈ **GUIDELINES FOR USE:** Take green tea supplements at meals with a full glass of water. Drink freshly brewed green tea on its own or with meals. To make tea, use 1 teaspoon of green tea leaves per cup of very hot water. Let the brew steep for three to five minutes; then strain and drink it.

Possible side effects

Green tea is very safe, both as a supplement and as a beverage. People who are sensitive to caffeine, however, may not want to drink too much green tea, because each cup contains about 40 mg of caffeine. (Indeed, for this reason, pregnant women and those who are breast-feeding should limit their consumption to two cups a day.) Green tea supplements, however, have very little caffeine. The recommended dose of green tea supplements provides the same amount of polyphenols as four cups of green tea, but generally contains only 5 to 6 mg of caffeine.

- Green tea leaves contain hefty amounts of vitamin K, but a cup of brewed tea or green tea supplements have virtually none. This means that people taking anticoagulant drugs for heart disease (who may have been told to avoid large servings of foods rich in vitamin K because of the vitamin's influence on blood clotting) can enjoy green tea with no fear of side effects.

- Drinking boiling hot green tea can damage your throat and esophagus and may over time increase your cancer risk. Try the traditional Asian method: Heat cold water until just before it boils (or boil it and let it cool for a few minutes), then pour the hot-but-not-boiling water over the tea leaves. This method also helps accent the delicate flavor of green tea.

- Imported from China, gunpowder tea is simply green tea presented in tiny pellets resembling gunpowder. When placed in hot water, the leaves slowly unfold.

LATEST FINDINGS

- According to researchers at the University of Kansas, green tea's main antioxidant (EGCG) is 100 times more powerful than vitamin C and 25 times more potent than vitamin E in protecting DNA from the kind of damage thought to increase cancer risk.

Green tea can be taken in supplement form or enjoyed as a soothing beverage.

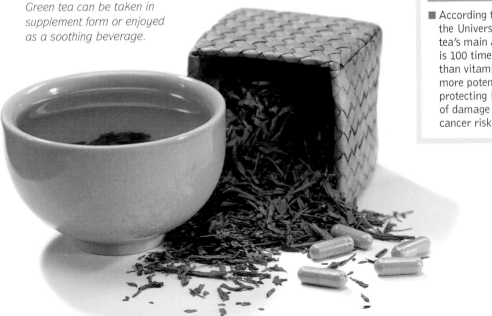

gugulipid

Commiphora mukul

Since antiquity, the gum resin of the mukul myrrh tree has been used in India to treat obesity and arthritis. Now a modern purified extract called gugulipid has been found to be as effective as some prescription drugs for lowering cholesterol and triglyceride levels in the blood.

COMMON USES

- *Helps lower high blood cholesterol and high blood triglycerides.*
- *Reduces heart disease risk.*
- *Treats arthritis inflammation.*
- *May aid weight loss.*

FORMS

- Capsule
- Tablet

CAUTION!

- Never use the crude gum guggul, or guggulu, which can cause rashes, diarrhea, stomach pain, and loss of appetite. Opt for standardized gugulipid instead.
- Pregnant women should not use gugulipid.
- Reminder: If you have a medical condition, talk to your doctor before taking supplements.

What it is

Gugulipid comes from the gummy resin of the small thorny mukul myrrh tree native to India. The tree's resin is closely related to the richly perfumed Biblical myrrh, traditionally used for purification purposes.

Called gum guggul ("guggulu"), the resin itself has been part of Ayurveda, the traditional medicine of India, for thousands of years. Guggulu, however, has toxic compounds. Fortunately, modern Indian pharmacologists have devised a way to extract the active components in the resins and leave the toxic substances behind. The result is the standardized extract called gugulipid.

What it does

The active ingredients in gugulipid, known as guggulsterones, appear to affect the way the body metabolizes fat and cholesterol. They also have anti-inflammatory and antioxidant properties.

PREVENTION: If you have high blood cholesterol levels, you are at increased risk for developing coronary heart disease. Studies suggest that gugulipid can lower these levels; it is the guggulsterones, in particular, that seem to stimulate the liver to break down potentially harmful LDL cholesterol. In addition, gugulipid sometimes elevates the levels of protective HDL cholesterol. A study of 205 people in India found that gugulipid, in combination with a low-fat diet, reduced total cholesterol by an average of 24% in more than three-quarters of the participants. In another study comparing the efficacy of gugulipid with that of clofibrate, a prescription cholesterol-lowering medication, total cholesterol dropped by 11% in the gugulipid group and by 10% in the clofibrate group. In addition,

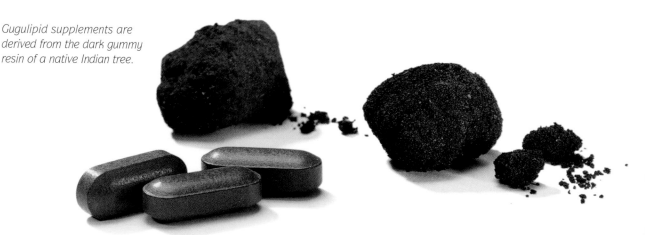

Gugulipid supplements are derived from the dark gummy resin of a native Indian tree.

nearly two-thirds of those taking gugulipid experienced increases in HDL cholesterol levels on average; however, no change in HDL was seen in those using clofibrate.

In animal studies, gugulipid has been shown to prevent the formation of artery-blocking plaque, and even to help reverse existing plaque. In addition, it inhibits blood platelets from sticking together, and thus may protect against blood clots, which often trigger heart attacks.

✳ **ADDITIONAL BENEFITS:** Studies lend support to two of the traditional uses for guggul: arthritis and obesity. Results from animal studies indicate that the anti-inflammatory action of guggulsterones may be as powerful as that of over-the-counter pain medications, such as ibuprofen, making it useful in treating arthritis. This action suggests that gugulipid may also be effective for acne; in fact, one study showed it had a beneficial effect on this condition.

There is some evidence that gugulipid stimulates the production of thyroid hormones, increasing the rate at which the body burns calories. In one small study, Indian researchers reported that in overweight patients, gugulipid supplements sparked significant weight loss. Much of the weight loss came from a reduction in fat around the abdomen, which is associated with an increased risk of heart disease and diabetes. Any effective long-term weight control program, of course, must begin with a low-fat, high-fiber diet and a regular exercise program.

How to take it

⊘ **DOSAGE:** To lower cholesterol, take a supplement that supplies 25 mg of guggulsterones per dose, three times a day.

◉ **GUIDELINES FOR USE:** Take gugulipid with or without meals. Pregnant women should avoid gugulipid; it should be used with caution by those with liver disease, inflammatory bowel disease, or diarrhea.

Possible side effects

Rarely, gugulipid may cause minor gastrointestinal problems, such as mild nausea, gas, or hiccups. In a few cases, headaches have also been reported.

Did You Know?

As early as 600 B.C., Ayurvedic physicians in India described a disease marked by the overeating of fatty foods, lack of exercise, an impaired metabolism, and the "coating and obstruction of channels." They called it "medoroga" (today it's known as atherosclerosis); to treat it they used guggul, a precursor to gugulipid.

hawthorn

Crataegus oxyacantha

If your doctor confirms that you have any form of heart disease, you'll want to know all about hawthorn. This herb, historically used both as a diuretic and as a treatment for kidney and bladder stones, is presently one of the most widely prescribed heart remedies in Europe.

COMMON USES

- *Relieves chest pain of angina.*
- *Lowers high blood pressure.*
- *Helps the heart pump more efficiently in people with congestive heart failure.*
- *Corrects irregular heartbeat (cardiac arrhythmia).*

FORMS

- Tablet
- Capsule
- Tincture
- Powder
- Dried herb/Tea

CAUTION!

- In people who don't have heart disease, large doses of hawthorn can cause very low blood pressure, which can lead to dizziness and fainting.
- Reminder: If you have a medical condition, talk to your doctor before taking supplements.

What it is

For centuries, hawthorn, a shrub that grows to 30 feet, has been trimmed to hedge height and planted along the edges of fields or property lines. As a divider, it looks attractive and discourages trespassers: It produces pretty white flowers and vibrant red berries, but it also sports large thorns, and the flowers on some varieties smell like rotting meat. What's more, the plant has long been associated with bad luck and death, because the crown of thorns that Christ wore at the Crucifixion is widely believed to have been woven from hawthorn twigs.

Given this reputation, it's surprising that anyone got close enough to discover hawthorn's cardioprotective benefits. But obviously a number of people in different eras and locations—from the ancient Greeks to the Native Americans—did consider the herb a potent tonic for the heart. The modern use of hawthorn originated with a nineteenth-century Irish physician who treated heart disease quite successfully. Because he closely guarded his heart formula, not until after his death in the 1890s was his secret remedy revealed to be tincture of hawthorn berry.

What it does

Hawthorn is an herb that directly benefits the workings of the heart. It can dilate blood vessels, increase the heart's energy supply, and improve its pumping ability. These powerful cardiac effects can probably be traced to its abundant supply of plant compounds called flavonoids—especially procyanidolic oligomers (PCOs)—which function as potent antioxidants.

Hawthorn supplements are derived from the plant's leaves and flowers, its red berries (right), or a combination of all three.

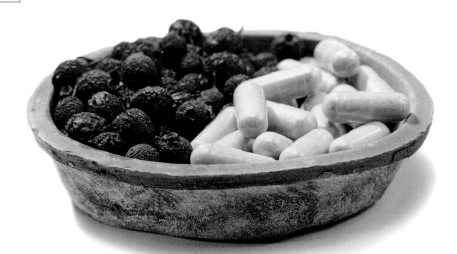

✪ **MAJOR BENEFITS:** Hawthorn seems to be an all-purpose heart drug. It widens arteries by interfering with an enzyme called ACE (angiotensin-converting enzyme), which constricts blood vessels. This action improves blood flow through the arteries, making the herb a good remedy for people with angina. In addition, chronically constricted arteries can lead to high blood pressure (because the heart must work harder to pump blood through inflexible arteries), so hawthorn may reduce blood pressure in those with mild hypertension.

Hawthorn also seems to block enzymes that weaken the heart muscle, thereby strengthening its pumping power. This property is especially useful for individuals with mild congestive heart failure who don't require strong heart medications, such as digitalis. Moreover, the antioxidant properties of hawthorn may help protect against damage associated with the buildup of plaque in the coronary arteries.

✱ **ADDITIONAL BENEFITS:** Hawthorn has a long history as a treatment for other conditions as well. It seems to exert a calming effect and functions as a sleeping aid in some who suffer from insomnia. Several researchers have also noted that hawthorn preserves collagen—the protein that composes connective tissue—which is damaged in such diseases as arthritis.

How to take it

🕖 **DOSAGE:** The recommended dose of hawthorn extract ranges from 300 to 450 mg a day in pill form, and from 1 teaspoon to 1 tablespoon (5 to 15 ml) of the tincture, depending on the type of heart condition. People at risk for heart disease may wish to take a 100 to 150 mg supplement or 1 teaspoon of the tincture daily as a heart disease preventive.

◈ **GUIDELINES FOR USE:** If you're on large doses, hawthorn works best when the daily amount is divided and taken at three different times during the day. Hawthorn may take a couple of months to build up in your system and produce noticeable results.

Possible side effects

Hawthorn is widely regarded as one of the safest herbal preparations. Though there have been reports of nausea, sweating, fatigue, and skin rash, these side effects are uncommon. Hawthorn appears to be safe to use with drugs prescribed for heart disease. You may even need less of some heart medications while you're taking hawthorn. Still, talk with your doctor before trying hawthorn, and never stop taking a drug that's been prescribed for you (or reduce the dose) without your doctor's consent.

SHOPPING HINTS
■ When buying hawthorn, look for standardized extracts that contain at least 1.8% vitexin, sometimes called vitexin-2"-rhamnoside. This is the main heart-protective substance in the herb.

LATEST FINDINGS

■ In an eight-week German study of 136 people with mild to moderate congestive heart failure, those who took hawthorn extract reported less shortness of breath, less ankle swelling, and better exercise performance than those given a placebo. Physical exams and laboratory tests confirmed that the condition of the hawthorn group improved while the condition of the placebo group worsened.

Did You Know?

Hawthorn varieties grow in Europe, eastern Asia, northern Africa, and the United States. It is also known as whitethorn and mayflower—in fact, the Pilgrim ship the *Mayflower* was named after the hawthorn blossom.

iodine

Many people associate iodine with the orange-brown topical antiseptic their mothers swabbed on their childhood scrapes and bruises. But the real value of this potent trace mineral is its role in thyroid health, where it is involved in numerous biological functions we couldn't live without.

COMMON USES

- *Corrects an iodine deficiency.*
- *Ensures proper functioning of the thyroid gland.*
- *May help treat fibrocystic breasts.*

FORMS

- Tablet
- Capsule
- Liquid

CAUTION!

- Because iodine deficiency is rare in developed countries, take iodine supplements only if prescribed by your physician.
- Reminder: If you have a medical or psychiatric condition, talk to your doctor before taking supplements.

What it is

Although the body needs just tiny amounts of iodine, this mineral is so crucial to an individual's overall health that in the 1920s government officials decided it should be added to a foodstuff common to nearly everyone—namely, table salt. The introduction of iodized salt to the American diet virtually eliminated one severe form of mental retardation called cretinism. Despite the recognized importance of this vital mineral, however, about 1.6 billion people in the world, mostly in underdeveloped countries, still suffer from iodine deficiency.

What it does

Unique among minerals, iodine has only one known function in the body: It is essential to the thyroid gland for manufacturing thyroxine, a hormone that regulates metabolism in all the body's cells.

PREVENTION: By getting enough iodine, pregnant women can prevent certain types of mental retardation in their developing fetus.

ADDITIONAL BENEFITS: Unlike many other minerals, iodine does not seem to help in the treatment of specific diseases; however, it does play a fundamental role in assuring the health of the thyroid, the butterfly-shaped gland that surrounds the windpipe (trachea). When your iodine intake is adequate, your body contains about an ounce of it, and 75% of that amount is stored in the thyroid. This organ controls the body's overall metabolism, which determines how quickly and efficiently calories are burned. It also regulates growth and development in children, reproduction, nerve and muscle function, the breakdown of proteins and fats, the growth of nails and hair, and the use of oxygen by every cell in the body. There is some evidence that iodine derived from an organic source may be effective in reducing the pain of fibrocystic breasts, but patients should discuss this type of supplementation with their doctor first.

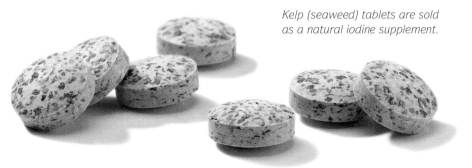

Kelp (seaweed) tablets are sold as a natural iodine supplement.

How much you need

The RDA for iodine is 150 mcg daily for adult men and women. Most people meet or exceed this amount by using iodized salt (1 teaspoon of iodized salt contains more than 300 mcg of iodine).

⊟ **IF YOU GET TOO LITTLE:** Thanks to the widespread use of iodized salt, not a single case of iodine deficiency has been reported in the United States since the 1970s. Among the first signs of iodine deficiency, now rarely seen, is an enlarged thyroid gland, known as a goiter. Lack of iodine can cause the gland to expand in an attempt to increase its surface area and trap as much of the iodine in the bloodstream as possible. If your iodine intake is low, your thyroid hormone level may well be low too. This condition can lead to fatigue, dry skin, a rise in blood fats, a hoarse voice, delayed reflexes, and reduced mental clarity. See your doctor if you have these symptoms.

⊞ **IF YOU GET TOO MUCH:** There is very little risk of iodine overdose, even at levels 10 to 20 times the RDA. However, if you ingest 30 times the RDA, you are likely to experience a metallic taste, mouth sores, swollen salivary glands, diarrhea, vomiting, headache, a rash, and difficulty in breathing. Ironically, a goiter can also develop if you consistently take extremely large amounts of iodine.

How to take it

⊘ **DOSAGE:** You probably get all the iodine you need from your daily intake of iodized salt or from regular servings of seafood. Iodine is also a standard ingredient in many multivitamin and mineral supplements. Even if you are on a severely restricted salt diet for high blood pressure, you probably don't require extra iodine, though you can safely take 150 mcg a day. People on a thyroid hormone should always discuss their condition with a doctor before taking individual iodine supplements.

◉ **GUIDELINES FOR USE:** When prescribed, iodine supplements can be taken at any time of the day, with or without food.

Other sources

Although the most abundant source of iodine is iodized table salt, the mineral can also be found in saltwater fish and in sea vegetation, such as kelp. Soil in coastal areas also tends to be iodine-rich, as are the dairy products produced by cows grazing there. The same is true for fruits and vegetables grown in soil high in iodine. Commercial baked goods—such as breads and cakes—are other good sources of iodine. Though iodized salt is not used in commercial baking, these products are often made with dough conditioners that contain iodine.

FACTS
& Tips

■ Even though health-food stores frequently promote sea salt as a healthier alternative to table salt, sea salt is not iodized, and therefore is not a good source of iodine.

■ If you're thinking the pretzels or potato chips you eat probably provide all the iodine you need, guess again. Iodized salt isn't used to flavor popular salty snacks.

LATEST FINDINGS

■ An analysis of 10 different studies, performed in countries where iodine deficiency is common, found evidence that an iodine deficiency can affect motor skills, decreasing reaction time, manual dexterity, coordination, and muscle strength. The analysis, headed by UNICEF researchers, also revealed that the IQ of people who were iodine deficient was some 13 points below that of those with adequate iodine.

iron

A surprising number of Americans get too little iron—and few realize that lack of this vital mineral can make them weak, unable to concentrate, and more susceptible to infection. Too much iron, however, can be dangerous. A blood test can show whether you would benefit from an iron supplement.

COMMON USES

- *Treats iron-deficiency anemia.*
- *Often needed during pregnancy; by women with heavy menstrual periods; or in other situations determined by your doctor.*

FORMS

- Tablet
- Capsule
- Softgel
- Liquid

CAUTION!

- Never take an iron supplement unless you are following your doctor's recommendation. More than 1 million Americans have an inherited disease called hemochromatosis, which causes them to absorb too much iron, and most don't even know it. (Early symptoms include fatigue and aching joints.)
- Taking iron on your own could also mask a cause of anemia, such as a bleeding ulcer, and prevent your doctor from making an early, lifesaving diagnosis.
- Reminder: If you have a medical condition, talk to your doctor before taking supplements.

What it is

Needed throughout the body, iron is an essential part of hemoglobin, the oxygen-carrying component of red blood cells. The mineral is also found in myoglobin, which supplies oxygen to the muscles, and is part of many enzymes and immune-system compounds. The body, which gets most of the iron it requires from foods, carefully monitors its iron status, absorbing more of the mineral when demand is high (during periods of rapid growth, such as pregnancy or childhood) and less when stores of it are adequate. Because the body loses iron when bleeding, menstruating women may often have low levels. Dieters, vegetarians, and endurance athletes may experience iron shortfalls as well.

What it does

By helping the blood and muscles deliver oxygen, iron supplies energy to every cell in the body. Yet iron deficiency is surprisingly common in the United States. According to federal statistics, 9% of adolescent girls and 11% of women under age 50 are deficient in this mineral. Though it is very difficult to develop an iron deficiency from poor nutrition (iron is found in many foods), women with heavy menstrual periods and people with certain medical conditions may need supplements to prevent or correct the severe condition known as iron-deficiency anemia.

⭐ **MAJOR BENEFITS:** Keeping your body well supplied with iron provides energy, helps your immune system function at its best, and gives your mind an edge. Studies show that even mild iron deficiency—well short of the levels commonly associated with anemia—can cause adults to have a short attention span and teens to do poorly in school.

How much you need

The RDA for iron in men of all ages and women over age 50 is 10 mg a day. For younger women, it's 15 mg daily (in pregnancy, 30 mg a day). To combat anemia, additional iron—either through diet or supplements—is typically needed for a period of weeks or months.

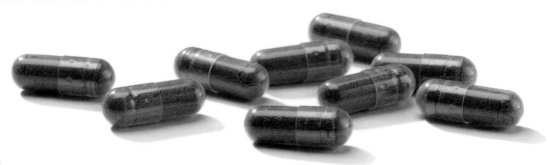

⊖ **IF YOU GET TOO LITTLE:** If you get too little iron in your diet or lose too much through heavy menstrual periods, stomach bleeding (commonly caused by arthritis drugs), or cancer, your body draws on its iron reserve. Initially, there are no symptoms, but as your iron supply dwindles, so does your body's ability to produce healthy red blood cells. The result is iron-deficiency anemia, marked by weakness, fatigue, paleness, breathlessness, palpitations, and increased susceptibility to infection.

⊕ **IF YOU GET TOO MUCH:** Some studies link too much iron to an increased risk of chronic diseases, including heart disease and colon cancer. Excess iron can be particularly dangerous in adults with a genetic tendency to overabsorb it (hemochromatosis), and in children who are especially susceptible to iron overdose.

How to take it

▨ **DOSAGE:** Iron supplements should be taken only under your doctor's supervision; self-treatment can be dangerous. Anemia requires a careful diagnosis and treatment to correct the underlying cause. When a doctor recommends it, iron is typically taken in a form called ferrous salts—usually ferrous sulfate, ferrous fumarate, or ferrous gluconate. A typical prescribed dose provides about 30 mg of iron one to three times daily. Most men and postmenopausal women do not need iron supplements and should make sure iron is not included in their daily multivitamin.

◪ **GUIDELINES FOR USE:** Iron is best absorbed when taken on an empty stomach. However, if iron upsets your stomach, have it with meals, preferably with a small amount of meat and a food or drink rich in vitamin C, such as broccoli or orange juice, to help boost the amount of iron your body absorbs. Never take iron for more than six months without having your blood iron levels rechecked by your doctor.

Other sources

Iron-rich foods include liver, beef, and lamb. Clams, oysters, and mussels also contain iron. Vegetarians can get plenty of iron from beans and peas, leafy greens, dried fruits (apricots, raisins), seeds (pumpkin, squash, sunflower), and fortified breakfast cereals. Brewer's yeast, kelp, blackstrap molasses, and wheat bran are also exceptionally good sources. Cooking tomatoes or other acidic foods in a cast-iron pot adds iron to meals as well; a healthful amount leaches out of the cookware into the food.

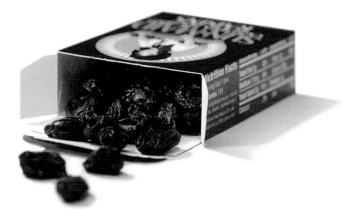

kava

Piper methysticum

When English explorer Captain James Cook sailed the South Pacific in the 1700s, the kava his crew sampled along the way may have eased the stress of the journey. The herb has long been appreciated for its calming effects, and today it continues to attract new enthusiasts.

COMMON USES

- *Combats anxiety.*
- *Eases panic attacks.*
- *Helps induce sleep.*
- *Relieves pain.*

FORMS

- Capsule
- Tablet
- Softgel
- Liquid
- Tincture
- Dried herb/Tea

CAUTION!

- Pregnant or breast-feeding women should not use kava.
- Don't take kava if you have Parkinson's disease. It may make symptoms worse.
- Reminder: If you have a medical or psychiatric condition, talk to your doctor before taking supplements.

What it is

A member of the pepper family, kava (also known as kava-kava) is a shrub that thrives on many South Pacific islands. The name "kava" refers not only to the herb but also to a traditional beverage made by crushing the root into a pulp, adding coconut milk or water, and straining it into coconut shells. For thousands of years, kava has played a major role in social events and religious rituals among Pacific islanders. In fact, island ceremonies—whether those welcoming royalty or simply hosting a neighborhood get-together—wouldn't be complete without kava, which serves a purpose similar to that of alcohol in other societies, namely, inducing a sense of well-being and fostering social discourse.

The kava plant, with its heart-shaped leaves, bears sterile flowers and can be propagated only by dividing the roots, which are thick and gnarled. These can weigh up to 22 pounds. Today, in many parts of the South Pacific, kava is widely cultivated for the medicinal properties of its roots and is exported to herb shops throughout the world.

What it does

Kava root contains a number of compounds (the most prominent are known as kavalactones), which have a wide range of therapeutic effects. In many European countries, doctors currently prescribe kava for the treatment of anxiety, stress, restlessness, and insomnia. Scientists aren't sure how it works but believe that kava targets the limbic system, a primitive part of the brain that (among other things) regulates emotions.

⭐ **MAJOR BENEFITS:** Kava is known primarily for its anxiety-relieving benefits. It can be useful for reducing general stress and nervousness, as well as for warding off the intense bouts of anxiety known as panic

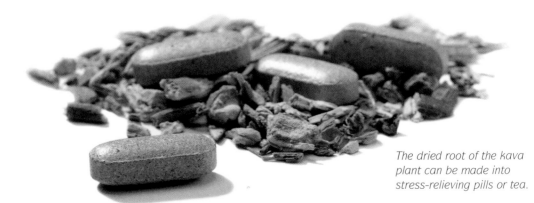

The dried root of the kava plant can be made into stress-relieving pills or tea.

attacks. Kava can also have a calming effect on individuals who are trying to stop smoking or wean themselves off alcohol. Its relaxing properties may help insomniacs fall asleep. And those with mild to moderate depression, who often suffer from anxiety, may likewise benefit from the herb. Unlike conventional tranquilizers, kava doesn't appear to dull the mind. Some studies even show that it improves mental reaction time. Surprisingly, people taking kava rarely seem to develop a tolerance to the herb. In addition, kava generally doesn't seem to be addictive.

✳ **ADDITIONAL BENEFITS:** Kava has pain-relieving qualities that may be of value in treating muscle aches as well as chronic pain affecting any part of the body. It also appears to have muscle-relaxing properties, and so may be beneficial for easing muscle spasms. In some people with epilepsy, kava seems to prevent seizures as effectively as some prescription anticonvulsants; its effects may be related to its power to relieve stress and anxiety, which can trigger epileptic attacks. Furthermore, preliminary studies suggest the herb may help stroke patients recover by minimizing the amount of permanent brain damage that can occur.

How to take it

◐ **DOSAGE:** The recommended dose is 250 mg of a standardized extract, two or three times a day. Consult your doctor if you have been taking kava for more than three months because prolonged use increases the chance of side effects (see below).

◆ **GUIDELINES FOR USE:** Do not exceed the recommended dose. Higher dosages can lead to intoxication or disorientation. (One man in Utah was convicted of driving under the influence after spending the evening consuming 16 cups of kava tea, which caused him to stagger, slur his speech, and drive as if drunk on alcohol.)

In addition, unless your doctor recommends it, avoid this herb if you are regularly taking other drugs that affect the central nervous system, such as antidepressants, sedatives, or tranquilizers. It's also a good idea to avoid drinking alcohol when using kava. Kava is, however, sometimes combined with herbal supplements that affect the brain, such as the antidepressant St. John's wort. Kava usually acts within minutes, though for some people with severe anxiety, the full benefits may not be apparent until up to eight weeks after first consuming the herb.

Possible side effects

Stomach upset is the most common side effect. Occasionally, people who are on very high doses for extended periods (as little as three months, though usually much longer) may find that their skin turns yellow (first their face, then the rest of their body) and becomes dry and scaly. Other side effects of very high doses include loss of appetite, labored breathing, blurred vision, bloodshot eyes, walking difficulties, and intoxication; if these occur, stop taking the herb. There have also been reports of allergic skin rashes, but these are quite uncommon.

Did You Know?

During South Pacific welcoming ceremonies, Lyndon and Lady Bird Johnson, Hillary Rodham Clinton, Queen Elizabeth, and Pope John Paul II all drank kava.

lecithin and choline

These closely related nutrients with the scientific-sounding names are actually essential for every cell in your body. They're particularly important for the liver and nerves. No wonder so many nutritionists urge Americans to get more of them.

COMMON USES

- *Help in preventing gallstones.*
- *Strengthen the liver, making them useful in the treatment of hepatitis and cirrhosis.*
- *Aid the liver in ridding the body of toxins in patients undergoing chemotherapy for cancer.*
- *Diminish heartburn symptoms.*
- *May boost memory and enhance brain function.*

FORMS

- Capsule
- Tablet
- Softgel
- Powder
- Liquid

CAUTION!

- Reminder: If you have a medical condition, talk to your doctor before taking supplements.

What it is

Lecithin (pronounced LESS-a-thin) is a fatty substance found in many animal- and plant-based foods, including liver, eggs, soybeans, peanuts, and wheat germ. It is also often added to processed foods—including ice cream, chocolate, margarine, and salad dressings—to help blend, or emulsify, the fats with water. In addition, the body manufactures it.

Lecithin is considered an excellent source of the B vitamin choline, primarily in the form called phosphatidylcholine. Once in the body, the phosphatidylcholine breaks down into choline, so that when you take lecithin, or absorb lecithin from foods, your body gets choline. However, only 10% to 20% of the lecithin found in plants and other natural sources consists of phosphatidylcholine. You can buy lecithin supplements that contain higher concentrations of phosphatidylcholine, but they can be very expensive. For most situations, just taking plain lecithin, rather than the more costly phosphatidylcholine, works fine.

Though dietary lecithin is a primary source of choline, choline is also found in liver, soybeans, egg yolks, grape juice, peanuts, cabbage, cauliflower, and other foods. You can also buy choline supplements, and it is often included as an ingredient in B-complex vitamins or other combination formulas.

What it does

Lecithin and choline are needed for a range of body functions. They help build cell membranes and facilitate the movement of fats and nutrients in and out of cells. They aid in reproduction and in fetal and infant development; they're essential to liver and gallbladder health; and they may help the heart. Choline is also a key component of the brain chemical acetylcholine, which plays a major role in memory and muscle control. As a result of these far-flung effects, lecithin and choline have been touted for almost everything—from curing cancer and AIDS to lowering cholesterol.

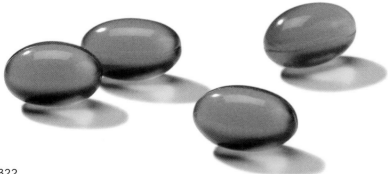

Lecithin is good for the brain and liver, and helps you digest fats. Softgels are a popular form of lecithin supplement.

And even though the evidence for some of these claims is weak, these nutrients should not be dismissed out of hand.

⊛ **MAJOR BENEFITS:** Lecithin and choline may be especially helpful in the treatment of gallbladder and liver diseases. Lecithin is a key component of bile, the fat-digesting substance, and low levels of this nutrient are known to precipitate gallstones. Taking supplements with lecithin or its purified extract, phosphatidylcholine, may treat or prevent this disorder. Lecithin may also be beneficial for the liver: The results of a 10-year study on baboons showed that it prevented severe liver scarring and cirrhosis caused by alcohol abuse; other studies have indicated that it helps liver problems associated with hepatitis.

Choline is often included in liver complex formulas along with other liver-strengthening supplements, such as the amino acid methionine, the B vitamin inositol, and the herbs milk thistle and dandelion. These preparations, often called lipotropic combinations or factors, can protect against the buildup of fats within the liver, improve the flow of fats and cholesterol through the liver and gallbladder, and help the liver rid the body of dangerous toxins. They may be especially helpful for liver or gallbladder diseases, such as hepatitis, cirrhosis, or gallstones, as well as for conditions that benefit from good liver function, such as endometriosis (the leading cause of female infertility) or side effects from chemotherapy. Choline, along with the B vitamins pantothenic acid and thiamin, may also help treat heartburn.

⊛ **ADDITIONAL BENEFITS:** These two nerve-building nutrients may be useful for improving memory in those with Alzheimer's disease, preventing neural tube birth defects (spina bifida), boosting performance in endurance sports, and treating twitches and tics (tardive dyskinesia) caused by antipsychotic drugs. They have also been proposed as possible remedies against high cholesterol and even cancer. However, more studies are needed to define their role in these and other diseases.

How to take it

⦿ **DOSAGE:** Lecithin is usually given in a dosage of two 1,200 mg capsules twice a day. It can also be taken in a granular form: 1 teaspoon contains 19 grains, or 1,200 mg of lecithin. Choline can be obtained from lecithin, although phosphatidylcholine (500 mg three times a day) or plain choline (500 mg three times a day) may be a better source. Choline can also be taken as part of a lipotropic combination product. Lecithin and choline have no RDAs, although recently, the scientific group that sets nutritional standards established what's called an Adequate Intake for choline: 550 mg for men and 425 mg for women.

◈ **GUIDELINES FOR USE:** Lecithin and choline should be taken with meals to enhance absorption. Granular lecithin has a nutty taste and can be sprinkled over foods or mixed into drinks.

Possible side effects

In high doses, lecithin and choline may cause sweating, nausea, vomiting, bloating, and diarrhea. Taking very high dosages of choline (10 grams a day) may produce a fishy body odor or a heart rhythm disorder.

Did You Know?

Lecithin and choline have no RDAs, but deficiencies are rare. Most Americans get enough of these nutrients in their daily diet—about 6 grams of lecithin and up to 1 gram of choline.

licorice

Glycyrrhiza glabra

In ancient Greece, licorice calmed coughs and soothed stomachs. In China, it's thought to lengthen life. Modern research finds that this herb boosts immunity, fights viruses, treats ulcers, reduces inflammation, protects the liver, eases menopause, and applied topically, relieves eczema.

COMMON USES

- *Reduces symptoms of chronic fatigue and fibromyalgia.*
- *Helps digestive problems.*
- *Helps treat eczema.*
- *Promotes hepatitis recovery.*
- *Enhances immunity.*
- *Eases respiratory illnesses.*
- *May be useful for menstrual disorders and menopause.*

FORMS

- Capsule
- Tablet
- Tincture
- Wafer (DGL)
- Lozenge
- Cream
- Dried herb/Tea

CAUTION!

- Glycyrrhizin, a key compound in licorice, raises blood pressure. Avoid licorice if you have heart, kidney, or liver disease; high blood pressure; are pregnant; or are taking diuretics or digitalis. DGL licorice, however, is fine.
- Reminder: If you have a medical condition, talk to your doctor before taking supplements.

What it is

One of the most extensively used and thoroughly studied herbal remedies, licorice has a long medicinal history. It was one of the first foods investigated by the National Cancer Institute's experimental food program.

Cultivated in Turkey and Greece, the licorice plant—a member of the pea family—is a tall shrub with bluish flowers. Its medicinal properties are in the root, or rhizome, which contains glycyrrhizin. Licorice is also a source of hundreds of other potentially beneficial substances, including plant estrogens and flavonoids.

Licorice root is made into capsules, tablets, tinctures, and cream for therapeutic use. Because it has a sweet, musty taste, licorice root is frequently combined with other herbs to mask their bitterness. Another form, DGL, or deglycyrrhizinated licorice, has had the glycyrrhizin removed; it is available in capsules and chewable wafers. The two types of licorice have different uses and effects on the body.

What it does

The glycyrrhizin in licorice stimulates the adrenal glands to produce certain hormones, reduces inflammation, and increases the levels of interferon, a virus-fighting substance manufactured by the immune system. Other compounds in licorice are potent antioxidants and may also mimic the effects of estrogen in the body. DGL has a beneficial effect on the digestive tract.

★ **MAJOR BENEFITS:** Licorice is helpful for respiratory problems because it fights the viruses that attack the respiratory tract, relieves symptoms such as coughing and sore throat, and works to thin mucus. Because of its action on the adrenal glands, licorice is often used by nutritionally

Licorice root is readily available in capsule form.

oriented physicians to treat chronic fatigue syndrome, fibromyalgia, and other disorders affected by the body's levels of cortisol, the main adrenal hormone. The herb can also be taken for virtually any condition involving inflammation. It's especially beneficial for hepatitis, combating inflammation in the liver and fighting the virus that often triggers the disease.

The DGL form does not work the same way licorice root does: DGL enhances the body's production of substances that coat the esophagus and stomach, protecting them from the corrosive effects of stomach acid. Therefore, DGL is helpful in cases of heartburn, ulcers, and inflammatory bowel disease. In fact, in several studies, DGL was more effective than standard prescription antiulcer medications. It works only when mixed with saliva, however, which is why the chewable wafer form of DGL is preferred for digestive problems. These wafers can also speed the healing of canker sores.

✳ **ADDITIONAL BENEFITS:** Licorice may be useful for menstrual problems and for menopause. Though glycyrrhizin inhibits the effect of the body's own estrogens, licorice's plant estrogens exert a mild estrogenic effect. A woman susceptible to PMS may find that taking licorice for 10 days leading up to her period eases some symptoms. In addition, topical licorice creams soothe skin irritations, such as eczema.

How to take it

⊘ **DOSAGE:** *For most disorders:* Take licorice root three times a day in 200 mg pills (standardized to contain 22% glycyrrhizinic acid or glycyrrhizin) or 45 drops of the fluid extract. *For heartburn and other digestive troubles:* Chew two to four 380 mg DGL wafers three times a day. *For eczema:* Apply cream to the affected area three or four times a day.

◉ **GUIDELINES FOR USE:** Licorice root supplements can be taken at any time of day. When using DGL, be sure to chew the wafers well and take them about 30 minutes before a meal. For sore throat, lozenges containing licorice work best.

Possible side effects

Because of its effect on the adrenal glands, licorice root can increase your blood pressure. For this reason, do not exceed recommended dosages. If you need to take licorice for more than a month, have your blood pressure monitored. True licorice candy and even chewing tobacco (which often contains licorice as a flavoring) can raise your blood pressure if they are used excessively. DGL does not raise blood pressure and has no other side effects.

Did You Know?

Licorice candy in the United States is typically flavored with anise oil, not licorice root, and red licorice isn't really licorice at all. True licorice candies (below) come from Europe. Don't overindulge; they can elevate blood pressure just like licorice root.

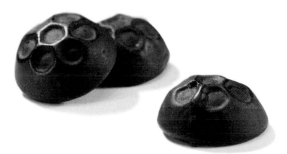

magnesium

Although little heralded, magnesium may be one of the most important health-promoting minerals. Studies suggest that besides enhancing some 300 enzyme-related processes in the body, magnesium may help prevent or combat many chronic diseases.

COMMON USES

- *Helps protect against heart disease and irregular heartbeat (arrhythmia).*
- *Eases fibromyalgia symptoms.*
- *Lowers high blood pressure.*
- *May reduce the severity of asthma attacks.*
- *Improves symptoms of premenstrual syndrome (PMS).*
- *Aids in preventing the complications of diabetes.*

FORMS

- Capsule
- Tablet
- Powder

CAUTION!

- People with kidney disease should consult their physicians before taking magnesium.
- Magnesium can make tetracycline antibiotics less effective. Consult your doctor.
- Reminder: If you have a medical condition, talk to your doctor before taking supplements.

What it is

The average person's body contains just an ounce of magnesium, but this small amount is vital to a number of bodily functions. Many people do not have adequate stores of magnesium, often because they rely too heavily on processed foods, which contain very little of this mineral. In addition, magnesium levels are easily depleted by stress, certain diseases or medications, and intense physical activity. For this reason, nutritional supplements may be necessary for optimal health. They are available in several forms, including magnesium aspartate, magnesium carbonate, magnesium gluconate, magnesium oxide, and magnesium sulfate.

What it does

One of the most versatile minerals, magnesium is involved in energy production, nerve function, muscle relaxation, and bone and tooth formation. In conjunction with calcium and potassium, magnesium regulates heart rhythm and clots blood; it also aids in the production and use of insulin.

PREVENTION: Recent research indicates that magnesium is beneficial for the prevention and treatment of heart disease. Studies show the risk of dying of a heart attack is lower in areas with "hard" water, which contains high levels of magnesium. Some researchers speculate that if everyone drank hard water, the number of deaths from heart attacks might decline by 19%. Magnesium appears to lower blood pressure and has also been found to aid recovery after a heart attack by inhibiting blood clots, widening arteries, and normalizing dangerous arrhythmias.

Preliminary studies suggest that an adequate intake of magnesium may prevent non-insulin-dependent (type 2) diabetes. Researchers at Johns Hopkins University measured magnesium levels in more than 12,000 people who did not have diabetes and tracked them for six years to see who developed the disease. Individuals with the lowest magnesium levels had a 94% greater chance of developing the disease than those with the highest levels. (These results, however, apply only to Caucasians; magnesium levels don't seem to affect diabetes in

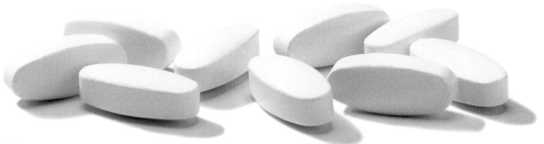

African-Americans.) Future studies are needed to see if magnesium supplements can prevent the disease.

⊕ **ADDITIONAL BENEFITS:** Because magnesium relaxes muscles, it's useful for sports injuries and fibromyalgia. It also seems to ease PMS and menstrual cramps, and may increase bone density in postmenopausal women, helping to stem the onset of osteoporosis. In addition, magnesium expands airways, which aids in the treatment of asthma and bronchitis. Studies are inconclusive about magnesium's role in preventing or treating migraines, but one study says it may improve the effect of sumatriptan, a prescription drug used for migraines.

How much you need

The RDA for magnesium is 350 mg for men and 280 mg for women daily. Higher doses are required for disease prevention or treatment, as well as for women who take oral contraceptives.

⊖ **IF YOU GET TOO LITTLE:** Even moderate deficiencies can raise the risk of heart disease and diabetes. Severe deficiencies can result in irregular heartbeat, fatigue, muscle spasms, irritability, nervousness, and confusion.

⊕ **IF YOU GET TOO MUCH:** Magnesium may cause diarrhea and nausea. More serious side effects—including muscle weakness, lethargy, confusion, and difficulty breathing—can develop if the body can't process high doses properly. Overdosing on magnesium, however, is rare because the kidneys are usually efficient at eliminating excess amounts.

How to take it

⊘ **DOSAGE:** *For heart disease prevention:* Take 400 mg a day. *For arrythmias, congestive heart failure, and asthma:* Use 400 mg twice a day. *For fibromyalgia:* Take 150 mg magnesium with 600 mg malic acid twice a day. *For high blood pressure:* Try 500 mg a day. *For diabetes:* Take 500 mg daily.

◑ **GUIDELINES FOR USE:** Magnesium is best absorbed when taken with each meal. If supplements cause diarrhea, lower the dose or use magnesium sulfate or gluconate, which are both easier on the digestive tract.

Other sources

Good food sources of magnesium are whole grains, nuts, legumes, dark green leafy vegetables, and shellfish.

FACTS & Tips

■ If you're taking magnesium supplements, be sure to take calcium supplements as well. Imbalances in the amounts of these two minerals can minimize their beneficial effects.

■ Research shows magnesium citrate is the form most readily absorbed by the body. Magnesium oxide may be the least expensive, but it's also the most poorly absorbed.

LATEST FINDINGS

■ A lack of magnesium can crimp a workout. In one study, women over age 50 needed more oxygen and had higher heart rates during exercise when magnesium levels were low.

■ Taking magnesium lowered blood pressure in a study of 60 men and women with hypertension. On average, systolic pressure (the top number) dropped 2.7 points; diastolic pressure (the bottom number) dropped 1.5 points. Declines of even a few points can reduce the risk of heart attack and stroke.

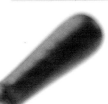

Did You Know?

You'd have to eat 3 cups of wild rice to meet the RDA requirement for a man—350 mg of magnesium.

melatonin

Hailed by some as a potent anti-aging hormone, melatonin has been credited with almost miraculous effects on a wide variety of ailments, including cancer. It is probably most effective, however, as a natural sleep aid to ease insomnia and overcome jet lag.

COMMON USES

- *Relieves insomnia.*
- *Promotes restful sleep, even during nighttime pain or stress-related sleep disturbances.*
- *Diminishes the effects and shortens the course of jet lag.*

FORMS

- Capsule
- Tablet
- Lozenge
- Softgel
- Liquid

CAUTION!

- Let your doctor know if you're taking melatonin. Adverse drug interactions have been reported in people taking common antidepressants (including Prozac or MAO inhibitors) or steroid or sedative drugs.
- Reminder: If you have a medical or psychiatric condition, talk to your doctor before taking supplements.

What it is

First identified in 1958, this naturally occurring hormone is manufactured by the pineal gland, a pea-size organ deep within the brain. All humans and most animals secrete melatonin throughout their lives, with the highest levels occurring during childhood. As we age, however, the production of melatonin declines, leading some researchers to theorize that melatonin supplementation might benefit all older people. Interestingly, natural melatonin levels vary widely: About 1% of the population have very low levels, and another 1% have levels 500 times above normal. There's no correlation, however, between these amounts and specific health concerns or sleep patterns.

What it does

One of the main functions of melatonin is to regulate cycles of sleep and wakefulness. It does so by helping to set the brain's internal clock, creating what are known as circadian rhythms—the body's daily biorhythms that govern everything from sleeping and waking times to digestive functions and the release of a variety of hormones linked to reproduction and other body processes. In order to produce melatonin, the body responds to light cues, making more when it's dark outside (production begins each evening around dusk and peaks between 2 A.M. and 4 A.M.) and less during the day. This daily cyclical melatonin secretion is what tells the body when to sleep and when to awaken.

⭐ **MAJOR BENEFITS:** Melatonin may be most effective as a sleep aid. Various studies of young and elderly adults indicate that in some people melatonin shortens the time needed to fall asleep and improves sleep quality by decreasing the number of times they awaken during the night. It may be beneficial when chronic pain or stress causes sleep disturbances. Melatonin can also help restore normal sleep patterns in people who do night shift work or in those suffering from jet lag as a result of crossing

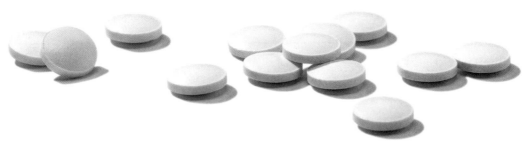

time zones. Moreover, it works without producing the addictive effects of conventional sleep medications.

✳ **ADDITIONAL BENEFITS:** Many other claims are made for melatonin. Interest in it as an anti-aging formula was sparked by an animal study in which nightly administration of the supplement to elderly mice prolonged their life by 25%. However, there have been no studies to show that melatonin supplementation delays aging in humans. Some research suggests that it may boost the immune system. And it may be an even stronger antioxidant than vitamins C or E or beta-carotene, hunting down and destroying the naturally occurring, cell-damaging compounds called free radicals that can lead to heart disease, cataracts, and other age-related degenerative changes. More research is needed to determine whether melatonin helps prevent these and other conditions.

Some studies suggest that when combined with certain cancer drugs, melatonin may help destroy malignant cells. Another study conducted in Holland in 1995 found that when taken in conjunction with birth control pills, melatonin has an estrogen-countering effect that may offer protection against some forms of breast cancer. In addition, reports indicate that melatonin may reduce some of the nerve damage associated with both Alzheimer's and Parkinson's diseases. And a 1997 study from Italy revealed it may also have beneficial effects on the blood vessels and thus play a role in reducing the risk of stroke and heart attack. More research is needed to determine the effectiveness and long-term safety of melatonin for these and other uses.

How to take it

⊘ **DOSAGE:** *For insomnia:* Take 1 to 3 mg before bedtime. *For jet lag:* Take a 3 mg dose on your day of travel, followed by 3 mg before bedtime for the first three or four nights at your final destination. *For shift work:* Take a 3 mg dose at your desired bedtime (at 8 A.M., for example) after working a night shift.

◑ **GUIDELINES FOR USE:** To combat insomnia, stick to a precise schedule, taking supplements at the same time every evening. Begin with the lowest dose and increase it as needed.

Possible side effects

No serious risks associated with melatonin use have been reported. In one study, patients who took very high doses (6,000 mg nightly) for one month had no major side effects. But long-term studies of six months or more are lacking.

For most people, melatonin causes drowsiness 30 minutes after taking it. This effect may last for several hours, so you should not drive or handle heavy machinery during this time. Other side effects can include headache, stomach upset, lethargy, or disorientation. Some individuals report that melatonin can cause fuzzy thinking upon waking, or vivid and sometimes unpleasant dreams, and even make insomnia worse. Others find that the effects wear off quickly with continued use.

LATEST FINDINGS

■ A study of 52 airline employees showed melatonin to be a very effective remedy against jet lag, significantly shortening the normal one-week adjustment period. Other studies with more than 400 people determined that the hormone reduces symptoms of jet lag by about 50%, on average, on both eastward and westward flights.

■ Preliminary studies at the Oregon Health Sciences University in Portland found tiny doses of melatonin may be effective for wintertime blues. Depressed patients who received several doses of 0.1 mg of melatonin in the afternoon showed significant mood improvements, compared with those who received no melatonin or a larger single dose in the morning. Scientists speculate small afternoon doses may better mimic the way melatonin is naturally released by the body, but caution against drawing conclusions until further studies are completed.

Did You Know?

In Canada, Britain, France, and a number of other countries, melatonin is classified as a drug and is available by prescription only.

milk thistle

Silybum marianum

The medicinal use of milk thistle can be traced back thousands of years to the times of the Greeks and the Romans. Today, researchers have completed more than 300 scientific studies that attest to the benefits of this herb, particularly for treating liver ailments.

COMMON USES

- Protects the liver from toxins, including drugs, poisons, and chemicals.
- Treats liver disorders, such as cirrhosis and hepatitis.
- Reduces liver damage from excessive alcohol.
- Aids in the treatment and prevention of gallstones.
- Helps clear psoriasis.

FORMS

- Tablet
- Capsule
- Softgel
- Tincture

CAUTION!

- Any liver disease requires careful evaluation and the supervision of a physician.
- Reminder: If you have a medical condition, talk to your doctor before taking supplements.

What it is

Known by its botanical name, *Silybum marianum,* as well as by its principal active ingredient, silymarin, milk thistle is a member of the sunflower family. The purple flowers and milky white leaf veins of this herb, which early settlers brought from Europe to North America, are a common sight along the East Coast and in California; the plant also grows as a weed in other parts of the United States and around the world. It blooms from June through August, and the shiny black seeds used for medicinal purposes are collected at the end of summer.

What it does

Milk thistle is one of the most extensively studied and documented herbs in use today. Scientific research continues to validate its healing powers, particularly for the treatment of liver-related disorders. Most of its effectiveness stems from a complex of three liver-protecting compounds, collectively known as silymarin, which constitutes 4% to 6% of the ripe seeds.

⭐ **MAJOR BENEFITS:** Among the most important benefits of milk thistle is its ability to fortify the liver, which is one of the body's most important organs, second in size only to the skin. The liver processes nutrients, including fats and other foods. In addition, it neutralizes, or detoxifies, many drugs, chemical pollutants, and alcohol. Milk thistle helps enhance and strengthen this vital organ by preventing the depletion of glutathione, an amino acid-like compound that is essential to the detoxifying process. What's more, studies show milk thistle can increase glutathione concentration by up to 35%. This herb is also an effective gatekeeper, limiting the number of toxins the liver processes at any given time.

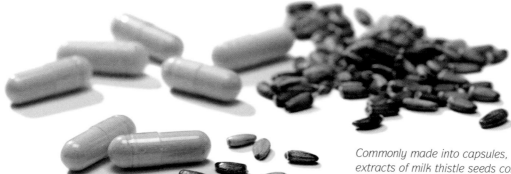

Commonly made into capsules, powdered extracts of milk thistle seeds contain a potent liver protector called silymarin.

Milk thistle is a powerful antioxidant as well. Even more potent than vitamins C and E, it helps prevent damage from highly reactive free-radical molecules. Furthermore, it promotes the regeneration of healthy, new liver cells, which replace old and damaged ones. Milk thistle eases a range of serious liver ailments, including viral infections (hepatitis) and scarring of the liver (cirrhosis). This herb is so potent that it's sometimes given in an injectable form in the emergency room to combat the life-threatening, liver-obliterating effects of poisonous mushrooms. In addition, because excessive alcohol depletes glutathione, milk thistle can aid in protecting the livers of alcoholics or those recovering from alcohol abuse.

✪ **ADDITIONAL BENEFITS:** In cancer patients, milk thistle limits the potential for drug-induced damage to the liver after chemotherapy treatments, and it speeds recovery by hastening removal of toxic substances that can accumulate in the body. The herb also reduces the inflammation and may slow the skin cell proliferation associated with psoriasis. It may be useful for endometriosis (the most common cause of infertility in women) because it helps the liver process the hormone estrogen, which at high levels can make pain and other symptoms worse. Finally, milk thistle can be beneficial in preventing or treating gallstones by improving the flow of bile, the cholesterol-laden digestive juice that travels from the liver through the gallbladder and into the intestine, where it helps to digest fats.

How to take it

⊘ **DOSAGE:** The recommended dose for milk thistle is up to 250 mg of standardized extract (containing 70% to 80% silymarin) three times a day. It is often combined with other herbs and nutrients, such as dandelion, choline, methionine, and inositol. This combination may be labeled "liver complex" or "lipotropic factors" ("lipotropic" refers to the formula's fat-metabolizing properties; it prevents the buildup of fatty substances in the liver). For proper dosage, follow package directions.

◆ **GUIDELINES FOR USE:** Milk thistle seems most effective when taken between meals. Its benefits may be noticeable within a week or two, though long-term treatment is often needed for chronic conditions. The herb appears to be safe, even for pregnant and lactating women. No interactions with other medications have been noted.

Possible side effects

Virtually no side effects have been attributed to the use of milk thistle, which is considered one of the safest herbs on the market. However, in some people it may have a slight laxative effect for a day or two.

SHOPPING HINTS

■ To be sure you're getting the proper dose, buy products made from standardized extracts that contain 70% to 80% silymarin, the active ingredient in milk thistle. You may also want preparations that contain milk thistle bound to phosphatidylcholine, a principal constituent of the natural fatty compound lecithin; studies show this combination may be better absorbed than regular milk thistle.

■ Be wary of alcohol-based tinctures. Some formulas contain high amounts of alcohol, which can be bad for the liver if taken in large doses.

LATEST FINDINGS

■ Milk thistle may one day prove to be an important weapon in the battle against skin cancer. Researchers at Case Western Reserve University in Cleveland found that when the active ingredient, silymarin, was applied to the skin of mice, 75% fewer skin tumors resulted following exposure to ultraviolet radiation. More studies are needed to see if it has a similar effect in humans.

Did You Know?

Milk thistle is not very soluble in water, so teas made from the seeds usually contain few of its liver-protecting ingredients.

mushrooms

Shiitake and maitake are more than just exotic-sounding words on a Japanese menu. In fact, they are members of a special group of medicinal mushrooms that Asians have heralded for centuries as longevity tonics and immune-system boosters.

Lentinus edodes (shiitake)
Grifola frondosa (maitake)
Ganoderma lucidum (reishi)
Coriolus versicolor (PSK)

COMMON USES

- *Build immunity.*
- *Help prevent cancer.*
- *Enhance cancer treatments.*
- *Alleviate bronchitis, sinusitis.*
- *Treat chronic fatigue syndrome.*
- *Help prevent heart disease.*

FORMS

- Capsule
- Tablet
- Liquid
- Powder
- Tea
- Dried mushrooms
- Fresh mushrooms

CAUTION!

- People taking anticoagulant drugs should avoid reishi supplements because the mushrooms contain compounds that also "thin" the blood.
- Reminder: If you have a medical condition, talk to your doctor before taking supplements.

What it is

For millennia, traditional Asian medicine has cherished certain mushrooms—including maitake, reishi, and shiitake—for their health-promoting effects. More recently, an extract from the mushroom *Coriolus versicolor*, called PSK, has been found to be a potent cancer fighter. Though other mushrooms—tree ear and oyster mushrooms, for instance—may also provide some health benefits, most of the attention, and research, has concentrated on the four types mentioned above.

These mushrooms are available as powders (in loose form for tea or in capsules or tablets) or as liquid extracts, which concentrate their potency. Dried reishi mushrooms and fresh and dried shiitake and maitake may be found in Asian groceries and some gourmet shops, but for therapeutic purposes, supplements are preferred. Maitake, reishi, and shiitake mushroom powders are sometimes combined in one capsule.

What it does

Medicinal mushrooms have varied effects, including boosting the body's immune system, lowering cholesterol, acting as an anticoagulant, and playing a supporting role in the treatment of cancer.

⭐ **MAJOR BENEFITS:** Maitake and *Coriolus versicolor* are commonly used in Japan to strengthen the immune systems of people undergoing chemotherapy treatment for cancer. Studies have shown that maitake extracts increase the effectiveness of lower chemotherapy doses while protecting healthy cells from the damage such drugs can cause. The Japanese have been employing the PSK extract from *Coriolus versicolor* as an adjunct to chemotherapy for many years. (In the United States, a similar product is labeled simply *Coriolus versicolor* extract.) Several studies have suggested that PSK can improve survival rates in people who have stomach, colon, or lung cancer.

Medicinal mushrooms appear to boost the immune system, assisting the body in fighting disease-causing organisms. Some studies indicate they may be powerful enough to help people with HIV infection and AIDS (who have very weak immune systems). For example, shiitake mushrooms contain a carbohydrate compound called lentinan, which promotes the

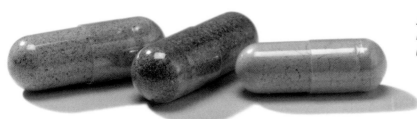

Supplements made from shiitake, reishi, and maitake mushrooms (left to right) come in capsule form.

body's production of T cells and other immune-system components. Laboratory studies show that *Coriolus versicolor* might be able to over-power HIV in the test tube; more research is needed to see if it can do the same in the human body. Other people with compromised immune systems—such as those with chronic fatigue syndrome—may benefit from medicinal mushrooms too.

✴ **ADDITIONAL BENEFITS:** Traditionally, reishi (known to the Chinese as "spirit plants") are used to help people relax, making them suitable for reducing stress and fatigue. Reishi also contain anti-inflammatory compounds that are beneficial for bronchitis and possibly for other respiratory ailments. In a Chinese study of 2,000 people with bronchitis, 60% to 90% of those given reishi tablets improved within two weeks. Shiitake, maitake, and reishi may also help fight heart disease by reducing the tendency of blood to clot, lowering blood pressure, and possibly reducing cholesterol levels.

How to take it

🕖 **DOSAGE:** *For immune-system support for cancer:* Take 500 mg of reishi, 400 mg shiitake, and 200 mg maitake mushrooms three times a day, and/or 3,000 mg of *Coriolus versicolor,* divided into two doses, a day. *For heart disease or HIV/AIDS:* Take 1,500 mg of reishi and 600 mg maitake daily. *For bronchitis or sinusitis:* Take 1,500 mg of reishi and/or 600 mg maitake daily during the illness.

◑ **GUIDELINES FOR USE:** The effects of medicinal mushrooms aren't dramatic, and may need several months to appear. For best results, divide the supplements into two or three daily doses and take with or without food.

Possible side effects

Shiitake, maitake, and reishi, as well as *Coriolus versicolor,* are all safe when used in appropriate doses. In fact, in the studies of cancer patients, the *Coriolus versicolor* was remarkably free of any adverse side effects.

In rare cases, long-term use of reishi mushrooms—three to six months of daily use—may cause dry mouth, a skin rash and itchiness, an upset stomach, nosebleeds, or bloody stools. Stop taking reishi if any of these symptoms arise. Pregnant or breast-feeding women should consult a physician before trying any of the mushrooms medicinally.

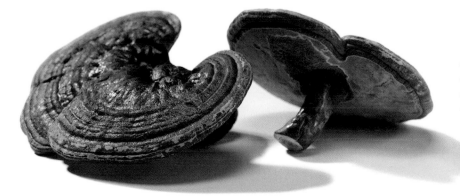

Helpful for stress, dried reishi mushrooms can be simmered in water to make a calming tea.

nettle

Urtica dioica

The healing powers of this herb date to the third century B.C., when it was used to remove venom from snakebites. Today, scientists are confirming that nettle has a valuable role to play in treating hay fever and prostate symptoms, as well as in easing the pain and inflammation of gout.

COMMON USES

- *Helps body remove excess fluid.*
- *Relieves allergy symptoms, particularly hay fever.*
- *Reduces inflammation.*
- *May ease prostate symptoms.*
- *Helps urinary tract infections.*

FORMS

- Capsule
- Tincture
- Liquid
- Dried herb/Tea

CAUTION!

- Reminder: If you have a medical condition, talk to your doctor before taking supplements.

What it is

Strange as it may sound, the original interest in using nettle for medicinal purposes probably was inspired by the plant's ability to irritate exposed skin. Nettle leaves are covered with tiny hairs—hollow needles actually—that sting and burn upon contact. This effect was believed to be beneficial for joint pain (stinging oneself with nettle is an old folk remedy for arthritis), and for centuries nettle leaf poultices were applied to draw toxins from the skin.

Also considered a nutritious food, nettle leaves taste like spinach. They're particularly high in iron and other minerals and are rich in carotenoids and vitamin C. (Opt for young shoots, which have no stingers.) The plant often grows up to five feet high in parts of the United States, Canada, and Europe.

What it does

Stinging yourself with nettle leaves probably won't help your joint pain, but nettle tea applied as a compress or nettle supplements taken orally may relieve inflamed joints, especially in people with gout. In addition, when taken internally, nettle has diuretic and antihistamine properties.

⭐ **MAJOR BENEFITS:** As a diuretic, nettle helps the body rid itself of excess fluid, and it may be useful as an adjunct treatment for many disorders. People suffering from urinary tract infections, for example, may find that it promotes urination, which flushes infection-causing bacteria out of the body. Women who become bloated just before their period may experience some relief after taking nettle supplements. The herb may also be

Supplements are a convenient way to get the diuretic and antihistamine effects of nettle leaves.

of value in some cases of high blood pressure—which can partly be attributed to excess fluid in the body—but it should be used for this purpose only under a doctor's supervision.

One of the tried-and-true benefits of nettle is its ability to control hay fever symptoms. Nasal congestion and watery eyes result when the body produces an inflammatory compound called histamine in response to pollen and other allergens. Nettle is a good source of quercetin, a flavonoid that has been shown to inhibit the release of histamine. In one study of allergy sufferers, over half of the participants rated nettle moderately to highly effective in reducing allergy symptoms when compared with a placebo.

✳ **ADDITIONAL BENEFITS:** Nettle may be suitable for men with an enlarged prostate not caused by cancer. This condition, called benign prostatic hyperplasia (BPH), occurs when the prostate enlarges and narrows the urethra (the tube that transports urine out of the bladder), making urination difficult. Nettle may aid in slowing prostate growth.

How to take it

⊘ **DOSAGE:** *For urinary tract infections:* Drink one cup of nettle tea a day. Use 1 teaspoon of the dried herb per cup of very hot water. *For allergies:* Take 250 mg standardized extract three times a day, as needed. *For BPH:* Use 250 mg standardized extract twice a day in combination with the herbs saw palmetto (160 mg twice a day) or pygeum africanum (100 mg twice a day). *For gout:* Take 250 mg three times a day. You can also apply a compress of nettle tea to painful joints.

◑ **GUIDELINES FOR USE:** In any of its forms, take nettle with food to minimize stomach upset. If you want to try the fresh leaves as a vegetable, keep in mind that the young shoots can be eaten raw, but older leaves (with mature, stinging hairs) must be cooked to inactivate the stingers.

Possible side effects

Generally, nettle is considered safe, with only a minimal risk of causing an allergic reaction. There have been some reports, however, that it may irritate the stomach, causing indigestion and diarrhea.

niacin

This B vitamin has been in the limelight as a potent cholesterol-lowering agent that rivals some prescription drugs in effectiveness. But niacin in its various forms also shows promise in the prevention and treatment of depression, arthritis, and a host of other ailments.

COMMON USES

- *Lowers cholesterol.*
- *May improve circulation.*
- *May ease symptoms of arthritis.*
- *May relieve depression.*
- *May prevent progression of type 1 diabetes.*

FORMS

- Capsule
- Tablet

CAUTION!

- Consult your doctor before using any form of niacin if you have any of the following conditions: diabetes, low blood pressure, bleeding problems, glaucoma, gout, liver disease, or ulcers. All can be aggravated by niacin.
- If you take a daily therapeutic dose of 1,000 mg or more of any form of niacin, see a doctor every three months to have your liver enzymes measured.
- Reminder: If you have a medical or psychiatric condition, talk to your doctor before taking supplements.

What it is

Also known as vitamin B_3, niacin is available as a supplement in three forms: nicotinic acid (or nicotinate), niacinamide, and inositol hexaniacinate (niacin bound to inositol, a member of the B-vitamin family). The body can also make niacin by converting the amino acid tryptophan—found in eggs, milk, and poultry—into the vitamin. About half of the niacin supplied by the average diet comes from the body's processing of tryptophan.

In supplement form, both nicotinic acid and niacinamide can satisfy your nutritional requirement for this B vitamin, but each of the three forms has its own specific role in treating disease.

What it does

Niacin is needed to release energy from carbohydrates. It is also involved in controlling blood sugar, keeping skin healthy, and maintaining the proper functioning of the nervous and digestive systems.

PREVENTION: High doses of niacin raise HDL ("good") cholesterol, while lowering LDL ("bad") cholesterol and triglyceride levels. In fact, studies show that niacin may be more effective than prescription cholesterol-lowering drugs in reducing the risk of heart disease, mainly because it is one of the few agents known to boost HDL. The cholesterol-lowering forms of niacin are nicotinic acid and inositol hexaniacinate. Although both are effective, inositol hexaniacinate is a safer form to use because it doesn't cause skin flushing and is less likely to cause liver damage.

ADDITIONAL BENEFITS: Niacin relaxes blood vessels, and so is useful for circulatory problems, such as intermittent claudication (a painful cramping in the calf caused by poor blood circulation that often occurs after walking), and Raynaud's disease (a disorder characterized by numbness and often pain in the hands or feet when exposed to cold). Inositol hexaniacinate is the preferred form to use for these conditions.

Niacin also helps foster healthy brain and nerve cells, and some evidence indicates that niacinamide can ease depression, anxiety, and insomnia. Niacinamide seems to have an anti-inflammatory effect, which

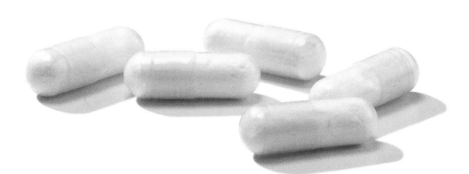

may benefit those with rheumatoid arthritis; it may also help heal damaged cartilage, potentially valuable for osteoarthritis. High doses of niacinamide may reverse the development of type 1 diabetes—the form that typically appears before age 30—if it is given early enough. This therapy should be tried only with medical supervision.

How much you need

The RDA for niacin is 14 mg for women and 16 mg for men daily. But far higher doses are required to lower cholesterol and treat other disorders.

⊖ **IF YOU GET TOO LITTLE:** A slight niacin deficiency will cause patches of irritated skin, appetite loss, indigestion, and weakness. Severe deficiencies (practically nonexistent in industrialized countries) result in pellagra, a debilitating disease. Symptoms include a rash in areas exposed to sunlight, vomiting, a bright red tongue, fatigue, and memory loss.

⊕ **IF YOU GET TOO MUCH:** Therapeutic doses of nicotinic acid may cause stomach upset, flushing and itching of the skin, and liver damage (at high doses, niacinamide may also harm the liver). To prevent these side effects, substitute inositol hexaniacinate whenever possible: It eliminates skin flushing and greatly reduces the risk of liver damage. But if you're taking any form of niacin for long periods, have your doctor do periodic blood tests to monitor your liver. Doses of inositol hexaniacinate higher than 2,000 mg a day may have a blood-thinning effect.

How to take it

⊘ **DOSAGE:** *For lowering cholesterol, or treating Raynaud's disease or intermittent claudication:* Take 500 mg of inositol hexaniacinate three times a day. When trying to reduce cholesterol, use the vitamin for two months; if your cholesterol levels are unchanged, stop taking the supplement. *For anxiety and depression:* Take 50 mg of niacin a day; this dosage can usually be found as part of a B-complex vitamin. *For insomnia:* Have 500 mg niacinamide one hour before bedtime. *For arthritis:* Use 1,000 mg niacinamide three times a day, but only under a doctor's supervision.

◈ **GUIDELINES FOR USE:** Take any form of niacin with meals or milk to decrease the likelihood of stomach upset. Do not take therapeutic doses of any form of niacin if you take cholesterol-lowering prescription drugs.

Other sources

Niacin is found in foods high in protein, such as chicken, beef, fish, and nuts. Breads, cereals, and pasta are also enriched with niacin. Though they're low in niacin, milk and other dairy products, as well as eggs, are good sources of the vitamin because they're high in tryptophan.

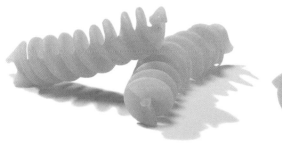
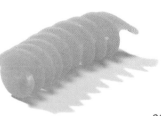

pau d'arco

Tabebuia impetiginosa

Rumored to have been prescribed by the Incas to treat serious ailments, the herb pau d'arco has recently been investigated as a remedy for infectious diseases and cancer. Though its anticancer properties are debatable, it may indeed combat a variety of infections.

COMMON USES

- *Treats vaginal yeast infections.*
- *Helps get rid of warts.*
- *Reduces inflammation of the airways in bronchitis.*
- *May be useful in treating such immune-related disorders as asthma, eczema, psoriasis, and bacterial and viral infections.*

FORMS

- Capsule
- Tablet
- Softgel
- Powder
- Tincture
- Dried herb/Tea

CAUTION!

- Pregnant or lactating women should avoid pau d'arco.
- Pau d'arco may amplify the effect of anticoagulant drugs.
- Reminder: If you have a medical condition, talk to your doctor before taking supplements.

What it is

Pau d'arco is obtained from the inner bark of a tree—*Tabebuia impetiginosa*—indigenous to the rain forests of South America. Native tribes have taken advantage of its healing powers for centuries. Pau d'arco is also known as *lapacho, taheebo,* or *ipe roxo.* In the United States, however, it's always sold as pau d'arco.

The therapeutic ingredients in pau d'arco include a host of potent plant chemicals called naphthoquinones. Of these, lapachol has been the most intensely studied.

What it does

Lapachol and other compounds in pau d'arco help destroy the microorganisms that cause diseases and infections, ranging from malaria and the flu to yeast infections. Most people, however, are interested in the potential cancer-fighting properties of this herb.

⭐ **MAJOR BENEFITS:** Pau d'arco appears to combat bacteria, viruses, and fungi; reduce inflammation; and support the immune system. One of its best-documented uses is for vaginal yeast infections; herbalists often recommend a pau d'arco tea douche to restore the normal environment of the vagina. In capsule, tablet, tincture, or tea form, pau d'arco may be effective in strengthening immunity in people with chronic fatigue syndrome, HIV or AIDS, or chronic bronchitis. The herb's anti-inflammatory properties likewise benefit acute bronchitis, which involves inflammation of the respiratory passages, as well as muscle pain. And a tincture of pau d'arco applied directly to warts is useful in eradicating them.

✳ **ADDITIONAL BENEFITS:** Pau d'arco's anticancer activity is subject to continuing debate. Because of the herb's traditional reputation as a cancer fighter, the National Cancer Institute (NCI) investigated it, identifying lapachol as its most active ingredient. In animal studies, pau d'arco

Pau d'arco can be taken as a supplement or brewed as a tea.

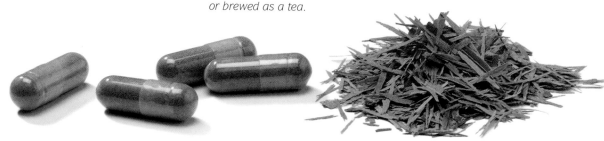

showed promise in shrinking tumors, and so the NCI began human trials using high doses of lapachol in the 1970s. Again, there was some evidence that lapachol was active in destroying cancer cells, but participants taking a therapeutic dose suffered serious side effects, including nausea, vomiting, and blood-clotting problems. As a result, research into lapachol and its source, pau d'arco, was abandoned.

Critics of this investigation believe that using therapeutic doses of pau d'arco—and not simply the isolated compound lapachol—would have produced similar benefits without the potentially dangerous blood-thinning effects. It's likely that lapachol interferes with the action of vitamin K, needed for the blood to clot properly. Some researchers suggest that other compounds in pau d'arco supply some vitamin K, so that use of the whole herb would not interfere with blood clotting. Others think that combining lapachol with vitamin K supplements might make it possible for people to take doses of lapachol high enough to permit its potential antitumor action to be further studied without provoking a reaction. Despite the controversy, many practitioners rely on the historical evidence of pau d'arco's anticancer action and often recommend it as a complement to conventional cancer treatment.

How to take it

⏣ **DOSAGE:** When using pau d'arco in capsule or tablet form, the typical daily dosage is 250 mg twice a day. This dose of pau d'arco is often recommended for chronic fatigue syndrome or HIV and AIDS in alternation with other immune-boosting herbs such as echinacea or goldenseal. Pau d'arco is also commonly consumed as a tea in dried herb form. To make it, steep 2 or 3 teaspoons of pau d'arco in two cups of very hot water; drink the tea over the course of a day.

◈ **GUIDELINES FOR USE:** Herbalists recommend whole-bark products (not only those that contain just lapachol) because they suspect the herb's healing properties come from the full range of plant chemicals in the bark. *For vaginal yeast infections:* Let pau d'arco tea cool to lukewarm before using it as a douche. *For warts:* Apply a tincture-soaked compress to the affected area at bedtime and leave it on all night. Repeat until the wart disappears.

Possible side effects

Whole-bark products are generally safe; they do not produce the side effects of high doses of lapachol. If pau d'arco tea or supplements cause stomach upset, take them with food.

peppermint

Mentha piperita

For centuries this powerfully aromatic herb has provided relief for indigestion, colds, and headache. Today, medicinal peppermint is most prized for its ability to soothe the digestive tract, easing indigestion, irritable bowel syndrome, and other complaints.

COMMON USES

- Relieves heartburn, nausea, and indigestion.
- Eases symptoms of diverticulosis and irritable bowel syndrome.
- Helps dissolve gallstones.
- Sweetens the breath.
- Soothes muscle aches.
- Eases coughs and congestion due to allergies or colds.

FORMS

- Capsule
- Oil
- Ointment/Cream
- Tincture
- Dried or fresh herb/Tea

CAUTION!

- Because peppermint oil relaxes gastrointestinal muscles, it may aggravate the symptoms of a hiatal hernia.
- Peppermint oil should not be applied to the nostrils or chest of infants and children under age 5 because it can cause a choking sensation.
- Reminder: If you have a medical condition, talk to your doctor before taking supplements.

What it is

Peppermint is cultivated worldwide for use as a flavoring agent and an herbal medicine. A natural hybrid of spearmint and water mint, peppermint has square stems and oval, pointed dark green or purple leaves and lilac-colored flowers. For medicinal purposes, the leaves and stems of the plant are harvested just before the flowers bloom in summer. The major active ingredient of peppermint is its volatile oil, which is made up of more than 40 different compounds. The oil's therapeutic effect comes mainly from menthol (35% to 55% of the oil), menthone (15% to 30%), and menthyl acetate (3% to 10%). Medicinal peppermint oil is made by steam-distilling the parts of the plant that grow above the ground.

What it does

Particularly effective in treating digestive disorders, peppermint relieves cramps and relaxes intestinal muscles. It freshens the breath and may clear up nasal congestion as well.

⭐ **MAJOR BENEFITS:** Peppermint oil relaxes the muscles of the digestive tract, helping to relieve intestinal cramping and gas. Its antispasmodic effect also makes it useful for alleviating the symptoms of irritable bowel syndrome, a common disorder characterized by abdominal pain, alternating bouts of diarrhea and constipation, and indigestion. The menthol in peppermint aids digestion because it stimulates the flow of natural digestive juices and bile. This action explains why peppermint oil is commonly

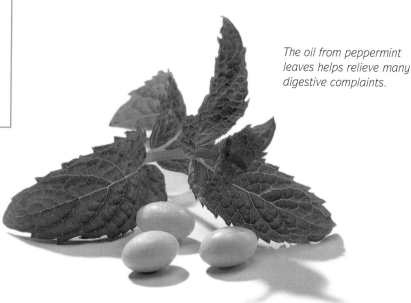

The oil from peppermint leaves helps relieve many digestive complaints.

included in over-the-counter antacids. Several studies indicate that the menthol in peppermint oil assists in dissolving gallstones as well, providing a possible alternative to surgery. Consult your doctor before trying the oil for this purpose. You can also put the oil directly on your tongue; it provides a minty antidote to bad breath.

As a tea or oil, peppermint serves as a mild anesthetic to the stomach's mucous lining, which helps reduce nausea and motion sickness. The tea may ease symptoms of diverticulosis as well, including gas and bloating.

✱ **ADDITIONAL BENEFITS:** When rubbed on the skin, peppermint oil relieves pain by stimulating the nerves that perceive cold while muting those that sense pain, making it a welcome remedy for aching muscles.

Findings are contradictory concerning peppermint's historical use in the treatment of colds and coughs. Some tests show the aromatic plant has no effect. But Commission E, a German health board recognized as an authority on the scientific investigation of herbs, found that peppermint was an effective decongestant that reduced inflammation of the nasal passageways. In addition, many people with colds report that inhaling peppermint's menthol enables them to breathe more easily. Drinking peppermint tea also may offer relief from the bronchial constriction of asthma.

How to take it

⬤ **DOSAGE:** *For the treatment of irritable bowel syndrome, nausea, and gallstones:* Try enteric-coated capsules containing peppermint oil because they release peppermint oil where it's most needed—in the small and large intestine rather than in the stomach. Take one or two capsules (containing 0.2 ml of oil per capsule) two or three times a day, between meals. *To freshen the breath:* Place a few drops of peppermint oil on the tongue. *To relieve gas and calm the stomach:* Make a tea by steeping 1 or 2 teaspoons of dried peppermint leaves in a cup of very hot water for between 5 and 10 minutes; be sure to cover the cup to keep the volatile oil from escaping. *For congestion:* Drink up to four cups of peppermint tea a day. *For pain relief:* Add a few drops of peppermint oil to ½ ounce of a neutral oil. Apply to the affected areas up to four times daily.

◀ **GUIDELINES FOR USE:** Take enteric-coated capsules between meals. If you prefer peppermint tea, drink a cup three or four times a day, after or between meals. Apply peppermint oil or ointments containing menthol no more than three or four times daily. To take peppermint tincture, put 10 to 20 drops in a glass of water. Avoid large doses during pregnancy.

Possible side effects

Even for prolonged periods, peppermint leaves in the recommended doses generally have no side effects. On rare occasions, enteric-coated peppermint oil capsules can cause skin rash and heartburn. Topical peppermint oil can produce allergic skin rashes, especially if applying heat as well. If side effects occur, stop using the herb.

phosphorus

If you compiled a list of nutrients the body could not live without, phosphorus would doubtless be near the top. Although its main function is building strong bones and teeth, this mineral is needed by virtually every cell. Fortunately, the chance of deficiency is very small.

COMMON USES

- *Builds strong bones and maintains skeletal integrity.*
- *Helps form tooth enamel and strengthens teeth.*

FORMS

- Capsule
- Tablet
- Powder
- Liquid

CAUTION!

- The greatest risk associated with phosphorus may be getting too much, which some experts caution may lead to a calcium deficiency. Never take phosphorus supplements without discussing it with your doctor first.
- In a rare instance of a phosphorus deficiency—such as from kidney or digestive disease or severe burns—phosphorus supplementation must be medically supervised.
- Reminder: If you have a medical condition, talk to your doctor before taking supplements.

What it is

Phosphorus is the second most abundant mineral in the body (after calcium), and up to one and a half pounds of it are found in the average person. Although 85% of this mineral is concentrated in the bones and teeth, the rest is distributed in the blood and in various organs, including the heart, kidneys, brain, and muscles. Phosphorus interacts with a variety of other nutrients, but its most constant companion is calcium. In the bones, the ratio of calcium to phosphorus is around 2:1. In other tissues, however, the ratio of phosphorus is much higher.

What it does

There is hardly a biological or cellular process that does not, directly or indirectly, involve phosphorus. In some instances, the mineral works to protect cells, strengthening the membranes that surround them. In other cases, it acts as a kind of biological escort, assisting a variety of nutrients, hormones, and chemicals in doing their jobs. There's also evidence that phosphorus helps activate the B vitamins, enabling them to provide all their benefits.

✪ MAJOR BENEFITS: One of phosphorus's most important functions is to team up with calcium to build bones and aid in maintaining a healthy, strong skeleton. The phosphorus-calcium partnership is also crucial for strengthening the teeth and keeping them strong. In addition, phosphorus joins with fats in the blood to make compounds called phospholipids, which, in turn, play structural and metabolic roles in cell membranes throughout the body. Furthermore, without phosphorus, the body could not convert the proteins, carbohydrates, and fats from food into energy. The mineral is needed to create the molecule known as adenosine triphosphate, or ATP, which acts like a tiny battery charger, supplying vital energy to every cell in the body.

✪ ADDITIONAL BENEFITS: Phosphorus serves as a cell-to-cell messenger. In this capacity, it contributes to the coordination of such body processes as muscle contraction, the transmission of nerve impulses from the brain

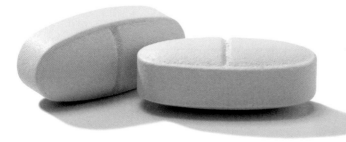

Some multivitamin pills contain phosphorus. But most people get enough of this mineral from their daily diet.

to the body, and the secretion of hormones. An adequate phosphorus supply may therefore enhance your physical performance and be effective in fighting fatigue. In addition, the mineral is necessary for maintaining the pH (the acid-base balance) of the blood and for manufacturing DNA and RNA, the basic components of our genetic makeup.

How much you need

Because phosphorus is found in so many foods, the need for supplements is virtually nonexistent. The RDA for phosphorus in men and women is the same, 700 mg daily. In the past, many nutritionists recommended that phosphorus and calcium be taken in a 1:1 ratio, but most recently, experts have advised that this ratio has little practical benefit. Most people today consume more phosphorus than calcium in their diets.

⊖ **IF YOU GET TOO LITTLE:** Although rare, a deficiency of phosphorus can lead to fragile bones and teeth, fatigue, weakness, a loss of appetite, joint pain and stiffness, and an increased susceptibility to infection. A mild deficiency may produce a modest decrease in energy.

⊕ **IF YOU GET TOO MUCH:** There are no immediate adverse effects from getting too much phosphorus. However, some experts caution that over the long term, excessive phosphorus intake may inhibit calcium absorption, though it's uncertain whether this can result in a calcium deficiency that threatens bone health.

How to take it

⊘ **DOSAGE:** Most people get all the phosphorus they require through their everyday diet. In addition, a small amount of phosphorus may be included in daily multivitamin and mineral supplements. If you have a medical condition that depletes this mineral, such as a bowel ailment or failing kidneys, your doctor will prescribe an appropriate dose.

◁ **GUIDELINES FOR USE:** Never take individual phosphorus supplements without a doctor's supervision.

Other sources

High-protein foods, such as meat, fish, poultry, and dairy products, contain a lot of phosphorus. It is also used as an additive in many processed foods. Soft drinks, particularly colas, often have large amounts. Phosphorus is present in grain products as well, although whole grain breads and cereals may include ingredients that partially reduce its absorption.

FACTS & Tips

■ The aluminum present in some antacids can diminish phosphorus levels in the body. If you habitually take antacids, talk to your doctor about the need for phosphorus supplements.

LATEST FINDINGS

■ One study showed teenage girls who regularly consume great amounts of phosphorus-rich cola beverages are at greater risk for bone fractures than non-soda drinkers. Experts disagree, however, on whether it's the phosphorus at work. They point out that soda drinkers are much less likely to drink milk—and therefore do not get enough of the bone-building mineral calcium in their diets.

■ Swiss researchers report that phosphorus supplementation may be especially beneficial for burn victims, who were found to have low phosphorus levels within a week of suffering severe burns. Thus supplements may be necessary to restore patients to full health following a major burn injury.

Did You Know?

The average American diet contains between 1,000 and 1,500 mg of phosphorus daily, well above the RDA for this mineral.

potassium

You're probably careful not to eat too much sodium, especially if you're watching your blood pressure. You might want to focus your efforts, however, on getting more potassium. For some people, this mineral may be as important in controlling blood pressure as sodium.

What it is

The third most abundant mineral in the body after calcium and phosphorus, potassium is an electrolyte—a substance that takes on a positive or negative charge when dissolved in the watery medium of the bloodstream. Sodium and chloride are electrolytes too, and the body needs a balance of these minerals to perform a host of essential functions. Almost all the potassium in the body is found inside the cells.

What it does

Along with the other electrolytes, potassium is used to conduct nerve impulses, initiate muscle contractions, and regulate heartbeat and blood pressure. It controls the amount of fluid inside the cells, and sodium regulates the amount outside, so the two minerals work to balance fluid levels in the body. Potassium also enables the body to convert blood sugar (glucose)—its primary fuel—into a stored form of energy (glycogen) that's held in reserve by the muscles and liver.

⬢ PREVENTION: Study after study has shown that people who get plenty of potassium in their diets have lower blood pressure than those who get very little. This effect holds true even when sodium intake remains high (though reducing sodium produces better results). In one study, 54 people on medication for high blood pressure were divided into two groups. Half followed their regular diet; the other half added three to six servings of potassium-rich foods a day. After a year, 81% of those getting extra potassium were able to reduce their drug dosages significantly, compared with only 29% of the individuals following their regular diets.

✳ ADDITIONAL BENEFITS: Through its effects on blood pressure, potassium may also decrease the risk of heart disease and stroke. In one study, a group of people with hypertension who ate one serving of a food high in potassium every day reduced their risk of fatal stroke by 40%. A 12-year investigation found that men who got the least amount of potassium

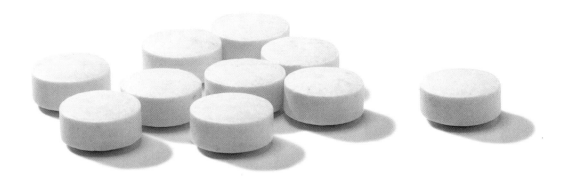

were two and a half times more likely to die from a stroke than men who consumed the most; for women with a low potassium intake, the risk of fatal stroke was nearly five times greater.

How much you need

There is no RDA for potassium, but most experts recommend 2,000 to 3,000 mg a day. More may be needed to control blood pressure.

⊟ **IF YOU GET TOO LITTLE:** Potassium is found in a wide variety of foods, so it is practically impossible not to get enough of this mineral to perform the basic body functions. But a serious deficiency can occur if an individual is taking a potent diuretic (a drug that reduces fluid levels in the body) or is suffering from an extreme case of diarrhea or vomiting. The first sign of deficiency is muscle weakness and nausea. If potassium is not replaced, low levels could lead to heart failure.

⊞ **IF YOU GET TOO MUCH:** Potassium toxicity is highly unlikely because most people can safely consume up to 18 grams a day. Toxicity usually occurs only if an individual has a kidney disorder or takes too many potassium supplements. Signs of potassium overload include muscle fatigue and an irregular heartbeat. Even in small doses, potassium supplements may cause stomach irritation and nausea.

How to take it

⊘ **DOSAGE:** Most people don't need potassium supplements unless they are taking certain diuretic medications. Try to get sufficient potassium in your daily diet; if you want extra insurance, take no more than 500 mg of potassium in supplement form a day. People who use ACE inhibitors (such as captopril or enalapril) for high blood pressure or angina and those who have kidney disease should not take potassium supplements at all.

◈ **GUIDELINES FOR USE:** If you use potassium supplements, take them with food to decrease stomach irritation.

Other sources

Fresh fruits and vegetables—such as bananas, oranges and orange juice, and potatoes—are very high in potassium. Meats, poultry, milk, and yogurt are also good sources.

F A C T S & Tips

■ Microwave or steam vegetables whenever possible—boiling them decreases their potassium content. For example, boiled potatoes lose 50% of their potassium; steamed potatoes lose less than 6%.

■ By law, over-the-counter potassium supplements cannot contain more than 99 mg per pill (this includes multivitamin and mineral preparations). If you think you need potassium supplements, talk to your doctor about higher-dose pills available by prescription.

LATEST FINDINGS

■ An analysis of the results of 33 studies confirms that potassium has a positive impact on blood pressure. People with normal blood pressure who added 2,340 mg of potassium a day—from foods, supplements, or a combination—to their normal diets had an average drop of 2 points in systolic blood pressure (the upper reading) and 1 point in diastolic pressure (the lower reading). If the figures sound insignificant, consider that even these small changes reduce the chance of developing hypertension by 25%. The extra potassium produced even greater benefits—a 4.4 point drop in systolic pressure and a 2.5 point drop in diastolic—in people who already had high blood pressure.

Did You Know?

A large navel orange supplies 250 mg of potassium, about a quarter of what most people get in a day.

psyllium

These tiny seeds are so rich in fiber that they've been prescribed for constipation and a wide range of other digestive ailments for more than 500 years. New research finds that psyllium offers an added benefit: It lowers blood cholesterol safely and effectively.

Plantago psyllium
P. ovata

COMMON USES

- *Relieves constipation, diarrhea.*
- *Treats diverticular disease and irritable bowel syndrome.*
- *Helps prevent gallstones.*
- *Reduces hemorrhoid pain.*
- *May lower cholesterol.*
- *Facilitates weight loss.*

FORMS

- Powder
- Capsule
- Wafer

CAUTION!

- Always take psyllium with plenty of liquid. Without lots of fluid, it is possible to develop an intestinal blockage, causing severe, painful constipation.
- Some people are allergic to psyllium. Reactions are often quick, marked by a rash, itching, and in severe cases, difficulty breathing or swallowing. Get immediate medical help.
- Reminder: If you have a medical condition, talk to your doctor before taking supplements.

What it is

Odorless and nearly tasteless, psyllium comes from the small, reddish brown to black seeds of the *Plantago psyllium* plant. Also known as the plantain, it should not be confused with the edible bananalike fruit of the same name *(Musa paradisiaca)* or with the herb plantain *(Plantago lanceolata)* sometimes used for coughs. *Plantago* grows as a weed in numerous places around the world and is commercially cultivated in Spain, France, India, Pakistan, and other countries. Various species of the plant are used in herbal medicine, most commonly the seeds of *Plantago psyllium* and *P. ovata.* These seeds, so tiny that they are sometimes called "flea seeds," are generally dried, ground, and sold in powder, capsule, or chewable tablet (wafer) form. Psyllium is sometimes added to breakfast cereals.

What it does

When mixed with water, the fibrous husks of psyllium seeds form a gel-like mass that absorbs excess water from the intestines and creates larger, softer stools. Psyllium helps to lower cholesterol by binding to cholesterol-rich bile in the digestive tract, causing the body to draw cholesterol from the bloodstream. As an inexpensive source of soluble fiber (the kind of fiber that blends with water), it's particularly suitable for those people who don't eat enough fiber-rich foods, such as whole grains (oats are particularly rich in soluble fiber), beans, fruits, and vegetables.

⭐ **MAJOR BENEFITS:** Psyllium can help normalize bowel function in a wide variety of disorders, including constipation, diarrhea, diverticulosis, hemorrhoids, and irritable bowel syndrome. It does so by a single mechanism: absorbing water, which lends bulk to stools. In the case of constipation, the added water and bulk help soften stools, making them easier to pass. And though it doesn't cure hemorrhoids, passing softer stools reduces irritation in the tender area. In one study, 84% of hemorrhoid

Psyllium seeds, commonly ground into powder and packed into capsules, are a potent remedy for various digestive ills.

sufferers receiving a supplement containing psyllium reported less bleeding and pain. Psyllium has also been reported to have a soothing effect on those with irritable bowel syndrome. In people with diverticular disease—in which small pockets in the intestine's lining trap fecal particles and become susceptible to infection—psyllium bulks the stools and speeds their passage through the intestine, helping to alleviate the problem. And psyllium's ability to absorb large amounts of excess water from loose stools is an effective treatment for diarrhea.

✳ **ADDITIONAL BENEFITS:** Although psyllium has been used for constipation for centuries, only in the 1980s did scientists discover another benefit: It reliably lowers blood cholesterol, especially the "bad" LDL cholesterol that can stick to artery walls and lead to heart disease. In several studies of men and women with high cholesterol levels, 10 grams or more of psyllium daily for six weeks or longer lowered LDL from 6% to 20% more than the cholesterol-lowering effect of a low-fat diet. Sometimes, simply adding psyllium to your diet is enough to eliminate the need for cholesterol-lowering medications.

This fiber source may also play a role in weight-loss programs. By absorbing water, it fills the stomach, providing a sense of fullness. It also delays the emptying of food from the stomach, thus extending the time you feel full. In a small British study, women who took psyllium with water three hours before a meal consumed less fat and fewer calories during the meal. Whether this effect persists and leads to long-term weight loss, however, is unknown. And psyllium can help stabilize levels of glucose (sugar) in the blood, which may control food cravings.

How to take it

🖊 **DOSAGE:** The usual dosage is 1 to 3 tablespoons (or up to 10 grams) two or three times a day. Some formulas are more concentrated, so check labels. Don't exceed 30 grams a day.

◉ **GUIDELINES FOR USE:** Relief of constipation usually occurs in 12 to 24 hours, although it can take as long as three days. Because psyllium absorbs water, always consume it with large amounts of fluid. Dissolve psyllium powder in water (or juice), drink it, and then drink another glass of water or juice. In addition, drink six to eight glasses of water a day. Take psyllium two hours or more after taking medications or other supplements so that it doesn't delay their absorption. If you are pregnant, check with your doctor first before using psyllium.

Possible side effects

Psyllium can cause temporary bloating and increased flatulence because it supplies fiber. Avoid these problems by slowly increasing psyllium intake over several days. Amounts of psyllium larger than the recommended doses may reduce the absorption of certain minerals. Allergic reactions, though rare, can be life-threatening; if you have trouble swallowing or breathing, seek immediate medical help.

FACTS & Tips

■ In 1998, the Food and Drug Administration (FDA) allowed breakfast cereals that contain psyllium to claim that they reduce the risk of heart disease as part of a diet low in saturated fat and cholesterol. To qualify, a cereal must contain 1.7 grams of soluble fiber from psyllium per serving. Four servings a day deliver 7 grams of soluble fiber, enough to lower blood cholesterol significantly. Combining a psyllium-enriched cereal with a whole-oat cereal may be an even more effective cholesterol-lowering strategy.

LATEST FINDINGS

■ Not only may psyllium aid in weight loss by suppressing appetite, but it may also prevent gallstones. A Mexican study of obese patients on very low calorie diets, which put them at increased risk for gallstones, found that psyllium helped avert this sometimes acutely painful condition.

■ Psyllium lowers cholesterol even in youngsters. In a study of 25 children ages 6 to 18 who had high cholesterol, adding a cereal containing psyllium to a low-fat diet reduced harmful LDL cholesterol by an additional 7%.

Did You Know?

In Europe during the Middle Ages, Arab physicians sold a constipation remedy called diagridium. Psyllium was one of its main ingredients.

riboflavin

For years riboflavin, also known as vitamin B_2, was overlooked. But thanks to exciting new research, this vitamin is now being praised for its potential powers in battling painful migraines, preventing sight-robbing cataracts, healing skin blemishes—and much more.

What it is

Looking through a microscope in 1879, scientists discovered a fluorescent yellow-green substance in milk, but not until 1933 was the substance identified as riboflavin. This water-soluble vitamin is part of the B-complex family, which is involved in transforming protein, fats, and carbohydrates into fuel for the body. Found naturally in many foods, riboflavin is also added to fortified breads and cereals. It is easily destroyed when exposed to light. Inadequate riboflavin intake often accompanies other B-vitamin deficiencies, which are a common problem in the elderly and alcoholics. Riboflavin is available as a single supplement, in combination with other B vitamins (vitamin B complex), or as part of a multivitamin.

What it does

The body depends on riboflavin for a wide range of functions. It plays a vital role in the production of thyroid hormone, which speeds up metabolism and helps assure a steady supply of energy. Riboflavin also aids the body in producing infection-fighting immune cells; it works in conjunction with iron to manufacture red blood cells, which transport oxygen to all the cells in the body. In addition, it converts vitamins B_6 and niacin into active forms so that they can do their work.

Riboflavin produces substances that assist powerful antioxidants, such as vitamin E, in protecting cells against damage from the naturally occurring, highly reactive molecules known as free radicals. It is essential for tissue maintenance and repair—the body uses extra amounts to speed the healing of wounds after surgery, burns, and other injuries. The vitamin is also necessary to maintain the function of the eye and may be important for healthy nerves as well.

◉ PREVENTION: By boosting antioxidant activity, riboflavin protects many body tissues—particularly the lens of the eye. It may therefore help prevent the formation of cataracts, the milky opacities in the lens that impair the vision of so many older people. Ophthalmologists urge everyone, especially those with a family history of this eye disorder, to get an adequate and steady supply of riboflavin throughout their lives.

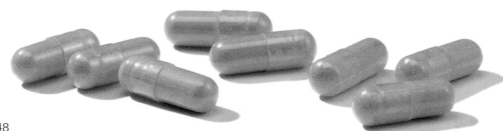

The vitamin has also been shown to be highly effective in reducing the frequency and severity of migraine headaches. Migraine sufferers are believed to have reduced energy reserves in the brain, and riboflavin may prevent attacks by increasing the energy supply to brain cells.

✴ **ADDITIONAL BENEFITS:** Riboflavin has proved valuable in treating skin disorders, including rosacea, which causes facial flushing and skin pustules in many adults. In combination with other B vitamins, including vitamin B_6 and niacin, it may help against a broad range of nerve and other ailments, including numbness and tingling, Alzheimer's disease, epilepsy, and multiple sclerosis, as well as anxiety, stress, and even fatigue. Some doctors prescribe extra riboflavin supplementation to treat sickle-cell anemia, because many of these patients have a riboflavin deficiency.

How much you need

The daily RDA for riboflavin is 1.3 mg for men and 1.1 mg for women. These amounts simply prevent general deficiencies; larger doses are usually prescribed for specific conditions.

⊖ **IF YOU GET TOO LITTLE:** Classic deficiency symptoms include cracking and sores in the corner of the mouth and increased sensitivity to light, with tearing, burning, and itchy eyes. The skin around the nose, eyebrows, and earlobes may peel, and there may be a skin rash in the groin area. A low red blood cell count (anemia), resulting in fatigue, can also occur.

⊕ **IF YOU GET TOO MUCH:** Excess riboflavin isn't dangerous because the body excretes any extra in the urine. However, high intakes of this vitamin can turn the urine bright yellow—a harmless but unsettling side effect.

How to take it

⊘ **DOSAGE:** *For cataract prevention:* The usual dosage is 25 mg a day. *For rosacea:* Dosages of 50 mg a day are recommended. *For migraines:* Even higher amounts may be needed—up to 400 mg a day. Many one-a-day vitamins meet the RDA for riboflavin; high-potency multivitamins may contain much higher amounts—30 mg or more. Mixed vitamin B formulas typically contain 50 or 100 mg of riboflavin along with other B vitamins, including niacin, thiamin, vitamins B_6 and B_{12}, and folic acid.

◉ **GUIDELINES FOR USE:** Consult your doctor if you are taking oral contraceptives, antibiotics, or psychiatric drugs, which can affect riboflavin needs. Don't take it with alcohol, which reduces absorption of riboflavin in the digestive tract.

Other sources

Good sources of riboflavin include milk, cheese, yogurt, liver, beef, fish, fortified breads and cereals, avocados, mushrooms, and eggs.

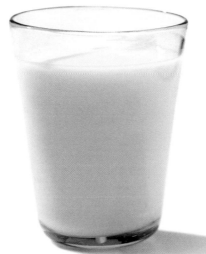

FACTS & Tips

■ Americans get about half their riboflavin from milk and other dairy products.

■ Milk stored in a clear glass bottle loses three-fourths of its riboflavin after just a few hours, because the vitamin is extremely sensitive to light. That's one reason why milk comes in opaque bottles or cardboard cartons.

■ A well-balanced diet is especially important in the case of the elderly, many of whom are deficient in riboflavin.

LATEST FINDINGS

■ In a recent European study, 55 patients who suffered two to eight migraines per month were given 400 mg of riboflavin a day. After three months, patients experienced, on average, 37% fewer headaches—a rate commonly achieved only with prescription migraine drugs. But riboflavin has far fewer side effects than those drugs, and at about 50 or 60 cents for a daily 400 mg dose, it's much cheaper.

Did You Know?

You'd have to drink approximately 72 8-ounce glasses of milk to get 30 mg of riboflavin, the amount found in many high-potency multivitamins.

saw palmetto

Serenoa repens

Native Americans regularly consumed this herb as a food, so they were probably not plagued by prostate problems. Now one of the ten best-selling supplements in the United States, saw palmetto is an herb with a man's troubles in mind.

CAUTION!

- Anyone finding blood in the urine or having trouble urinating should see a doctor before taking saw palmetto. These symptoms could be related to prostate cancer.
- Because saw palmetto affects hormone levels, men with prostate cancer or anyone taking hormones should discuss use of the herb with a doctor.
- Reminder: If you have a medical condition, talk to your doctor before taking supplements.

What it is

The saw palmetto, a small palm tree that grows wild from Texas to South Carolina, gets its name from the spiny saw-toothed stems that lie at the base of each leaf. With a life span of 700 years, the plant seems almost indestructible, resisting drought, insect infestation, and fire. Its medicinal properties are derived from the blue-black berries, which are usually harvested in August and September. This process is sometimes hazardous: Harvesters can easily be cut by the razor-sharp leaf stems, and they risk being bitten by the diamondback rattlesnakes that make their home in the shade of this scrubby palm.

What it does

Saw palmetto has a long history of folk use. Native Americans valued it for treating disorders of the urinary tract. Early colonists, noting the vitality of animals who fed on the berries, gave the fruits to frail individuals as a general tonic. Through the years, it's also been employed to relieve persistent coughs and improve digestion. Today, saw palmetto's claim to fame rests mainly on its ability to relieve the symptoms of an enlarged prostate gland—a use verified by a number of scientific studies.

✪ **MAJOR BENEFITS:** In Italy, Germany, France, and other countries, doctors routinely prescribe saw palmetto for the benign (noncancerous) enlargement of the prostate known medically as BPH, which stands for "benign prostatic hyperplasia," or "hypertrophy." When the walnut-size male prostate gland becomes enlarged, a common condition that affects more than half of men over age 50, it can press on the urethra, the tube that carries urine from the bladder through the prostate and out the penis. The resulting symptoms include frequent urination (especially at

The dried fruit of the saw palmetto tree, often processed into softgels, provides a potent remedy for prostate complaints.

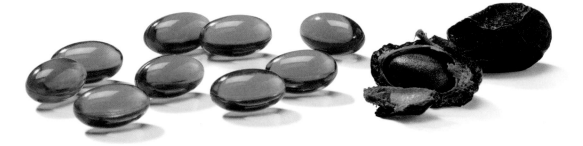

night), weak urine flow, painful urination, and difficulty emptying the bladder completely. Researchers believe that saw palmetto relieves the symptoms of BPH in various ways. Most importantly, it appears to alter levels of various hormones that cause prostate cells to multiply. In addition, the herb may act to curb inflammation and reduce tissue swelling.

Moreover, studies have found that saw palmetto produces fewer side effects (such as impotence) and quicker results than the conventional prostate drug finasteride (Proscar). And saw palmetto took only about 30 days to become effective, compared with at least six months for the prescription medication.

✴ **ADDITIONAL BENEFITS:** Although there is strong evidence that saw palmetto relieves the symptoms of BPH, other potential benefits of this herb are more speculative. Saw palmetto has been used to treat certain inflammations of the prostate (prostatitis). In the lab, it boosts the immune system's ability to kill bacteria, which suggests that it may be a potential treatment for prostate or urinary tract infections. Because saw palmetto affects levels of cancer-promoting hormones, scientists are also investigating its possible role in preventing prostate cancer.

How to take it

⊘ **DOSAGE:** The usual dosage is 160 mg twice a day. Be careful about taking higher amounts: Scientific studies have not examined the effects of daily doses above 320 mg. Choose supplements made from extracts standardized to contain 85% to 95% fatty acids and sterols—the active ingredients in the berries that are responsible for its therapeutic effects.

◆ **GUIDELINES FOR USE:** Because saw palmetto has a bitter taste, those using the liquid form may want to dilute it in a small amount of water. The herb can be taken with or without food. Although some healers recommend sipping tea made from saw palmetto, it may not contain therapeutic amounts of the active ingredients—and provide few benefits for the treatment of BPH.

Possible side effects

Relatively uncommon, side effects include mild abdominal pain, nausea, dizziness, and headache. Very rarely, men may develop breast enlargement. If side effects occur, lower the dose or stop taking it.

SHOPPING HINTS

■ Read the label carefully when buying a "Men's Formula." Although most contain saw palmetto, they usually also include a number of other herbs or nutrients, and some of these may not be right for you. In addition, the amount of saw palmetto in these products may be too small to be of any use.

LATEST FINDINGS

■ In an international study of 1,000 men with moderate BPH, two-thirds benefited from taking either a prescription prostate drug (Proscar) or saw palmetto for six months. Those using the herb had fewer problems with side effects associated with the drug, such as reduced libido and impotence. However, the conventional medication significantly reduced the size of the prostate, whereas the effect of saw palmetto was much less dramatic, particularly in men who had very large prostates. The study authors concluded the herb may be most appropriate when the gland is only slightly or moderately enlarged.

Did You Know?

The cost of daily doses of saw palmetto is one-third to one-half that of conventional prostate medications.

selenium

Although researchers didn't discover the importance of this trace mineral until 1979, selenium quickly gained prominence as a potentially powerful cancer fighter. Many experts now believe it could prove to be one of the most important disease-fighting nutrients.

COMMON USES

- *Works with vitamin E to help prevent cancer and heart disease.*
- *Protects against cataracts and macular degeneration.*
- *Fights viral infections; reduces the severity of cold sores and shingles; may slow the progression of HIV/AIDS.*
- *Helps relieve lupus symptoms.*

FORMS

- Capsule
- Tablet

CAUTION!

- Don't exceed recommended doses: In some people, taking selenium long term—as little as 900 mcg a day—can cause serious side effects, such as skin rashes, nausea, fatigue, hair loss, fingernail changes, and depression.
- Reminder: If you have a medical condition, talk to your doctor before taking supplements.

What it is

A trace mineral essential for many body processes, selenium is found in soil. In the body, selenium is present in virtually every cell but is most abundant in the kidneys, liver, spleen, pancreas, and testes.

What it does

Selenium acts as an antioxidant, blocking the rogue molecules known as free radicals that damage DNA. It's part of an antioxidant enzyme (called glutathione peroxidase) that protects cells against environmental and dietary toxins, and is often included in antioxidant "cocktails" with vitamins C and E. This combination may help guard against a range of disorders—from cancer, heart disease, cataracts, and macular degeneration to strokes and even aging—thought to be caused by free-radical damage.

⭐ **MAJOR BENEFITS:** Selenium has received a lot of attention recently for its role in combating cancer. A dramatic five-year study conducted at Cornell University and the University of Arizona showed that 200 mcg of selenium daily resulted in 63% fewer prostate tumors, 58% fewer colorectal cancers, 46% fewer lung malignancies, and a 39% overall decrease in cancer deaths. In other studies, selenium showed promise in preventing cancers of the ovaries, cervix, rectum, bladder, esophagus, pancreas, and liver, as well as against leukemia. Studies of cancer patients indicate that people with the lowest selenium levels developed more tumors, had a higher rate of disease recurrence, a greater risk of cancer spreading, and a shorter overall survival rate than those with high blood levels of selenium.

Additionally, selenium can protect the heart, primarily by reducing the "stickiness" of the blood and decreasing the risk of clotting—in turn, lowering the risk of heart attack and stroke. Moreover, selenium increases the ratio of HDL ("good") cholesterol to LDL ("bad") cholesterol, which is critical for a healthy heart. Smokers or those who've already had a heart attack or stroke may gain the greatest cardiovascular benefits from selenium supplements, though everyone can profit from taking selenium in a daily vitamin and mineral supplement.

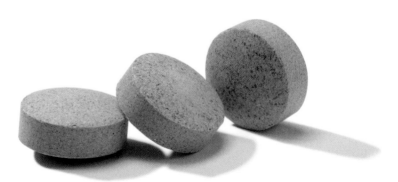

✳ **ADDITIONAL BENEFITS:** Selenium may be useful in preventing cataracts and macular degeneration, the leading causes of impaired vision or blindness in older Americans. It is also vital for converting thyroid hormone, which is needed for the proper functioning of every cell in the body, from a less active form (called T4) to its active form (known as T3). In addition, selenium is essential for a healthy immune system, assisting the body in defending itself against harmful bacteria and viruses, as well as cancer cells. Its immune-boosting effects may play a role in fighting the herpes virus that is responsible for cold sores and shingles, and it is also being studied for possible effectiveness against HIV, the virus that causes AIDS.

When combined with vitamin E, selenium appears to have some anti-inflammatory benefits as well. These two nutrients may improve chronic conditions such as rheumatoid arthritis, psoriasis, lupus, and eczema.

How much you need

The RDA for selenium is 70 mcg for men, and 55 mcg for women daily. To produce major benefits, up to 600 mcg a day may be needed.

➖ **IF YOU GET TOO LITTLE:** Most Americans consume enough selenium in their daily diet, so deficiencies are rare. Falling below the RDA, however, may lead to higher incidences of cancer, heart disease, immune problems, and inflammatory conditions of all kinds, particularly those affecting the skin. Insufficient amounts of selenium during pregnancy could increase the risk of birth defects (especially those involving the heart) or, possibly, sudden infant death syndrome (SIDS). Early symptoms of selenium deficiency include muscular weakness and fatigue.

➕ **IF YOU GET TOO MUCH:** It's hard to get too much selenium from your diet, but if you're taking this mineral in supplement form, it's important to remember that the margin of safety between a therapeutic dose of selenium (up to 600 mcg a day) and a toxic dose (as little as 900 mcg) is small compared with other nutrients. Symptoms of toxicity include nervousness, depression, nausea and vomiting, a garlicky odor to the breath and perspiration, and a loss of hair and fingernails.

How to take it

📋 **DOSAGE:** Most experts agree the optimum dose for long-term use of selenium should fall between 100 mcg and 400 mcg daily. Up to 600 mcg daily may be taken for a limited time as a treatment for viral infections or as part of a cancer treatment program.

◈ **GUIDELINES FOR USE:** Vitamin E greatly enhances selenium's effectiveness; be sure that you get 400 IU of it daily.

Other sources

The most abundant sources of selenium include Brazil nuts, seafood, poultry, and meats. Grains, particularly oats and brown rice, may also have significant amounts, depending on the selenium content of the soil in which they were grown.

shark cartilage

Sharks are finally getting a warm welcome, thanks to a tough, rubbery material in their skeletons. Though myriad claims are made for shark cartilage—most spectacularly that it cures cancer—its actual effect on disease remains uncertain.

COMMON USES

- *May help fight cancer.*
- *May ease arthritic joint pain, temper the skin lesions of psoriasis, and help heal cold sores.*

FORMS

- Tablet
- Capsule
- Powder

CAUTION!

- Because it may interfere with new blood vessel growth, shark cartilage should not be used by women who are pregnant or breast-feeding; by anyone who has suffered a heart attack or stroke; or by those who have had recent surgery.
- Reminder: If you have a medical condition, talk to your doctor before taking supplements.

What it is

Bone forms the framework of the human body. Cartilage does the same for sharks. This elastic substance, which is softer than bone but tough and fibrous, is found in people as well: in the nose, for example, and around the joints. In recent years, shark cartilage products have become popular worldwide as a much-hyped remedy for a variety of ills. Harvested from the head and fins, the cartilage is first cleaned and dried, and then ground into a fine white powder.

There is considerable debate, however, about whether the supplement is effective. Solid evidence proving its health benefits lags significantly behind the glowing testimonials. What's more, ecological concern is mounting because shark populations around the globe appear to be declining rapidly as a result of overfishing.

What it does

Most researchers greet the claims made for shark cartilage—from curing cancer and AIDS to healing arthritis and herpes—with skepticism. Some believe that stomach acids digest shark cartilage, rendering oral supplements ineffective; others say that even if the body does absorb the cartilage, it has no demonstrable therapeutic benefits. If shark cartilage does contain healing ingredients, they are present, at best, only in very small amounts. Though a few promising studies have been conducted, additional research is needed to confirm—or disprove—the effectiveness of this controversial supplement.

⊛ **MAJOR BENEFITS:** Research dating back to the 1980s sparked interest in this supplement's greatest claim to fame: its supposed ability to battle cancer. Observing that sharks rarely get cancer, investigators began studying various substances from sharks and noted that shark cartilage blocks the growth of new blood vessels. Because blood-vessel growth is

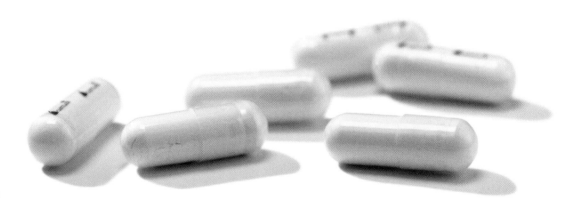

essential for tumors—providing them with an oxygen-rich blood supply that allows them to survive and grow—the researchers speculated that the cartilage might fight cancer. (Cancer therapies that inhibit blood vessel growth recently became headline news when two drugs that shrink tumors—called angiostatin and endostatin—were isolated in the lab.)

Other theories have been advanced for shark cartilage's supposed anticancer effects, and studies in test tubes and animals suggest that it may have some cancer-fighting benefits. But what works in the test tube or in animals is often a far cry from what works in people: Studies have generally failed to show any significant benefits to people with cancer, even when shark cartilage was given in very high doses. In fact, a leading maker of shark cartilage supplements recently admitted that the substance is "probably not effective" for cancer.

✱ **ADDITIONAL BENEFITS:** Shark cartilage may have anti-inflammatory properties, however, that make it useful for treating diseases such as rheumatoid arthritis and the skin ailment psoriasis. In one study, animals given a shark cartilage extract experienced less pain and inflammation from substances that irritate the skin.

Shark cartilage may also ease symptoms of osteoarthritis by facilitating the delivery of cartilage-building nutrients to the joints, thereby stimulating cartilage repair while reducing cartilage breakdown. (Most doctors, however, believe there are more effective remedies for this purpose, such as glucosamine.) Because of its possible immune-boosting effects, the supplement has also been proposed as a treatment for cold sores and other herpes infections.

How to take it

✐ **DOSAGE:** *For disorders such as arthritis:* Dosages of about 2,000 mg of shark cartilage three times a day are sometimes recommended. *For cancer:* Practitioners sometimes recommend doses as high as 1,000 mg per 2.2 pounds of body weight, which would mean 68,000 mg for someone weighing 150 pounds—a substantial expense for a supplement with unproven value.

◈ **GUIDELINES FOR USE:** Some researchers suggest taking the supplement on an empty stomach to minimize exposure to stomach acids that could destroy any active ingredients. Because of the large amounts recommended to treat cancer (in some cases the equivalent of more than 100 capsules a day), the powder form may be more convenient and inexpensive. However, those concerned about the fishy taste of many products may find tablets or capsules the best options.

Possible side effects

Even when taken in large amounts, shark cartilage does not seem to produce any toxic reactions.

· ·
SHOPPING HINTS
■ Many shark cartilage products contain few active ingredients because they are extensively diluted with binding agents and fillers. Read the label carefully to see what you're getting.
· ·

LATEST FINDINGS
■ According to a recent Canadian study, shark cartilage helps to treat psoriasis, a condition that's marked by excessive inflammation and growth of new blood vessels in the skin. To mimic the disease, investigators applied a chemical irritant to the arms of nine healthy volunteers. When spread on the skin prior to the application of the irritant, an extract of shark cartilage effectively curtailed inflammation. In a follow-up study, the extract also soothed the rashes of those with psoriasis.

■ Though shark cartilage is promoted for its cancer-fighting properties, the supplement appeared to have no effect in a recent study conducted by the Cancer Treatment Research Foundation. Some 60 patients with breast, colon, lung, prostate, and other advanced cancers took numerous spoonfuls of shark cartilage three times a day. Over 10 months, the supplement had no discernible effect on their tumors.

Did You Know?
In Japan, shark fin soup is considered a longevity booster.

siberian ginseng

Eleutherococcus senticosus

This ancient Chinese tonic, rediscovered by the Russians after World War II, helps an individual withstand stress. It appears to benefit the whole body, sharpening physical and mental performance and restoring vitality during times of overwork or illness.

COMMON USES

- Combats stress-related illness.
- Fights fatigue; restores energy.
- Enhances immunity and helps with chronic fatigue syndrome and fibromyalgia.
- Supports sexual function; may improve fertility in both sexes.
- Eases symptoms of menopause.
- May boost mental alertness in people with Alzheimer's disease.

FORMS

- Tablet
- Capsule
- Softgel
- Tincture
- Powder
- Dried herb/Tea

CAUTION!

- Siberian ginseng may interfere with heart medications. In one 74-year-old man, taking the herb along with digoxin caused the drug to accumulate in his body, reaching dangerous levels.
- Reminder: If you have a medical condition, talk to your doctor before taking supplements.

What it is

Also called eleuthero, Siberian ginseng is a distant botanical cousin of Panax ginseng, which is better known. Although not as revered (or expensive) as the Panax species, Siberian ginseng has been used in China for thousands of years to enhance the body's vital energy *(qi)*, restore memory, and prevent colds and flu. It is derived from *Eleutherococcus senticosus,* a plant native to eastern Russia, China, Korea, and Japan; supplements are usually made from the dried roots.

The herb gained prominence among Western doctors in the 1950s, after a Russian health researcher, I. I. Brekhman, completed experiments examining effects on thousands of men and women. His studies demonstrated that Siberian ginseng could help healthy people withstand physical stress, improve their immune systems, and increase their mental and physical performance. Subsequent research revealed the herb's potential for treating specific ailments.

What it does

Siberian ginseng contains substances that exert beneficial effects on the adrenals (the small glands on top of the kidneys that secrete stress-fighting hormones). It also raises energy levels and enhances immunity. Studies show that the herb is effective in protecting against all kinds of physical stresses: heat, cold, even radiation. It heightens mental alertness and allows the mind to focus in adverse situations. By reducing the effects of stress and supporting the immune system, Siberian ginseng may also be of value in decreasing the risk of many chronic illnesses.

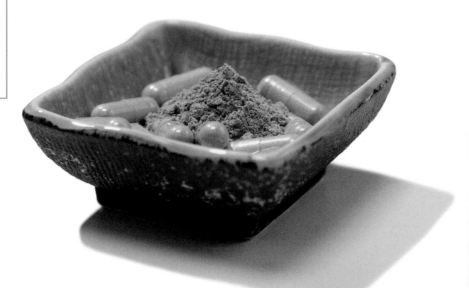

★ MAJOR BENEFITS: Siberian ginseng is often recommended as a general revitalizer for people who are fatigued (including those recovering from illness and those who are overworked). It's also suggested for people whose ability to work is impaired, or for those whose concentration is weak. Studies in Russia involving 2,100 healthy men and women ages 19 to 72 who were given extracts of the herb found that ginseng improved the following: physical labor performance; proofreading accuracy; radio telegraphists' speed and precision in noisy surroundings; the ability of humans to adapt to hot temperatures, as well as to a high-altitude, low-oxygen environment; and their ability to withstand motion sickness.

Because it also enhances immunity, Siberian ginseng is frequently included in nutritional support programs for people with chronic fatigue syndrome or fibromyalgia. In addition, it may benefit people in the early stages of Alzheimer's disease by increasing mental alertness.

✳ ADDITIONAL BENEFITS: By altering hormone levels and toning the uterus, Siberian ginseng may play a role in treating menstrual irregularities and the symptoms of menopause. Taken between menstrual periods, it may also be useful in preventing female infertility. The herb may be suitable as a fertility aid for men as well. When alternated with Panax ginseng, it may be of value for some cases of impotence.

Traditionally, the Chinese have utilized Siberian ginseng to suppress colds and flu; the herb's efficacy may partly be related to its ability to improve the immune system. Russian studies support this use. In a very large study, more than 13,000 auto workers who took the herb one winter reported suffering 40% fewer respiratory tract infections during that period than in previous winters. It has also been employed to treat certain heart conditions and to lower blood sugar; test-tube studies suggest that Siberian ginseng may help protect against some types of cancer or boost the effects of conventional chemotherapy drugs. More studies are needed to verify these and other potential benefits.

How to take it

⊘ DOSAGE: *For stress, fatigue, and other complaints:* Take 100 to 300 mg of a standardized extract of Siberian ginseng two or three times a day. *For menstrual disorders:* Mix Siberian ginseng with herbs such as chasteberry, dong quai, and licorice. Commercial combinations are available.

◖ GUIDELINES FOR USE: Siberian ginseng can be taken on a long-term basis. However, some authorities suggest using it for three months and then stopping for a week or two. German health authorities do not recommend it for people with high blood pressure, though there are few studies to indicate any adverse reactions in this group. Because Siberian ginseng may interact with prescription medications, including some heart drugs, check with your doctor before taking it.

Possible side effects

The herb appears to be very safe at recommended doses. In rare cases, it may cause mild diarrhea. Some people report feeling restless after taking Siberian ginseng, so do not have it too close to bedtime.

. . . .
SHOPPING HINTS

■ Buy standardized Siberian ginseng (eleuthero) extracts from a reputable company to be sure you're getting a quality product. These supplements contain specified amounts of the active ingredients, dubbed "eleutherosides." Look for extracts with an eleutheroside content of at least 0.8%.

■ Siberian ginseng is often added to "Adrenal Gland" formulas intended to combat stress. Look for the herb in combination with licorice, pantothenic acid, and other ingredients.

■ Avoid high-potency formulas of Siberian ginseng that exceed recommended daily doses. High doses (more than 900 mg a day) can cause insomnia, irritability, nervousness, and anxiety.
. . . .

LATEST FINDINGS

■ In Germany, Siberian ginseng is approved by medical authorities for use as an invigorating tonic for fatigue, weakness, an inability to work, impaired concentration, and convalescence from illness. But it may not be effective at enabling a fit, well-nourished American athlete to run any faster or longer. When 20 highly trained distance runners were given Siberian ginseng, they didn't perform any better in treadmill tests than their peers on placebos.

Did You Know?

After the Chernobyl nuclear accident, many Russians were offered Siberian ginseng to help minimize the effects of the radiation.

soy isoflavones

Soy has shown great promise in reducing the uncomfortable hot flashes of menopause, and new research indicates that it may also help protect against certain chronic diseases, including osteoporosis, heart disease, and some cancers.

What it is

Found in soybean products such as tofu and soy milk, and sold in supplement form, isoflavones are powerful compounds known as phytoestrogens. These plant-based substances are chemically similar to the hormone estrogen, produced in the body, but are much weaker. Phytoestrogens, however, can bind to estrogen receptors in the cells and produce various important health benefits. Most research on soy isoflavones has been done with people who regularly ate soy products, so even though most supplements contain the major isoflavones in soybeans, genistein and daidzein, it's not clear whether isoflavones are the only beneficial compounds in soy.

What it does

As phytoestrogens, soy isoflavones have two important effects. First, when estrogen levels are high, phytoestrogens can block the more potent forms of estrogen produced by the body and may help prevent hormone-driven diseases, such as breast cancer. Second, when estrogen levels are low, as they are after menopause, phytoestrogens can substitute for the body's own estrogen, possibly reducing hot flashes and preserving bones. Soy isoflavones may also have antioxidant and anticoagulant effects.

PREVENTION: Research indicates that soybean products help protect against heart disease by lowering LDL ("bad") cholesterol, and significantly increasing HDL ("good") cholesterol. Soy seems most effective in people with high cholesterol levels. In those with near-normal cholesterol levels, its effects are less powerful, and larger amounts are needed to produce the same benefits. Soy products may also inhibit the oxidation of LDL cholesterol, the first step in the accumulation of artery-clogging plaque. In addition, laboratory studies show the genistein in soy helps prevent blood clots from forming.

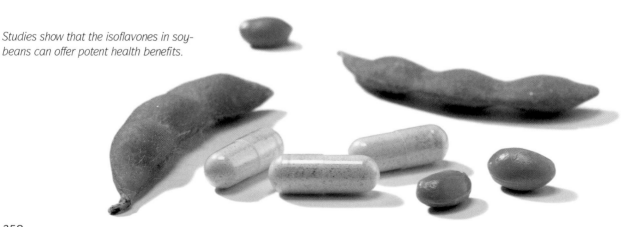

Studies show that the isoflavones in soybeans can offer potent health benefits.

In Asian countries where soy is a dietary staple, rates of certain cancers are much lower than they are in the United States. Preliminary studies indicate that regular consumption of soy foods or supplements may protect against cancers of the breast, prostate, and endometrium. And in animal studies, adding soy protein to the diet significantly reduces tumor formation and the likelihood that cancer, once developed, will spread. The phytoestrogens in the soy are most likely responsible for this effect. Researchers speculate that the isoflavone genistein may block a protein called tyrosine kinase, which promotes the growth and proliferation of tumor cells. This effect may be why soy is also associated with a lower risk of prostate cancer. Genistein has potent antioxidant properties as well, and for these reasons, it may one day prove useful against cancer—though more research is clearly needed.

✱ **ADDITIONAL BENEFITS:** Studies show that hot flashes and other symptoms of menopause are relatively rare in Asia, where women eat a lot of soy products. In addition, in one Western study, women who added 45 grams of soy flour to their daily diet experienced a 40% reduction in hot flashes.

Soy isoflavones may also help women maintain bone density. One study of postmenopausal women found that consuming 40 grams of soy protein a day resulted in a significant increase in bone mineral density in the spine, an area often weakened by osteoporosis.

How to take it

▱ **DOSAGE:** Experts don't know the amount of soy isoflavones needed to produce a therapeutic effect. In Asian countries, the isoflavone consumption ranges from 25 to 200 mg a day. Some researchers believe that an intake of 50 to 120 mg a day might be the minimum amount necessary. The supplements on the market vary in the types of isoflavones they contain and the total amount of isoflavones per pill. Choose a product that supplies a mixture of isoflavones—it should include both genistein and daidzein—and take enough pills to obtain 50 to 100 mg isoflavones a day.

◖ **GUIDELINES FOR USE:** Most experts recommend that you try to get your soy isoflavones from soy foods. In addition to their isoflavone content, these foods are good sources of protein, so they can replace red meat and other foods high in saturated fat.

The amount of isoflavones in soybeans—and therefore any product made from them—varies. In general, eating one to two servings of soy products a day is probably sufficient. (Λ serving equals: 3½ ounces tofu or miso, 1 cup soy milk, or ½ cup soy flour, cooked soybeans, or textured vegetable protein.) If eating this much soy is not to your taste, you might want to get your isoflavones from a combination of foods and supplements. Another alternative is soy powder, which contains both soy protein and isoflavones; mix it into juice, milk, or shakes. Take soy supplements with a large glass of warm water right before eating breakfast and dinner.

Possible side effects

Soy products, even in large quantities, are not known to produce side effects. However, the small percentage of people who are allergic to soybeans should avoid all soy supplements and soy-based foods.

spirulina and kelp

Health enthusiasts are looking to the lakes and seas for algae and plant proteins that are powerful food supplements. Spirulina and kelp have inspired hope as well as hype, but these aquatic plants actually do contain various beneficial substances.

COMMON USES

Spirulina
- Treats bad breath.
- Adds protein, vitamins, and minerals to the diet.

Kelp
- Treats underactive thyroid.
- Provides essential nutrients.

FORMS

- Capsule
- Tablet
- Powder
- Tincture
- Liquid

CAUTION!

- Kelp may aggravate the condition of patients taking medication for an overactive thyroid.
- Reminder: If you have a medical condition, talk to your doctor before taking supplements.

What it is

Spirulina and kelp are two very different types of aquatic algae. The smaller of the two, spirulina (also known as blue-green algae), is actually a single-celled microorganism, or microalga, that closely resembles a bacterium. Because its spiral-shaped filaments are rich in the plant pigment chlorophyll, spirulina turns the lakes and ponds where it grows a dark blue-green. Kelp is another beneficial protector—one that comes from the sea. Derived from various species of brown algae known as *Fucus* or *Laminaria*, this long-stemmed seaweed is a prime source of iodine, crucial in preventing thyroid problems.

What it does

Spirulina and kelp have been used medicinally for thousands of years in China. Their devotees make many claims—ranging from increased libido to reduced hair loss—but most of these remain highly speculative. The algae do, however, have some confirmed powers.

⚂ **MAJOR BENEFITS:** Because it is a prime source of chlorophyll, spirulina is ideal for combating one of life's most bothersome complaints: bad breath. It can be an extremely effective remedy, provided the condition is not due to gum disease or chronic sinusitis. Many commercial chlorophyll breath fresheners contain spirulina as a key ingredient.

The high iodine content of kelp makes it useful for treating an underactive thyroid that's caused by a shortage of iodine. This remedy is rarely necessary, however, because iodized salt supplies plenty of this mineral. Kelp is also marketed as a weight-loss aid, but it is probably effective only in the extremely rare cases when weight gain is secondary to an iodine-deficient, underactive thyroid. It should be taken only under a doctor's close supervision for the treatment of thyroid disorders.

Spirulina is the most popular of the blue-green algae supplements.

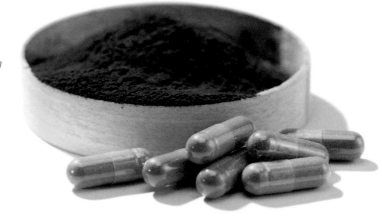

✳ ADDITIONAL BENEFITS: Sometimes spirulina and kelp are included in vegetarian and macrobiotic diets. Spirulina contains protein, vitamins (including B_{12} and folic acid), carotenoids, and other nutrients. In addition to iodine, kelp provides carotenoids, as well as fatty acids, potassium, magnesium, calcium, iron, and other nutrients. However, the concentrations of all these substances appear to be fairly low. There are many less expensive—and better tasting—sources of vitamins and minerals than spirulina and kelp, including an array of common garden vegetables.

Various other claims are made for kelp and spirulina—that they boost energy, relieve arthritis, enhance liver function, prevent heart disease and certain types of cancer, boost immunity, suppress HIV and AIDS, and protect cells against damage from X rays or heavy metals, such as lead. But most studies on these supplements have been done in test tubes or with animals, and more research is needed.

How to take it

⬤ DOSAGE: *To freshen the breath with spirulina:* Use a commercial, chlorophyll-rich "green" drink (the label will often say if the chlorophyll is derived in part from spirulina) or mix a teaspoon of spirulina powder in half a glass of water. Swish the liquid around the mouth, then swallow it. Alternatively, chew a tablet thoroughly, then ingest it. Repeat three or four times a day, or as needed.

To use kelp for an underactive thyroid: Use only when recommended by your doctor; if iodine is needed, your doctor can prescribe an appropriate dose. Powder forms dissolve easily in water, though some people don't like the taste. Tablets, capsules, and tinctures are equally effective.

◈ GUIDELINES FOR USE: Take with food to minimize the chances of digestive upset. Pregnant or lactating women may want to avoid kelp because of its high iodine content, though spirulina seems to be very safe.

Possible side effects

Occasionally, nausea or diarrhea develops in those taking spirulina or kelp; if this side effect occurs, lower the dose or stop using it. Up to 3% of the population is sensitive to iodine and may experience adverse reactions to long-term ingestion of kelp—including a painful enlargement of the thyroid gland that disappears once the kelp is discontinued. This condition is most common in Japan, where seaweed is a dietary staple.

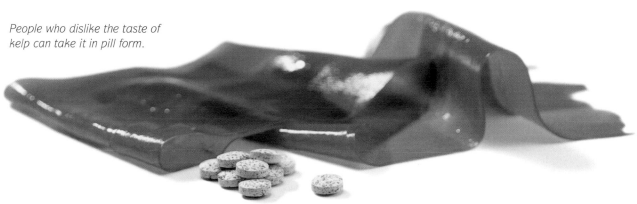

People who dislike the taste of kelp can take it in pill form.

st. john's wort

Hypericum perforatum

Ancient Greeks and Romans believed that this herb could deter evil spirits. Today, St. John's wort has found new and widespread popularity as a natural antidepressant—a gentle alternative to conventional medications, with far fewer side effects.

COMMON USES

- *Treats depression.*
- *Helps fight off viral and bacterial infections.*
- *May help treat premenstrual syndrome (PMS) and fibromyalgia.*
- *Helps relieve chronic pain.*
- *Soothes hemorrhoids.*
- *May aid in weight loss.*

FORMS

- Tablet
- Capsule
- Softgel
- Tincture
- Cream/Ointment

What it is

A shrubby perennial bearing bright yellow flowers, St. John's wort is cultivated worldwide. It was named for Saint John the Baptist because it blooms around June 24, the day celebrated as his birthday; "wort" is an old English word for plant. For centuries, St. John's wort was used to soothe the nerves and to heal wounds, burns, and snakebites. Supplements are made from the dried flowers, which contain a number of therapeutic substances, including a healing pigment called hypericin.

What it does

St. John's wort is most often used to treat mild depression. Scientists aren't sure exactly how the herb works, though it's believed to boost levels of the brain chemical serotonin, which is key to mood and emotions.

⭐ **MAJOR BENEFITS:** A careful recent analysis of 23 different studies of St. John's wort concluded that the herb was as effective as antidepressant drugs—and more effective than a placebo—in the treatment of mild to moderate depression. (Few studies have examined its usefulness for more serious depression, though it may prove beneficial for this as well.) St. John's wort may be helpful for many conditions associated with depression too, such as anxiety, stress, premenstrual syndrome (PMS), fibromyalgia, or chronic pain; it may even have some direct pain-relieving effects. This herb promotes sound sleep and may be especially valuable when depression is marked by fatigue, sleepiness, and low energy levels. It may also aid in treating "wintertime blues" (seasonal affective disorder), a type of depression that develops in the fall and winter and dissipates in the bright sunlight of spring and summer.

Some people are leery of conventional antidepressants because of their potential for causing undesirable side effects, especially reduced sexual function. St. John's wort has fewer bothersome side effects than

Whether you take softgels, capsules, or tablets, St. John's wort may be an effective natural remedy for depression.

these drugs. In addition, although St. John's wort may interact with anti-depressant medications, it doesn't appear to interact with most other conventional drugs, making it useful for older people taking multiple medications. The herb seems so promising that the National Institutes of Health (NIH) is now conducting a major study of its effectiveness.

✤ **ADDITIONAL BENEFITS:** St. John's wort fights bacteria and viruses as well. Research indicates that it may play a key part in combating herpes simplex, influenza, and Epstein-Barr virus (the cause of mononucleosis), and preliminary laboratory studies reveal a possible role for the herb in the fight against AIDS. When an ointment made from St. John's wort is applied to hemorrhoids, it relieves burning and itching. Taken along with the herb ephedra, St. John's wort may also be useful as a weight-loss aid.

How to take it

⌀ **DOSAGE:** The recommended dose is 300 mg of an extract standardized to contain 0.3% hypericin, three times a day. Supplements containing 450 mg are also available and can be taken twice a day.

◔ **GUIDELINES FOR USE:** Take St. John's wort close to mealtime to reduce stomach irritation. In the past, those using the herb were advised not to eat certain foods, including aged cheese and red wine—the same foods best avoided by those taking MAO inhibitors (a type of antidepressant). But recent studies suggest that these foods do not present a problem for those on St. John's wort.

Like a prescription antidepressant, the herb must build up in your blood before it becomes effective, so be sure to allow at least four weeks to determine whether it works for you. It can be used long term, as needed. Unless you are under the care of a doctor familiar with both conventional antidepressants and St. John's wort, the medication and the herb should not be taken together because of the potential for adverse reactions. Some doctors also recommend combining St. John's wort with the nutritional supplement 5-HTP.

Though no adverse effects have been reported in pregnant or lactating women using the herb, there have been few studies in this group of patients, so caution is advised.

Possible side effects

While uncommon, side effects can include constipation, upset stomach, fatigue, dry mouth, and dizziness. People with fair skin are advised to avoid prolonged exposure to sunlight while taking St. John's wort, but increased sensitivity to the sun doesn't appear to be much of a problem at recommended doses.

FACTS
& Tips

■ You can buy a 30-day supply of St. John's wort for under $10—less than a quarter of the cost of popular antidepressant drugs. Choose preparations that are standardized to contain 0.3% hypericin, the therapeutic ingredient found in the herb.

■ In Germany, where doctors prescribe herbal remedies routinely, St. John's wort is the most common form of antidepressant—and much more popular than conventional drugs such as Prozac and Zoloft.

LATEST FINDINGS

■ In one recent study, 50 participants with depression were given either St. John's wort or a placebo. After eight weeks, 70% of those on St. John's wort showed marked improvement, versus 45% of those receiving a placebo. No adverse reactions to the herb were noted.

■ Although used for mild and moderate depression, St. John's wort may one day prove effective for more severe cases. A study of 209 people with serious depression found the herb as effective as conventional antidepressants. But more research is needed before the supplement can be recommended for this purpose.

tea tree oil

Melaleuca alternifolia

For centuries, Australian aborigines relied on the leaves of the tea tree to fight infections. Today, tea tree oil is valued throughout the world as a potent antiseptic, and scientists have confirmed its powerful ability to combat harmful bacteria and fungal infections.

COMMON USES

- *Disinfects and promotes the healing of cuts and scrapes.*
- *Minimizes scarring.*
- *Speeds recovery from bug or spider bites and stings, including bee stings.*
- *Fights athlete's foot, fungal nail infections, and yeast infections.*

FORMS

- Oil
- Gel
- Cream
- Vaginal suppository

CAUTION!

- Tea tree oil is for topical use only. Do not ingest; it can be toxic. Keep it away from eyes.
- Consult your doctor before applying to deep, open wounds.
- Reminder: If you have a medical condition, talk to your doctor before using supplements.

What it is

A champion infection fighter, tea tree oil has a pleasant nutmeglike scent. It comes from the leaves of the *Melaleuca alternifolia,* or tea tree, a species that grows only in Australia (and is completely different from the *Camellia* species used to make black, oolong, and green drinking teas). Extracted through a steam-distillation process, quality tea tree oil contains at least 40% terpinen-4-ol—the active ingredient that is responsible for its healing effects—and less than 5% cineole, a substance that is believed to counteract the medicinal properties of the oil. With the rise of antibiotics after World War II, tea tree oil fell out of favor. Recently interest in it has revived, and more than 700 tons are now produced annually.

What it does

Tea tree oil is used topically to treat a variety of common infections. Once applied to the skin, the oil makes it impossible for many disease-causing fungi to survive. Several studies have shown that it fights various bacteria as well, including some that are resistant to powerful antibiotics. Experts think one reason tea tree oil is so effective is that it readily mixes with skin oils, allowing it to attack the infective agent quickly and actively.

⊛ **MAJOR BENEFITS:** Tea tree oil's antiseptic properties are especially useful for treating cuts and scrapes, as well as insect bites and stings. The oil promotes healing of minor wounds, helps prevent infection, and minimizes any future scarring.

As an antifungal agent, tea tree oil fights the fungus *Trichophyton,* the culprit in athlete's foot, jock itch, and some nail infections. It may also be effective against *Candida albicans* and *Trichomonas vaginalis,* two of the organisms that cause vaginal infections. Unfortunately, some fungal infections can be stubborn to treat; in these cases, your doctor may have to prescribe a more potent conventional antifungal medication.

✳ **ADDITIONAL BENEFITS:** Tea tree oil may be beneficial in the treatment of acne. In one study, a gel containing 5% tea tree oil was shown to be as effective against acne as a lotion with 5% benzoyl peroxide, the active ingredient in most over-the-counter acne medications. But there were fewer side effects with tea tree oil: It caused less scaling, dryness, and itching than the benzoyl peroxide formula. Another study found that a solution containing 0.5% tea tree oil offered protection against *Pityrosporum ovale,* a common dandruff-causing fungus. Sometimes tea tree oil is suggested as a treatment for warts, which are caused by viruses, though studies have not confirmed this use.

How to take it

🅿 **DOSAGE:** *To treat athlete's foot, skin wounds, or nail infections:* Apply a drop or two of pure, undiluted tea tree oil to affected areas of the skin or nails two or three times a day. Tea tree oil creams and lotions can also be used. *To treat vaginal yeast infections:* Insert a commercially available tea tree oil vaginal suppository every 12 hours, for up to five days.

◉ **GUIDELINES FOR USE:** Tea tree oil is for topical use only. Never take tea tree oil orally. If you or a child ingests it, call your doctor or a poison control center right away. Rarely, tea tree oil can cause an allergic skin rash in some people. Before using the oil for the first time, dab a small amount onto your inner arm with a cotton swab. If you are allergic, your arm will quickly become red or inflamed. If this response occurs, dilute the oil by adding a few drops to a tablespoon of bland oil, such as vegetable oil or almond oil, and try the arm test again. If you have no skin reaction, it's safe to apply the diluted oil elsewhere.

Possible side effects

Although tea tree oil can cause minor skin irritation, it otherwise appears to be safe for topical use. Like many herbal oils in pure, undiluted form, it can irritate the eyes and mucous membranes.

Skin-care products such as soap and cosmetics often contain tea tree oil due to its germ-fighting ability.

thiamin

Concerns about getting enough thiamin disappeared in the 1940s, when a law was passed requiring that the B vitamins removed during the milling of refined grains be added back. Although severe thiamin deficiency is a thing of the past, even a moderate deficit has health consequences.

COMMON USES

- *Aids energy production.*
- *Promotes healthy nerves.*
- *May improve mood.*
- *Strengthens the heart.*
- *Soothes heartburn.*

FORMS

- Tablet
- Capsule

What it is

An often overlooked but key member of the B-complex vitamin family, thiamin is known as vitamin B_1 because it was the first B vitamin discovered. Most people get enough thiamin in their diets to meet their basic needs; however, experts believe some people, especially older adults, are mildly deficient in this nutrient. Thiamin is available as an individual supplement, but it's best to get it from a B-complex supplement, because it works closely with the other B vitamins.

What it does

Thiamin is essential for converting the carbohydrates in foods into energy. It also plays a role in promoting healthy nerves and may be useful in treating certain types of heart disease.

⭐ **MAJOR BENEFITS:** In people with congestive heart failure (CHF), thiamin can improve the pumping power of the heart. Thiamin levels in the body are depleted by long-term treatment with diuretic drugs, which are often prescribed for CHF patients to reduce the fluid buildup associated with the disease. In one study, CHF patients who took furosemide (a diuretic) were given either 200 mg a day of thiamin or a placebo. After six weeks, the thiamin group showed a 22% improvement.

By helping to maintain healthy nerves, thiamin may minimize numbness and tingling in the hands and feet. This problem frequently plagues people with diabetes or other diseases that cause nerve damage.

✴ **ADDITIONAL BENEFITS:** In combination with choline and pantothenic acid (also B vitamins), thiamin can enhance the digestive process and provide relief from heartburn. Some researchers think that a thiamin deficiency is linked to mental illnesses, including depression, and that high-dose thiamin supplementation may be beneficial. Thiamin may also boost memory in people with Alzheimer's disease—but evidence is far from conclusive. However, the confusion that is common in older adults

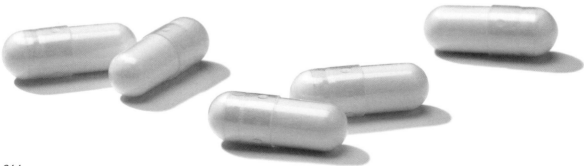

after surgery may be prevented by additional doses of thiamin in the weeks before an operation. Doctors also use thiamin to treat the psychosis related to alcohol withdrawal. Antiseizure medications interfere with the vitamin's absorption, so people taking them may need extra thiamin; this may also reduce the fuzzy thinking that such drugs can cause.

How much you need

To maintain good health and to prevent a thiamin deficiency, the RDA of 1.2 mg a day for men and 1.1 mg a day for women is sufficient. However, higher doses are recommended for therapeutic use.

⊖ **IF YOU GET TOO LITTLE:** A mild thiamin deficiency may go unnoticed. Its symptoms are irritability, weight loss, depression, and muscle weakness. A severe thiamin deficiency causes beriberi, a disease that leads to mental impairment, the wasting away of muscle, paralysis, nerve damage, and eventually death. Once rampant in many countries, beriberi is rare today. It is seen only in parts of Asia where the diet consists mainly of white rice, which is stripped of thiamin and other nutrients during milling. In the U.S., thiamin is added to white bread, cereals, pasta, and white rice.

⊕ **IF YOU GET TOO MUCH:** There are no adverse effects associated with high doses of thiamin, because the body is efficient at eliminating excess amounts through the urine.

How to take it

◐ **DOSAGE:** Specific disorders can benefit from supplemental thiamin. *For congestive heart failure:* Take 200 mg of thiamin daily. *For numbness and tingling:* Take 100 mg of thiamin a day (50 mg as part of a B-complex supplement, 50 mg of extra thiamin). *For depression:* Take 50 mg daily as part of a B complex. *For heartburn:* Take 500 mg a day in the morning. *For alcoholism:* Take 150 mg daily (50 mg as part of a B complex and an extra 100 mg).

◐ **GUIDELINES FOR USE:** Thiamin is best absorbed in an acid environment. Take it with meals, when stomach acid is produced to digest food. Divide your dose and have it twice a day, because high doses are readily flushed out of the body through urine.

Other sources

Lean pork is probably the best dietary source of thiamin, followed by whole grains, dried beans, and nuts and seeds. Enriched grain products also contain thiamin.

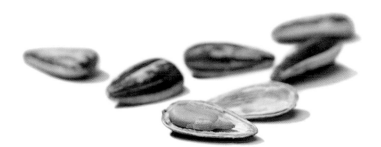

trace minerals

The old adage that good things come in small packages certainly is true for trace minerals. Though some of these tiny nutritional powerhouses are poorly understood, some of them are known to be essential for everything from strong bones to a healthy heart.

COMMON USES

Boron, silicon, and fluoride
- *Aid in building strong bones, teeth, and nails.*

Manganese
- *Treats heart arrhythmias, osteoporosis, epileptic seizures, sprains, and back pain.*

Vanadium
- *May aid people with diabetes.*

Molybdenum
- *Helps the body use iron.*

FORMS

- Tablet
- Capsule
- Powder
- Liquid

CAUTION!

- Molybdenum may aggravate symptoms of gout.
- Boron can affect hormone levels and should be used with care by those at risk for cancer of the breast or prostate.
- Manganese may be toxic for anyone with liver or gallbladder disease.
- Reminder: If you have a medical condition, talk to your doctor before taking supplements.

What it is

Trace minerals are those the body needs in only minuscule amounts. For example, though the average-size person carries around approximately 3 pounds of calcium, the trace mineral manganese weighs in at only 1/2,500 of an ounce. Some trace minerals, such as copper, iron, magnesium, selenium, and zinc, have been studied extensively and are included elsewhere in this book. Others, discussed here, include **boron, fluoride, manganese, molybdenum, silicon,** and **vanadium.**

What it does

The vast majority of trace minerals act as coenzymes, which—in partnership with the proteins known as enzymes—facilitate chemical reactions throughout the body. They aid in forming bones and other tissues, assist in growth and development, make up part of the genetic material DNA, and help the body burn fats and carbohydrates.

PREVENTION: Preliminary evidence suggests that some trace minerals are (like their big brother calcium) good for the bones and may be effective against osteoporosis. Along with silicon, manganese helps build strong bones and connective tissue, the durable substance that holds much of the body together. Boron may enhance bone health by preventing calcium loss and activating the bone-maintaining hormone estrogen, whereas vanadium seems to stimulate bone-building enzymes. And although fluoride is known mainly for its ability to prevent cavities, some studies suggest that it may also aid in protecting against bone fractures.

ADDITIONAL BENEFITS: In addition to strengthening bones, manganese is part of the enzyme superoxide dismutase—a potent antioxidant that plays a role in protecting cells throughout the body. Furthermore, some evidence suggests that manganese may benefit people with epilepsy by reducing the likelihood of seizures. Researchers are investigating the possibility that silicon may be useful in guarding against heart disease. Blood vessel walls concentrate this mineral, and people who get more silicon in

Trace minerals are often part of daily multivitamin and mineral supplements.

their diet may have a decreased risk of this disease. Because silicon also strengthens connective tissue, it is sometimes used to nourish hair, skin, and nails. Molybdenum helps the body use its stores of iron and assists in the burning of fat for energy. And, vanadium may be beneficial for people with diabetes because of its ability to enhance or mimic the effects of the hormone insulin, which regulates blood sugar (glucose) levels.

How much you need

There is no RDA for many trace minerals, because scientific evidence is too scanty to provide a firm requirement. Instead, a few have what's called an Estimated Safe and Adequate Daily Dietary Intake: For manganese, it's 2.0 to 5.0 mg; for fluoride, 3.1 to 3.8 mg; for silicon, 5 to 10 mg; for boron, about 1 mg; for molybdenum, 150 to 500 mcg; and for vanadium, 10 mcg.

⊟ **IF YOU GET TOO LITTLE:** A fluoride deficiency makes people more prone to cavities, and a low boron intake may weaken bones. Deficiencies of manganese, vanadium, and silicon (determined mostly from animal studies) can result in poor growth and development, imbalances in cholesterol levels, and problems making insulin.

⊞ **IF YOU GET TOO MUCH:** In most cases, there is no reason to take high doses of these trace minerals. However, the majority do not cause serious adverse reactions when ingested in large amounts. Manganese toxicity, which has been noted in people inhaling the metal in mines, can cause severe psychiatric disorders, violent rages, poor coordination, and stiff muscles. High doses of boron (more than 500 mg a day) may produce diarrhea, vomiting, nausea, and fatigue. Too much vanadium (more than 10 mg daily) can cause cramping, diarrhea, and a green tongue.

How to take it

⊘ **DOSAGE:** Many bone-building formulas and multivitamin and mineral supplements contain varying doses of trace minerals, including up to 3 mg of boron, 10 mg of manganese, 25 mg of silicon, and 5 mg of vanadium. Most people don't need to take individual trace minerals, though single supplements such as manganese (up to 100 mg a day) are available.

◈ **GUIDELINES FOR USE:** Whether certain factors affect absorption and whether one supplement form is preferable to another is unclear. Boron is probably best taken as part of a bone-building supplement that also contains calcium, manganese, magnesium, and other minerals. Manganese absorption may be impaired by a high iron intake.

Other sources

Manganese is present in whole grains, pineapple, nuts, and leafy greens. Nuts and leafy greens also supply boron, as do broccoli, apples, and raisins. Vanadium is found in whole grains, shellfish, mushrooms, soy products, and oats. Silicon is available in whole grains, turnips, beets, and soy products.

Did You Know?

Processed foods, such as white bread, contain less silicon than their whole grain counterparts.

valerian

Valeriana officinalis

It's 3 A.M., and you're wide awake—again. You wish there was something that you could safely take to help you fall asleep. Valerian may be just what you need, because this herb gently induces slumber, without the unpleasant side effects of conventional drugs.

COMMON USES

- *Promotes restful sleep.*
- *Soothes stress and anxiety.*
- *Improves the symptoms of some digestive disorders.*

FORMS

- Capsule
- Tablet
- Softgel
- Tincture
- Dried herb/Tea

CAUTION!

- If taken during the day, valerian may cause drowsiness.
- If you are pregnant or breast-feeding, do not use valerian.
- Reminder: If you have a medical or psychiatric condition, talk to your doctor before taking supplements.

What it is

In Germany, Great Britain, and other European countries, valerian is officially approved as a sleep aid by medical authorities. A perennial plant native to North America and Europe, valerian has pinkish-colored flowers that grow from a tuberous rootstock, or rhizome. Harvested when the plant is two years old, the rootstock contains a number of important compounds—valepotriates, valeric acid, and volatile oils among them—that at one time or another were each thought to be responsible for the herb's sedative powers. Many experts believe that valerian's effectiveness may be the result of synergy among the various compounds.

What it does

Taken for centuries as an aid to sleep, valerian can also act as a calming agent in stressful daytime situations. It is used in treating anxiety disorders and conditions worsened by stress, such as diverticulosis and irritable bowel syndrome.

⭐ **MAJOR BENEFITS:** Compounds in valerian seem to affect brain receptors for a nerve chemical (neurotransmitter) called gamma-aminobutyric acid, or GABA. It's through this interaction that valerian promotes sleep and eases anxiety. Unlike benzodiazepines—drugs such as diazepam (Valium) or alprazolam (Xanax) commonly prescribed for these disorders—valerian is not addictive and does not make you feel drugged. Rather than inducing sleep directly, valerian calms the brain and body

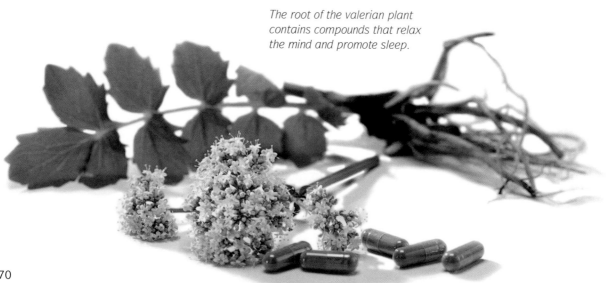

The root of the valerian plant contains compounds that relax the mind and promote sleep.

so sleep can occur naturally. One of the benefits of valerian for insomniacs is that when taken at recommended doses, it doesn't make you feel groggy in the morning as some prescription drugs do.

According to various studies, valerian works as well as prescription drugs for many individuals, and when compared with a placebo, appears to lull a person to sleep. In one study, 128 people were given one of two valerian preparations or a placebo. It was found that the herb improved sleep quality: Those taking valerian fell asleep more quickly and woke up less often than those receiving a placebo. In another study involving insomniacs, nearly all reported improved sleep when taking valerian, and 44% classified their sleep quality as perfect.

Although modern interest in valerian as an anti-anxiety aid is relatively recent, the herb is increasingly recommended by herbalists and nutritionally oriented physicians for this purpose.

✱ **ADDITIONAL BENEFITS:** Valerian helps relax the smooth muscle of the gastrointestinal tract, making it valuable for the treatment of irritable bowel syndrome and diverticulosis, both of which often involve painful spasms of the intestine. In addition, because flare-ups of these disorders are sometimes triggered by stress, valerian's calming action may also account for its effectiveness.

How to take it

⊘ **DOSAGE:** *For insomnia:* Take 250 to 500 mg of the powdered extract in pill form or 1 teaspoon of the tincture 30 to 45 minutes before bedtime. Studies show that for most people, higher doses produce no additional benefit. However, if the low dose does not work for you, you can safely use as much as 900 mg (or 2 teaspoons of the tincture). *For anxiety:* Consume 250 mg twice a day and 250 to 500 mg prior to bedtime.

◐ **GUIDELINES FOR USE:** If you opt for the tincture, try blending it with a little honey or sugar to make this herb, which is a bit unpleasant tasting, more palatable. Although valerian is not addictive, it is not a good idea to rely on any substance, herbal or not, to fall asleep every night. Therefore, don't take valerian nightly for more than two weeks in a row. And make sure you don't combine it with prescription tranquilizers or sleeping pills. It is safe, however, to take valerian with other herbs, such as chamomile, hops, melissa (also known as lemon balm), or passionflower, which may increase its effectiveness as a sleep aid. Valerian can also be used with St. John's wort if you're depressed, and with kava if you're anxious.

Possible side effects

Studies have shown that even in amounts 20 times higher than recommended, valerian has no dangerous side effects. However, extremely large doses can cause dizziness, restlessness, blurred vision, nausea, headache, giddiness, and grogginess in the morning.

....
SHOPPING HINTS
■ When buying valerian, look for a product made from a standardized extract that contains 0.8% valeric (or valerenic) acid.
....

LATEST FINDINGS

■ Prescription sleep aids often cause grogginess the morning after they are taken and can impair a person's ability to drive or perform other tasks requiring concentration. Valerian does not, according to a German study. Researchers compared the effects of valerian; valerian and hops; a benzodiazepine drug; and a placebo. The herbal preparations and the drug all improved sleep quality. The benzodiazepine drug reduced performance the next morning, but the herbs did not. However, performance was slightly impaired for two or three hours after taking the herbs, so avoid driving or performing hazardous tasks for a time after you take valerian.

Did You Know?

Valerian preparations have a very disagreeable odor—so much so that inexperienced users may think they have a bad batch. Don't be put off by the smell; it's completely normal.

vitamin A

One of the first vitamins to be discovered, this essential nutrient keeps your eyesight keen, your skin healthy, and your immune system strong. And so it follows that an extra dose of vitamin A may help treat various eye problems, a number of skin disorders, and a wide range of infections.

COMMON USES

- *Fights colds, flu, and other types of infections.*
- *Treats skin disorders.*
- *Heals wounds, burns, and ulcers.*
- *Maintains eye health.*
- *Enhances chemotherapy.*
- *Eases inflammatory bowel disease.*

FORMS

- Tablet
- Capsule
- Softgel
- Liquid

CAUTION!

- Like vitamin D (another fat-soluble vitamin), vitamin A can build up to toxic levels, so be careful not to get too much.
- If you're pregnant or considering pregnancy, don't take more than 5,000 IU of vitamin A daily; higher doses may cause birth defects. Practice effective birth control when taking doses higher than 5,000 IU and for at least a month afterward.
- Reminder: If you have a medical condition, talk to your doctor before taking supplements.

What it is

Vitamin A, a fat-soluble nutrient, is stored in the liver. The body gets part of its vitamin A from animal fats and makes part in the intestine from beta-carotene and other carotenoids in fruits and vegetables. Vitamin A is present in the body in various chemical forms called retinoids—so named because the vitamin is essential to the health of the retina of the eye.

What it does

This vitamin prevents night blindness; maintains the skin and cells that line the respiratory and gastrointestinal tracts; and helps build teeth and bones. It is vital for normal reproduction, growth, and development too. In addition, vitamin A is crucial to the immune system, including the plentiful supply of immune cells that line the airways and digestive tract and form an important line of defense against disease.

✱ **MAJOR BENEFITS:** Vitamin A is perhaps best known for its ability to maintain vision, especially night vision, assisting the eye in adjusting from bright light to darkness. It can also alleviate such specific eye complaints as "dry eye," in addition to its many other benefits.

By boosting immunity, vitamin A greatly strengthens resistance to infections, including sore throat, colds, flu, and bronchitis. It may also combat cold sores and shingles (caused by a herpes virus), warts (a viral skin infection), eye infections, and vaginal yeast infections—and perhaps even control allergies. The vitamin may help the immune system battle against breast and lung cancers and improve survival rates in those with leukemia; in addition, animal studies suggest it inhibits melanoma, a deadly form of skin cancer. Another benefit for cancer patients is that vitamin A may enhance the effectiveness of chemotherapy.

✱ **ADDITIONAL BENEFITS:** Vitamin A was first used in the 1940s to treat skin disorders, including acne and psoriasis, but the doses were high and toxic. Scientists later developed safer vitamin A derivatives (notably retinoic acid); now sold as prescription drugs, these include the acne and antiwrinkle cream Retin-A. Lower doses of vitamin A (25,000 IU a day) can be used to treat a range of skin conditions, including acne, dry skin,

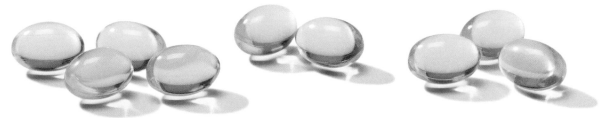

eczema, rosacea, and psoriasis. Vitamin A also promotes healing of skin wounds and can be applied to cuts, scrapes, and burns; it may hasten recovery from sprains and strains. The therapeutic effects of vitamin A extend to the lining of the digestive tract, where it helps treat inflammatory bowel disease and ulcers. In addition, getting enough of this vitamin will speed recovery in people who have had a stroke. Women with heavy or prolonged menstrual periods are sometimes deficient in this vitamin, so supplements may be of value in treating this condition as well.

How much you need

The RDA for vitamin A is 4,000 IU a day for women, and 5,000 IU a day for men. Higher doses are typically given for specific ailments.

⊖ **IF YOU GET TOO LITTLE:** Although quite rare in the United States, a vitamin A deficiency can cause night blindness (even total blindness) and a greatly lowered resistance to infection. Milder cases of deficiency do occur, especially in the elderly, who often have vitamin-poor diets. Infections such as pneumonia can deplete vitamin A stores.

⊕ **IF YOU GET TOO MUCH:** An overabundance of vitamin A can be a real problem. A single dose of 500,000 IU may induce weakness and vomiting. And as little as 25,000 IU a day for six years has been reported to cause serious liver disease (cirrhosis). Signs of toxicity include dry, cracking skin and brittle nails, hair that falls out easily, bleeding gums, weight loss, irritability, fatigue, and nausea.

How to take it

Ⓓ **DOSAGE:** Multivitamins supply vitamin A, sometimes in the form of beta-carotene. For specific complaints in adults, up to 10,000 IU a day is generally safe for long-term use (except for pregnant women and those considering pregnancy, who should not exceed 5,000 IU a day). As a broad guideline, it's safe to take 25,000 IU a day for up to a month or 100,000 IU for up to a week, though in some cases higher doses may be needed.

◉ **GUIDELINES FOR USE:** Take supplements with food; a little fat in the diet aids absorption. Vitamin E and zinc help the body use vitamin A, which in turn boosts absorption of iron from foods.

Other sources

Vitamin A is richly represented in fish, egg yolks, butter, organ meats such as liver (3 ounces provide more than 9,000 IU), and fortified milk (check the label to be sure). Dark green, yellow, orange, and red fruits and vegetables have large amounts of beta-carotene and many other carotenoids, which the body makes into vitamin A on an as-needed basis.

FACTS & Tips

■ You can't overdose on vitamin A by eating carotenoid-rich fruits and vegetables, such as apricots, leafy greens, or cantaloupe. Although your body converts some carotenoids to vitamin A, it makes only as much as it needs. Unless you eat a lot of liver or oily fish, it's almost impossible to get too much vitamin A from your diet.

■ Vitamin A doses can be given as retinol equivalents (RE) rather than international units (IU). One RE is equivalent to 3.3 IU.

■ If you're heading to the North Pole, watch what you eat: A quarter pound of polar bear liver contains an acutely toxic dose of vitamin A—more than 2,000,000 IU.

LATEST FINDINGS

■ Vitamin A shows promise in the treatment of diabetes. In two recent studies, up to 25,000 IU of vitamin A daily improved insulin's ability to control blood sugar. (Poor blood sugar control is a prime problem in people with diabetes.)

■ A Brazilian study found that vitamin A may combat chronic lung diseases. After 30 days of taking supplements, men who received 5,000 IU a day could breathe better than those who were given a placebo.

Did You Know?

You'd have to eat more than 10 large eggs to meet the daily RDA for vitamin A. Most people get enough from other animal sources and from carotenoid-rich fruits and vegetables.

vitamin B₆

This remarkable nutrient is probably involved in more bodily processes than any other vitamin or mineral. Government surveys indicate, however, that one-third of all adults—and half of all women—are not getting enough of this key vitamin in their diets.

What it is

Vitamin B_6, unequivocally the "workhorse" of nutrients, performs more than 100 jobs innumerable times a day. It functions primarily as a coenzyme, a substance that acts in concert with enzymes to speed up chemical reactions in the cells.

Another name for vitamin B_6 is pyridoxine. In supplement form, it is available as pyridoxine hydrochloride or pyridoxal-5-phosphate (P-5-P). Either form satisfies most needs, but some nutritionally oriented physicians prefer P-5-P because it may be better absorbed.

What it does

Forming red blood cells, helping cells make proteins, manufacturing brain chemicals (neurotransmitters) such as serotonin, and releasing stored forms of energy are just a few of the functions of vitamin B_6. There is also evidence that vitamin B_6 plays a role in preventing and treating many diseases.

PREVENTION: Getting enough B_6 through the diet or supplements may help prevent heart disease. Working with folic acid and vitamin B_{12}, this vitamin assists the body in processing homocysteine, an amino acid-like compound that has been linked to an increased risk of heart disease and other vascular disorders when large amounts are present in the blood.

ADDITIONAL BENEFITS: Some women suffering from premenstrual syndrome (PMS) report that vitamin B_6 provides relief from many of the symptoms. This beneficial effect probably occurs because of the vitamin's involvement in clearing excess estrogen from the body. And in its role as a building block for neurotransmitters, vitamin B_6 may be useful in reducing the likelihood of having epileptic seizures, as well as lifting depression. In fact, up to 25% of people with depression may be deficient in vitamin B_6.

In addition, the vitamin maintains nerve health. People with diabetes, who are at risk for nerve damage, can also benefit from B_6. Furthermore, it is effective in easing the symptoms of carpal tunnel syndrome, which involves nerve inflammation in the wrist. And for people with asthma, vitamin B_6 may reduce the intensity and frequency of attacks; it is especially important for those taking the asthma drug theophylline.

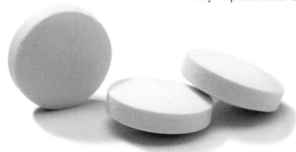

How much you need

The RDA for vitamin B_6 is 1.3 mg a day for women and men younger than age 50, and 1.5 mg (for women) to 1.7 mg (for men) a day for those older than age 50. Therapeutic doses are higher.

⊖ **IF YOU GET TOO LITTLE:** A recent survey found that half of all women fail to meet the RDA for vitamin B_6. Women taking oral contraceptives may have especially low levels of this vitamin. Mild deficiencies of B_6 can raise homocysteine levels, increasing the risk of heart and vascular diseases. Symptoms of severe deficiency, which is rare, are skin disorders such as dermatitis, sores around the mouth, and acne. Neurological signs include insomnia, depression, and in extreme cases, seizures and brain wave abnormalities.

⊕ **IF YOU GET TOO MUCH:** High doses of vitamin B_6 (more than 2,000 mg a day) can cause nerve damage when taken for long periods. In rare cases, prolonged use at lower doses (200 to 300 mg a day) can have the same consequence. Fortunately, nerve damage is completely reversible once you discontinue the vitamin. If you're using B_6 for nerve pain, call your doctor if you experience any new numbness or tingling and stop taking the vitamin. Doses up to 100 mg a day are safe, even for long-term use.

How to take it

⊘ **DOSAGE:** You can keep homocysteine levels in check with just 3 mg of B_6 a day, but a daily dose of 50 mg is often recommended. Higher doses are needed for therapeutic uses. *For PMS:* Take 100 mg of B_6 a day. *For acute carpal tunnel syndrome:* Try 50 mg of B_6 or P-5-P three times a day. *For asthma:* Take 50 mg of B_6 twice a day.

◉ **GUIDELINES FOR USE:** Vitamin B_6 is best absorbed in doses of no more than 100 mg at one time. When taking higher doses, this more gradual intake will also decrease your chances of nerve damage.

Other sources

Fish, poultry, meats, chickpeas, potatoes, avocados, and bananas are all good sources of vitamin B_6.

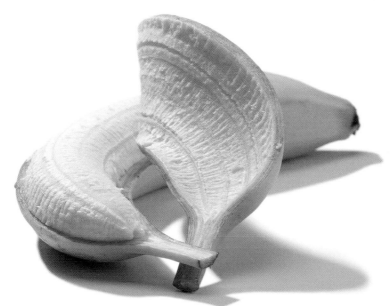

vitamin B$_{12}$

Although this vitamin is plentiful in most people's diets, after age 50 some individuals have a limited ability to absorb it from food. Supplements are usually recommended, because even mild deficiencies may increase the risk of heart disease, depression, and possibly Alzheimer's.

COMMON USES

- *Prevents a form of anemia.*
- *Helps reduce depression.*
- *Thwarts nerve pain, numbness, and tingling.*
- *Lowers the risk of heart disease.*
- *May improve multiple sclerosis and tinnitus.*

FORMS

- Tablet
- Capsule

CAUTION!

- If you take a vitamin B$_{12}$ supplement, you must also have a folic acid supplement: A high intake of one can mask a deficiency of the other.
- Reminder: If you have a medical or psychiatric condition, talk to your doctor before taking supplements.

What it is

Also known as cobalamin, vitamin B$_{12}$ was the last vitamin to be discovered. In the late 1940s it was identified as the substance in calf's liver that cured pernicious anemia, a potentially fatal disease primarily affecting older adults. Vitamin B$_{12}$ is the only B vitamin the body stores in large amounts, mostly in the liver. The body absorbs B$_{12}$ through a very complicated process: Digestive enzymes in the presence of enough stomach acid separate B$_{12}$ from the protein in foods. The vitamin then binds with a substance called intrinsic factor (a protein produced by cells in the stomach lining) before being carried to the small intestine, where it is absorbed. Low levels of stomach acid or an inadequate amount of intrinsic factor—both of which occur with age—can lead to deficiencies. However, because the body has good reserves of B$_{12}$, it can take several years for a shortfall to develop.

What it does

Vitamin B$_{12}$ is essential for cell replication and is particularly important for red blood cell production. It maintains the protective sheath around nerves (myelin), assists in converting food to energy, and plays a critical role in the production of DNA and RNA, the genetic material in cells.

⬛ **PREVENTION:** Moderately high blood levels of homocysteine, an amino acid-like substance, have been linked to an increased risk of heart disease. Working with folic acid, vitamin B$_{12}$ helps the body process homocysteine and so may lower that risk. Because of its beneficial effects on the nerves, vitamin B$_{12}$ may help prevent a number of neurological disorders, as well as the numbness and tingling often associated with diabetes. It may also play a part in treating depression.

✱ **ADDITIONAL BENEFITS:** Research shows that low levels of vitamin B$_{12}$ are common in people with Alzheimer's disease. Whether this deficiency is a contributing factor to the disease or simply a result of it is unknown. The nutrient does, however, keep the immune system healthy. Some studies suggest that it lengthens the amount of time between infection with the HIV virus and the development of AIDS. Other research indicates

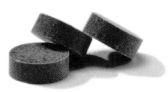

adequate B_{12} intake improves immune responses in older people. With its beneficial effect on nerves, vitamin B_{12} may lessen ringing in the ears (tinnitus). As a component of myelin, it is valuable in treating multiple sclerosis, a disease that involves the destruction of this nerve covering. And through its role in cell replication, B_{12} may improve symptoms of rosacea.

How much you need

The RDA for vitamin B_{12} is 2.4 mcg a day for adults. But, many experts recommend that you get 100 to 400 mcg. Supplements of vitamin B_{12} are very important for older people and vegans (who eat no meat products).

⊟ **IF YOU GET TOO LITTLE:** Symptoms of a vitamin B_{12} deficiency include fatigue, depression, numbness and tingling in the extremities caused by nerve damage, muscle weakness, confusion, and memory loss. Dementia and pernicious anemia can develop; both are reversible if caught early.

The level of B_{12} in the blood decreases with age. People with ulcers, Crohn's disease, or other gastrointestinal disorders are at risk, as are those taking prescription medication for epilepsy (seizures), chronic heartburn, or gout. Excessive alcohol also hinders absorption of vitamin B_{12}.

⊞ **IF YOU GET TOO MUCH:** Excess vitamin B_{12} is readily excreted in urine; there are no known adverse effects from a high intake of vitamin B_{12}.

How to take it

⊘ **DOSAGE:** A general dose of 1,000 mcg of vitamin B_{12} a day is useful for heart disease prevention, pernicious anemia, numbness and tingling, tinnitus, multiple sclerosis, and rosacea. If you're deficient in B_{12}, higher doses may be needed. Or if you do not produce enough intrinsic factor, B_{12} shots or a prescription nasal spray may be necessary; ask your doctor.

◈ **GUIDELINES FOR USE:** Take vitamin B_{12} once a day, preferably in the morning, along with at least 400 mcg of folic acid. Most multivitamins contain at least the RDA of vitamin B_{12} and folic acid; B-complex supplements have higher amounts. For larger, therapeutic amounts, look for a supplement with just vitamin B_{12} or B_{12} with folic acid. Using a sublingual (under-the-tongue) form enhances absorption.

Other sources

Animal foods are the primary source of B_{12}. These include organ meats, brewer's yeast, oysters, sardines and other fish, eggs, meat, and cheese. Some breakfast cereals are fortified with this vitamin as well.

vitamin C

This vitamin is probably better known and more widely used than any other nutritional supplement. But even if you think you're familiar with vitamin C, read on. You may be surprised to discover exactly how versatile and health-enhancing this nutrient truly is.

COMMON USES

- *Enhances immunity.*
- *Minimizes cold symptoms; shortens duration of illness.*
- *Speeds wound healing.*
- *Promotes healthy gums.*
- *Treats asthma.*
- *Helps prevent cataracts.*
- *Protects against some forms of cancer and heart disease.*

FORMS

- Tablet
- Capsule
- Liquid
- Powder

CAUTION!

- Don't take more than 500 mg a day if you have kidney stones, kidney disease, or hemochromatosis, a genetic tendency to store excess iron (vitamin C enhances iron absorption).
- Vitamin C can distort the accuracy of medical tests for diabetes, colon cancer, and hemoglobin levels. Let your doctor know if you're taking it.
- Reminder: If you have a medical condition, talk to your doctor before taking supplements.

What it is

As early as 1742 lemon juice was known to prevent scurvy, a debilitating disease that often plagued long-distance sailors. But not until 1928 was the healthful component in lemon juice identified as vitamin C. Its antiscurvy, or antiscorbutic, effect is the root of this vitamin's scientific name: ascorbic acid. Today, interest in vitamin C is based less on its ability to cure scurvy than on its potential to protect cells. As the body's primary water-soluble antioxidant, vitamin C helps fight damage caused by unstable oxygen molecules called free radicals—especially in those areas that are mostly water, such as the interior of cells.

What it does

Vitamin C is active throughout the body. It helps strengthen the capillaries (the tiniest blood vessels) and cell walls and is crucial for the formation of collagen (a protein found in connective tissue). In these ways, vitamin C prevents bruising, promotes healing, and keeps ligaments (which connect muscle to bone), tendons (which connect bone to bone), and gums strong and healthy. It also aids in producing hemoglobin in red blood cells and assists the body in absorbing iron from foods.

PREVENTION: As an antioxidant, vitamin C offers protection against cancer and heart disease; several studies have shown that low levels of this vitamin are linked to heart attacks. In addition, vitamin C may actually lengthen life. In one study, men who consumed more than 300 mg of vitamin C a day (from food and supplements) lived longer than men who consumed less than 50 mg a day.

Another study found that over the long term, vitamin C supplements protect against cataracts, a clouding of the lens of the eye that interferes with vision. Women who took vitamin C for 10 years or more had a 77% lower rate of early "lens opacities," the beginning stage of cataracts, than women who didn't use supplements.

ADDITIONAL BENEFITS: Does vitamin C prevent colds? Probably not, but it can help lessen symptoms and may shorten the duration of this illness. In a 1995 analysis of studies exploring the connection between

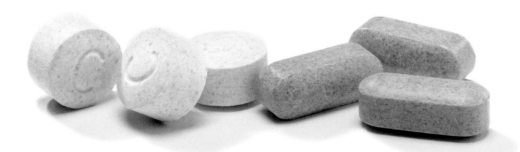

vitamin C and colds, the researchers concluded that taking 1,000 to 6,000 mg a day at the onset of cold symptoms reduces the cold's duration by 21%, about one day. Other studies have shown that vitamin C helps elderly patients fight severe respiratory infections. Vitamin C also appears to be a natural antihistamine. High doses of the vitamin can block the effect of inflammatory substances produced by the body in response to pollen, pet dander, or other allergens.

The vitamin is an effective asthma remedy as well. Numerous studies have found that vitamin C supplements helped prevent or improve asthmatic symptoms. For people with type 1 diabetes, which interferes with the transport of vitamin C into cells, supplementing with 1,000 to 3,000 mg a day may prevent complications of the disease, such as eye problems and high cholesterol levels.

How much you need

The RDA for vitamin C for men and women is 60 mg a day (for smokers, it's 100 mg). However, even conservative experts think an optimal intake is at least 200 mg a day, and they recommend higher doses for the treatment of specific diseases.

⊖ **IF YOU GET TOO LITTLE:** You'd have to consume less than 10 mg a day to get scurvy, but receiving less than 50 mg of vitamin C a day has been linked with an increased risk of heart attack, cataracts, and a shorter life.

⊕ **IF YOU GET TOO MUCH:** Large doses of vitamin C—more than 2,000 mg a day—can cause loose stools, diarrhea, gas, and bloating; all can be corrected by reducing your daily dose. At this level, the vitamin may interfere with the absorption of copper and selenium, so make sure you consume enough of these minerals in foods or supplements.

How to take it

▨ **DOSAGE:** *For general health:* Get 500 mg of vitamin C a day through foods and supplements. *For the treatment of various diseases:* Depending on the condition, 1,000 to 6,000 mg a day may be appropriate.

◈ **GUIDELINES FOR USE:** Large amounts are best absorbed in 1,000 mg doses, taken with meals throughout the day. The vitamin works very well when combined with other antioxidants, such as vitamin E.

Other sources

Citrus fruits and juices, broccoli, red peppers, dark greens, strawberries, and kiwifruits are all good sources of vitamin C.

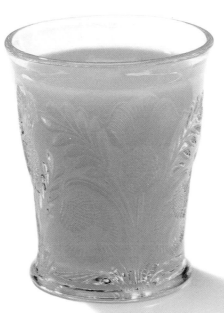

LATEST FINDINGS

■ Vitamin C may help prevent reblockage (restenosis) of arteries after angioplasty (an alternative to bypass surgery). A study of 119 angioplasty patients found that restenosis occurred in just 24% of those who took 500 mg of vitamin C a day for four months, compared with 43% of those who did not take the vitamin.

■ In addition to being an antioxidant, vitamin C helps the body recycle other antioxidants. In one study, vitamin E concentrations were 18% higher in those who got more than 220 mg of vitamin C a day, compared with people who got 120 mg or less.

■ Vitamin C recently came under attack when a small test-tube study found that it may cause genetic damage, potentially increasing the risk of cancer. But scientists have since identified serious flaws in the study. Many better studies show that vitamin C provides numerous benefits, including preventing certain cancers.

Did You Know?

An 8-ounce glass of fresh-squeezed orange juice supplies 124 mg of vitamin C, which is more than twice the RDA for this vitamin.

vitamin D

Called the sunshine vitamin (because your body makes all it needs with enough sunlight), vitamin D is essential for bone health and may slow the progression of arthritis. It is also believed to strengthen the immune system and possibly prevent some cancers.

COMMON USES

- *Aids in the body's absorption of calcium.*
- *Promotes healthy bones.*
- *Strengthens teeth.*
- *May protect against some types of cancer.*

FORMS

- Tablet
- Capsule
- Softgel
- Liquid

CAUTION!

- Overuse of vitamin D supplements can result in elevated blood levels of calcium, leading to weight loss, nausea, and heart and kidney damage.
- Reminder: If you have a medical condition, talk to your doctor before taking supplements.

What it is

Technically a hormone, vitamin D is produced within the body when the skin is exposed to the ultraviolet B (UVB) rays in sunlight. Theoretically, spending a few minutes in the sun each day supplies all the vitamin D your body needs, but many people don't get enough sun to generate adequate vitamin D, especially in the winter.

What's more, the body's ability to manufacture vitamin D declines with age, so vitamin D deficiencies are common in older people. But even young adults may not have sufficient vitamin D stores. One study of nearly 300 patients (of all ages) hospitalized for a variety of causes found that 57% of them did not have high enough levels of vitamin D. Of particular concern was the observation that a vitamin D deficiency was present in a third of the people who obtained the recommended amount of vitamin D through diet or supplements. This finding suggests that current recommendations for vitamin D may not be high enough.

What it does

The basic function of vitamin D is to regulate blood levels of calcium and phosphorus, helping to build strong bones and healthy teeth.

PREVENTION: Studies have shown that vitamin D is important in the prevention of osteoporosis, a disease that causes porous bones and thus an increased risk of fractures. Without sufficient vitamin D, the body cannot absorb calcium from food or supplements—no matter how much calcium you consume. When blood calcium levels are low, the body will move calcium from the bones to the blood to supply the muscles—especially the heart—and the nerves with the amount they need. Over time, this reallocation of calcium leads to a loss of bone mass.

Vitamin D is available as softgels (below) or tablets. It may also be added to calcium supplements.

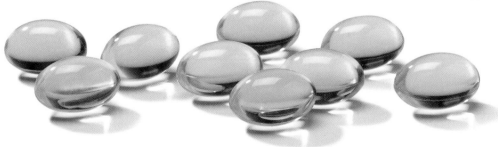

ADDITIONAL BENEFITS: Scientists are continuing to discover more about the functions of vitamin D in the body. Some studies suggest that it is important for a healthy immune system. Others indicate that it may help prevent prostate, colon, or breast cancer. One study found that adequate vitamin D slowed the progression of osteoarthritis in the knees, although it did not prevent the disease from developing in the first place.

How much you need

The RDA for vitamin D is 200 IU a day for people under age 50; 400 IU for those ages 51 to 70; and 600 IU for those over age 70. Many experts, however, think the recommendations for people over age 50 are too low.

IF YOU GET TOO LITTLE: A vitamin D deficiency can harm the bones, causing a bone-weakening disease in children (rickets) and increasing the risk of osteoporosis in adults. A deficiency can also cause diarrhea, insomnia, nervousness, and muscle twitches. The likelihood of a child developing rickets today is remote, however, because vitamin D is added to milk. In addition, children typically spend enough time in the sun to generate ample vitamin D.

IF YOU GET TOO MUCH: Although your body effectively rids itself of any extra vitamin D it makes from sunlight, overloading on supplements may create problems. Daily doses of 1,000 to 2,000 IU over six months can cause constipation or diarrhea, headache, loss of appetite, nausea and vomiting, heartbeat irregularities, and extreme fatigue. Continued high doses weaken the bones and allow calcium to accumulate in soft tissues, such as the muscles.

How to take it

DOSAGE: As little as 10 to 15 minutes of midday sunlight on your face, hands, and arms two or three times a week can supply all the vitamin D you need. But if you are over age 50; if you don't drink milk (which is fortified with vitamin D); if you don't get outdoors much between the hours of 8 A.M. and 3 P.M.; or if you always wear sunscreen, you might want to consider vitamin D supplements. Many experts recommend 400 to 600 IU a day for people over age 50 and 800 IU for those over age 70; 200 to 400 IU a day is probably sufficient for younger adults.

GUIDELINES FOR USE: Supplements can be taken at any time of day, with or without food. Most daily multivitamins contain up to 400 IU of vitamin D. It is also often found in calcium supplements.

Other sources

Vitamin D is added to milk; one cup contains 100 IU. Some breakfast cereals are fortified with 40 to 100 IU of vitamin D in each serving. Fatty fish, such as herring, salmon, and tuna, are naturally rich in the vitamin.

vitamin E

A superstar nutrient with antioxidant capability, vitamin E offers a multitude of preventive benefits, including protection against heart disease, cancer, and a broad range of other disorders. Working at the body's cellular level, vitamin E may even slow the aging process.

COMMON USES

- *Helps protect against heart disease, certain cancers, and various other chronic ailments.*
- *May delay or prevent cataracts.*
- *Enhances the immune system.*
- *Protects against secondhand smoke and other pollutants.*
- *Aids in skin healing.*

FORMS

- Capsule
- Tablet
- Softgel
- Cream
- Oil
- Liquid

CAUTION!

- People on prescription blood-thinning drugs (anticoagulants) or aspirin should consult their doctor before using vitamin E.
- Do not take vitamin E two days before or after surgery.
- Reminder: If you have a medical condition, talk to your doctor before taking supplements.

What it is

Vitamin E is a generic term for a group of related compounds called tocopherols, which occur in four major forms: alpha-, beta-, delta-, and gamma-tocopherols. Alpha-tocopherol is the most common and most potent form of the vitamin. Because it is fat-soluble, vitamin E is stored for relatively long periods in the body, mainly in fat tissue and the liver. Vitamin E is found in only a few foods, and many of these are high in fat, which makes it difficult to get the amount of vitamin E you require while on a healthy low-fat diet. Therefore, supplements can be very useful in obtaining optimal amounts of this nutrient.

What it does

One of vitamin E's basic functions is to protect cell membranes. It also helps the body use selenium and vitamin K. But vitamin E's current reputation comes from its disease-fighting potential as an antioxidant—meaning it assists in destroying or neutralizing free radicals, the unstable oxygen molecules that cause damage to cells.

PREVENTION: By safeguarding cell membranes and acting as an antioxidant, vitamin E may play a role in preventing cancer. Some of the most compelling research to date suggests that vitamin E can help protect against cardiovascular disease, including heart attack and stroke, by reducing the harmful effects of LDL ("bad") cholesterol and by preventing blood clots. In addition, vitamin E may offer protection because it works to reduce inflammatory processes that have been linked to heart disease. Findings from two large studies suggest that vitamin E may reduce the risk of heart disease by 25% to 50%—and it may prevent chest pain (angina) as well. And recent findings suggest that taking vitamin E with vitamin C may help block some of the harmful effects of a fatty meal.

ADDITIONAL BENEFITS: Because it protects cells from free-radical damage, some experts think that vitamin E may retard the aging process. There is also evidence to suggest that it improves immune function

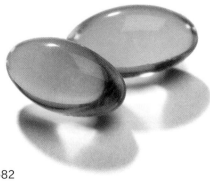
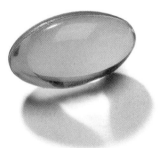

in the elderly, combats toxins from cigarette smoke and other pollutants, treats Parkinson's disease, postpones the development of cataracts, and slows the progression of Alzheimer's disease.

Other research found that vitamin E can relieve the severe leg pain caused by a circulatory problem called intermittent claudication. It may alleviate premenstrual breast pain and tenderness as well. In addition, many people report that applying creams or oils containing vitamin E to skin wounds helps promote healing.

How much you need

The RDA for vitamin E is 8 mg for women and 10 mg for men daily—which is equal to 12 to 15 IU. Although this amount may be enough to prevent deficiency, higher doses are needed to provide the full antioxidant effect.

⊖ **IF YOU GET TOO LITTLE:** Intakes of vitamin E below the RDA can lead to neurological damage and shorten the life of red blood cells. If you are eating a balanced diet, however, you are probably not at risk.

⊕ **IF YOU GET TOO MUCH:** No toxic effects from large doses of vitamin E have been discovered, even at levels as high as 3,200 IU a day. Minor effects, such as headaches and diarrhea, have rarely been reported. But, large doses of vitamin E can interfere with the absorption of vitamin A.

How to take it

⊘ **DOSAGE:** To obtain the disease-fighting potential of vitamin E, many experts recommend 400 to 800 IU daily in capsule or tablet form. (This total includes amounts you get in a multivitamin.) Doses of up to 1,200 IU have been recommended for people at high risk for heart disease and certain cancers. It may be particularly effective when taken with vitamin C.

◉ **GUIDELINES FOR USE:** Try to take vitamin E supplements at the same time each day. Combining it with a meal decreases stomach irritation and increases the absorption of this fat-soluble vitamin. For topical use, break open a capsule and apply the oil directly to your skin, or use a commercial cream containing vitamin E as needed.

Other sources

Wheat germ is an outstanding dietary source of vitamin E: 1 ounce (about 2 tablespoons) contains the equivalent of 54 IU. Beneficial amounts of vitamin E are also found in vegetable oils, nuts and seeds (hazelnuts, almonds, sunflower seeds), green leafy vegetables, and whole grains.

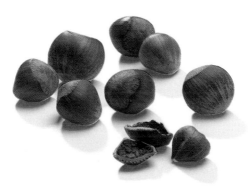

vitamin K

Doctors have long used vitamin K, which promotes blood clotting, to help heal incisions in surgical patients and to prevent bleeding problems in newborns. This vitamin also aids in building strong bones and may be useful for combating the threat of osteoporosis.

What it is

In the 1930s Danish researchers noted that baby chickens fed a fat-free diet developed bleeding problems. They eventually solved the problem with an alfalfa-based compound that they named vitamin K, for *Koagulation*. Scientists now know that most of the body's vitamin K needs are met by bacteria in the intestines that produce this vitamin, and only about 20% comes from foods. Deficiencies are rare in healthy people, even though the body doesn't store vitamin K in high amounts. Natural forms of vitamin K come from chlorophyll—the same substance that gives plants such as alfalfa their green color. Synthetic supplements are also available by prescription. Other names for vitamin K are phytonadione and menadiol.

What it does

This single nutrient sets in motion the entire blood-clotting process as soon as a wound occurs. Without it, we might bleed to death. Researchers have discovered vitamin K plays a protective role in bone health as well.

PREVENTION: Doctors often recommend preventive doses of vitamin K if bleeding or hemorrhaging is a concern. Even when no deficiency exists, surgeons frequently order vitamin K before an operation to reduce the risk of postoperative bleeding. Under medical supervision, it can also be prescribed for excessive menstrual bleeding. Though not yet a widely accepted treatment, vitamin K may provide great benefits for those suffering from osteoporosis. Some studies show it helps the body make use of calcium and decreases the risk of fractures. Vitamin K may be especially important for bone health in older women. Not surprisingly, it is included among the ingredients in many bone-building formulas.

ADDITIONAL BENEFITS: Vitamin K may play a role in cancer prevention and help those undergoing radiation therapy. Recent findings also put vitamin K in the arsenal of heart-smart nutrients: Some evidence suggests it may halt the buildup of disease-causing plaque in arteries and reduce the blood level of LDL ("bad") cholesterol. But more research is needed to define the role of vitamin K in these and other disorders.

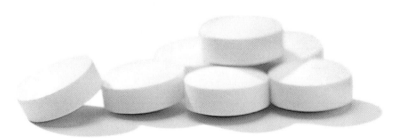

How much you need

Because vitamin K needs are met by the body, the daily RDA is low: 80 mcg for men over age 25 and 65 mcg for women over age 25.

⊖ **IF YOU GET TOO LITTLE:** In healthy people, a vitamin K deficiency is rare, because the body manufactures most of what it requires. In fact, deficiencies are found only in those with liver disease or intestinal illnesses that interfere with fat absorption. However, vitamin K levels can wane as a result of using antibiotics long term. One of the first signs of a deficiency is a tendency to bruise easily. Those at risk need careful medical monitoring because they could bleed to death in the event of a serious injury.

⊕ **IF YOU GET TOO MUCH:** It's hard to get too much vitamin K because it's not abundant in any one food (except leafy greens). Although even megadoses are not toxic, high doses can be dangerous if you're taking anticoagulants. Large doses also may cause flushing and sweating.

How to take it

⊘ **DOSAGE:** Multivitamins often contain between 25 and 60 mcg of vitamin K. Bone-building formulas provide around 300 mcg a day, the equivalent of adding a large leafy salad to your daily diet. Higher doses (such as those in prenatal multivitamins) may be prescribed under medical supervision for those with specific medical needs.

◆ **GUIDELINES FOR USE:** When prescribed, vitamin K should be taken with meals to enhance absorption.

Other sources

Leafy green vegetables, including—per cup of vegetable—kale (547 mcg), Swiss chard (299 mcg), and turnip greens (138 mcg), are richest in vitamin K. Broccoli, spring onions, and brussels sprouts are also good sources. Other foods with some vitamin K are pistachios, vegetable oils, meats, and dairy products.

A cup of kale provides the equivalent of more than five 100 mcg tablets of vitamin K.

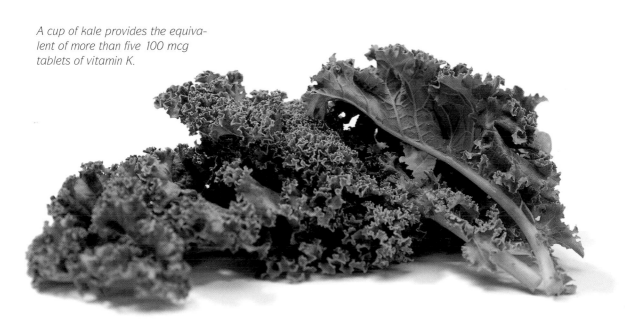

white willow bark

Salix alba

Used for thousands of years to treat fevers and headaches, white willow bark contains a chemical forerunner of today's most popular painkiller—aspirin. The herb is sometimes called "herbal aspirin" but has few of that drug's side effects.

COMMON USES

- *Relieves acute and chronic pains, including back and neck pain, headaches, and muscle aches.*
- *Reduces arthritis inflammation.*
- *May lower fevers.*

FORMS

- Capsule
- Tablet
- Tincture
- Powder
- Dried herb/Tea

CAUTION!

- Anyone who has been told to avoid aspirin should also refrain from using white willow bark. This advice applies to people allergic to aspirin, those with ulcers or other gastrointestinal disorders, and teens or children with a fever.
- Pregnant or breast-feeding women should consult their doctors before taking white willow bark, because its safety has not been established in these situations.
- Reminder: If you have a medical condition, talk to your doctor before taking supplements.

What it is

White willow bark comes from the stately white willow tree, which can grow up to 75 feet tall. In China, its medicinal properties have been appreciated for centuries. But not until the eighteenth century was the herb recognized as a pain reliever and fever reducer in the West. European settlers brought the white willow tree to North America, where they discovered local tribes were using native willow species to alleviate pain and fight fevers.

In 1828 the plant's active ingredient, salicin, was isolated by German and French scientists, and ten years later, European chemists manufactured salicylic acid, a chemical cousin to aspirin, from it. Aspirin, or acetylsalicylic acid, was later created from a different salicin-containing herb called meadowsweet. By the end of the nineteenth century, the Bayer Company had begun commercially producing aspirin, which was marketed as a new and safer pain reliever than wintergreen and black birch oil, the herbs commonly employed at that time for reducing pain.

All parts of the white willow contain salicin, but concentrations of this chemical are highest in the bark, which is collected in early spring from trees that are two to five years old. *Salix alba,* or white willow, is the most popular species for medicinal use, but other types of willow are also rich in salicin, including *Salix fragilis* (crack willow), *Salix purpurea* (purple willow), and *Salix daphnoides* (violet willow). These species are often sold simply as willow bark in health-food stores.

What it does

In the body, the salicin from white willow bark is metabolized to form salicylic acid, which reduces pain, fever, and inflammation. Though the herb is slower acting than aspirin, its beneficial effects last longer, and it causes

Bark from the white willow tree—dried, concentrated, and packaged into pills—is the source of a potent natural pain reliever.

fewer adverse reactions. Most notably, it does not promote stomach bleeding—one of aspirin's most potentially serious side effects.

✱ **MAJOR BENEFITS:** White willow bark can be very effective for relieving headaches, as well as acute muscle aches and pains. It can also alleviate all sorts of chronic pain, including back and neck pain. When recommended for arthritis, especially if there is pain in the back, knees, and hips, it can reduce swelling and inflammation and increase joint mobility. In addition, it may help ease the pain of menstrual cramps—the salicin interferes with the action of hormonelike chemicals called prostaglandins that can contribute to inflammation and cause pain.

✱ **ADDITIONAL BENEFITS:** White willow bark, like aspirin, may be useful for bringing down fevers.

How to take it

⊘ **DOSAGE:** Take one or two pills three times a day, or as needed to relieve pain, lower a fever, or reduce inflammation (follow package instructions). Look for preparations that are standardized to contain 15% salicin. This dosage provides between 60 and 120 mg a day of salicin. Standardized extracts can also be taken in tincture or powder form. White willow bark teas are likely to be less effective than standardized extracts, because they supply only a small amount of pain-relieving salicin.

◑ **GUIDELINES FOR USE:** White willow bark is safe to use long term. It has a bitter, astringent taste, so the most convenient way to take it is probably in pill form. Do not consume white willow bark with aspirin because it can amplify the side effects of aspirin.

In addition, do not give the herb to a child or teen under age 16 who has a cold, the flu, or chicken pox. Taking aspirin puts these youngsters at risk for a potentially fatal brain and liver condition called Reye's syndrome. Salicin, the therapeutic ingredient in white willow bark, is not likely to cause this problem because it is metabolized differently than aspirin. However, its similarities to the painkiller warrant this course of action. Acetaminophen is a better choice than white willow bark or aspirin for children and teens.

Possible side effects

This herb rarely causes side effects at recommended doses. However, higher doses can lead to an upset stomach, nausea, or tinnitus (ringing in the ears). If any of these occur, lower the dosage or stop taking the herb. See your doctor if side effects persist.

wild yam

Dioscorea villosa

Misconceptions about the active ingredients in wild yam have led to much marketing hype. The herb has been hailed as a natural alternative to hormone replacement therapy for menopause. Even though it's not been proved effective for this purpose, wild yam does have other benefits.

COMMON USES

- *Relieves menstrual cramps.*
- *May ease the pain of endometriosis.*
- *Reduces inflammation.*

FORMS

- Capsule
- Tablet
- Softgel
- Tincture
- Dried herb/Tea

CAUTION!

- **Pregnant women should not use wild yam.**
- **Reminder: If you have a medical condition, talk to your doctor before taking supplements.**

What it is

Wild yam is not related, even distantly, to the familiar vegetable most commonly served at Thanksgiving. (In fact, these orange tubers aren't true yams at all but sweet potatoes.) A native plant of North and Central America, the wild yam was first used medicinally by the Aztecs and Mayans because of its pain-relieving qualities. Later, European settlers took advantage of the wild yam's therapeutic properties and utilized it for treating joint pain and colic. The root is the part of the plant that has medicinal value. It is available as a dried herb for use in tea, and is also sold in capsule, tablet, softgel, and tincture forms.

What it does

In recent years, wild yam has been extolled for its ability to mimic certain hormones—especially progesterone—and said to relieve menopausal or PMS symptoms. Most of these claims, however, remain scientifically unproved. It is true that wild yam contains a substance called diosgenin that can be converted to progesterone in the laboratory, but the human body is unable to make this conversion.

Some holistic practitioners, however, have reported that patients suffering from premenstrual syndrome (PMS) and menopausal symptoms experienced good results with wild yam cream—which is applied to the

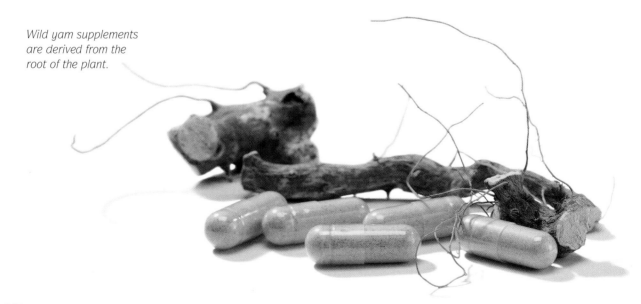

Wild yam supplements are derived from the root of the plant.

soft areas of the body (belly and thighs). How the cream helps is unclear. Sometimes manufacturers of the creams add laboratory-synthesized progesterone, which could well account for some of the therapeutic effects. (This progesterone is not always listed on the product label.) At this time, despite the positive patient reports, the value of pure wild yam creams has yet to be scientifically proved.

When taken in capsule, tincture, or tea form, however, wild yam does have other medicinal effects. Some herbalists believe that crude forms of this herb may help hormonal imbalances associated with PMS and menopause because it contains estrogenlike substances. In addition, it acts as a muscle relaxant, antispasmodic, and anti-inflammatory, which may explain why it eases menstrual complaints in some women.

✳ **MAJOR BENEFITS:** Wild yam contains substances called alkaloids, which are muscle relaxants that especially target muscles in the abdomen and pelvis. This action suggests that wild yam may be of particular value for digestive disorders, such as diverticulitis, Crohn's disease, and irritable bowel syndrome. It can also improve menstrual cramps and the pain associated with endometriosis. Some women find that wild yam combined with other herbs, such as chasteberry, produces a mild sedative effect that can relieve symptoms of PMS.

✳ **ADDITIONAL BENEFITS:** Other active ingredients found in wild yam, known as steroidal saponins, play a role in alleviating muscle strains, chronic muscle pain, and arthritis.

How to take it

🖉 **DOSAGE:** In order to receive the therapeutic benefits of wild yam, take ½ teaspoon of tincture three or four times a day or 500 mg of wild yam in capsule form twice a day. If you prefer, drink a cup of wild yam tea three times a day.

◉ **GUIDELINES FOR USE:** Have wild yam supplements or tincture with food to minimize stomach upset. To make wild yam tea, pour a cup of very hot water over 1 or 2 teaspoons of the dried herb and let steep for 15 minutes. You can also add other soothing herbs to this tea—valerian or peppermint, for example—when using it for digestive disorders.

Possible side effects

In extremely large amounts, wild yam supplements and tinctures can cause nausea and diarrhea.

Did You Know?

The first birth control pill was derived from diosgenin, the hormonelike compound found in wild yam.

zinc

Everyone needs zinc. This mineral fuels enzymes that do everything from manufacturing DNA to healing wounds. It's a crucial component of a strong immune system, and it fights the common cold. Yet a surprising number of Americans don't get enough of this vital nutrient.

CAUTION!

- Don't take too much zinc: More than 100 mg daily can, over the long term, impair immunity. It can also interfere with copper absorption, leading to anemia.
- Reminder: If you have a medical condition, talk to your doctor before taking supplements.

What it is

An essential mineral required by every cell in the body, zinc is concentrated in the muscles, bones, skin, kidneys, liver, pancreas, eyes, and, in men, the prostate. It is plentiful in drinking water and in some foods, including meat. Because your body does not produce zinc, it depends on external sources for its supply.

What it does

Zinc plays a critical role in hundreds of body processes—from cell growth to sexual maturation and immunity, even for taste and smell. Consequently, everyone who takes a daily multivitamin and mineral supplement should be certain that it contains zinc. Individual supplements are also available for specific complaints.

✪ **MAJOR BENEFITS:** Necessary for the proper functioning of the immune system, zinc helps to protect the body against colds, flu, conjunctivitis, and other infections. In a study of 100 people in the initial stages of a cold, those who sucked on zinc lozenges every couple of hours recovered from their illness about three days earlier than those who sucked on placebo lozenges. Zinc lozenges may also speed the healing of canker sores and sore throat. Taken in pill form, zinc may aid in treating more serious illnesses, such as rheumatoid arthritis, lupus, fibromyalgia, and possibly multiple sclerosis, as well as other conditions, such as AIDS, which are associated with an improperly functioning immune system.

✪ **ADDITIONAL BENEFITS:** Zinc exerts beneficial effects on various hormones, including the sex and thyroid hormones. It shows promise for enhancing fertility in both women and men. Zinc may also shrink an enlarged prostate. In addition, it may be effective for those with an underactive thyroid and, because it improves insulin levels, it may help people with diabetes.

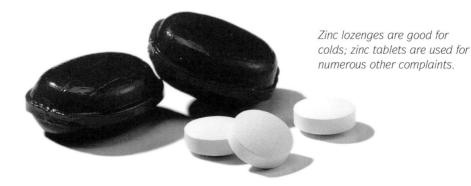

Zinc lozenges are good for colds; zinc tablets are used for numerous other complaints.

Because zinc affects so many body systems, it has many other uses. It stimulates the healing of wounds and skin irritations, making it useful for acne, burns, eczema, psoriasis, and rosacea, and promotes the health of the hair and scalp. Zinc has also been shown to slow vision loss in people with macular degeneration, a common cause of blindness in those over age 50. And in a recent Japanese study, tinnitus (ringing in the ears) improved with zinc supplementation. Zinc may also be useful for osteoporosis, hemorrhoids, inflammatory bowel disease, and ulcers.

How much you need

The RDA for zinc is 12 mg for women and 15 mg for men daily. Higher doses are usually reserved for specific complaints.

⊖ **IF YOU GET TOO LITTLE:** Severe zinc deficiency is rare in the United States, but a mild zinc deficiency can lead to poor wound healing, more colds and flu, a muted sense of taste and smell, and skin problems such as acne, eczema, and psoriasis. It can result in impaired blood sugar tolerance (and an increased diabetes risk) and a low sperm count.

⊕ **IF YOU GET TOO MUCH:** Long-term use of more than 100 mg a day has been shown to impair immunity and lower the level of HDL ("good") cholesterol. One study reported a connection between excess zinc and Alzheimer's, though evidence is scant. Larger doses (more than 200 mg a day) can cause nausea, vomiting, and diarrhea.

How to take it

⊘ **DOSAGE:** The usual dosage is 30 mg once a day. Taking zinc for longer than a month may interfere with copper absorption, so add 2 mg of copper for every 30 mg of zinc. For short-term use (colds or flu), use zinc lozenges every two to four hours for a week; don't exceed 150 mg a day.

◈ **GUIDELINES FOR USE:** Take zinc an hour before or two hours after a meal; if it causes stomach upset, have it with a low-fiber food. If you also use iron supplements, do not take them at the same time as zinc. Take zinc at least two hours after taking antibiotics.

Other sources

When looking for foods rich in zinc, think protein. It's abundant in beef, pork, liver, poultry (especially dark meat), eggs, and seafood (especially oysters). Cheese, beans, nuts, and wheat germ are other good sources, but the zinc in these foods is less easily absorbed than the zinc in meat.

Did You Know?

Almonds are a rich source of zinc for vegetarians, who may be deficient in it: 4 ounces provide about 6 mg—half the RDA of zinc for women.

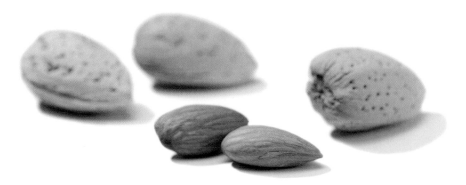

drug interactions

Many people believe that herbs and other "natural" supplements are safe to use under any circumstances. But some supplements may interact adversely with prescription or over-the-counter (OTC) drugs, intensifying the action of the medications or even producing dangerous side effects.

This section lists most of the popular drug classes and highlights possible reactions that may occur when specific supplements interact with them. Unfortunately, few studies have been done to determine the risks involved in taking supplements and medications together. Obviously further research is needed, and caution is always advised when combining any herbs or other supplements with drugs.

To check for possible adverse reactions, begin by scanning the general categories listed alphabetically below, finding any drug you are taking and noting if an interaction with a particular supplement may present a potential problem. The most popular members of each drug class are listed by generic name, but not every drug in the group is included. (If you have any questions, check with your doctor or pharmacist.) Remember that all drugs within a class are likely to have similar interactions. Even if you don't see the name of your particular medication listed, the interaction may still apply to all the drugs in that class.

In addition, avoid taking drugs and supplements that have similar effects unless your doctor recommends it. For example, if you are using an herb such as kava or valerian to treat insomnia, it may induce excessive sleepiness when combined with a conventional sleep aid or with any drug that can cause drowsiness—a narcotic pain reliever, an OTC antihistamine, or even alcohol. Similarly, a nutritional supplement that affects brain chemicals and enhances mood, such as melatonin or 5-HTP, is best tried only under the supervision

of a doctor if you're already taking a prescription antidepressant.

Furthermore, if you are using any type of prescription drug, do not stop taking it without your doctor's consent. And always consult your doctor or pharmacist before trying any herb or supplement if you have a medical or psychiatric condition or are on any prescription or OTC medication. To find out more about the specific supplements listed here, refer to the individual entries elsewhere in the book; general cautions for a number of supplements are noted below.

General cautions

Listed below are specific supplements that require special caution if you're taking certain conventional drugs.

- **Betaine HCl** Increases levels of digestive acids in the stomach. It's essential that people taking aspirin or other anti-inflammatory medicines (NSAIDs) avoid this supplement, because in combination they increase the risk of stomach bleeding.
- **Ephedra** Stimulates the nervous system and raises blood pressure. It is important to avoid taking it with medications that have a similar effect, including blood pressure drugs, caffeine, and other stimulants.
- **Forskolin** Should be used with caution by patients on asthma or blood pressure medications because it can intensify the effects of these drugs.
- **GABA** May cause excessive drowsiness in those also using sedatives or drugs that have sedative effects.
- **Gymnema sylvestre** May alter requirements for insulin or oral diabetes drugs; check with your doctor

before taking this herb with any diabetes medication.
- **Licorice** Can increase blood pressure and should be avoided by those taking blood pressure drugs or any medication that alters blood pressure.
- **Melatonin** Affects hormone levels and the brain. Caution is advised in those using drugs with similar effects, including antidepressants and hormone drugs. May cause excessive drowsiness if taken with drugs that cause sedation.
- **Psyllium** Should not be used within 2 hours of taking any medication because it may delay drug absorption.
- **Valerian** May cause excessive drowsiness in those also using sedatives or drugs that have sedative effects.

Acne drugs
Isotretinoin and other acne drugs
Supplement Interaction:
- **Vitamin A** When taken together, may cause high blood levels of vitamin A, increasing the chance of side effects.

Antacids
All antacids
Supplement Interactions:
- **Iron** May make the medication less effective. Take iron supplements 2 hours before or after an antacid.
- **Vitamin D** When used with antacids containing magnesium, may result in high blood levels of magnesium.

Antibiotics
All oral antibiotics
Supplement Interaction:
- **Iron** May make the antibiotic less effective. Take iron supplements 2 hours before or after the drug.

Doxycycline, minocycline, tetracycline
Supplement Interactions:
- **Calcium** May decrease the absorption of the drug. Don't take calcium within 1 to 3 hours of these antibiotics.
- **Iron** May make the antibiotic less effective. Take iron supplements 2 hours before or after the drug.

- **Magnesium** May make the drug less effective. Take magnesium supplements 1 to 3 hours before or after the drug.
- **Psyllium** May make the antibiotic less effective; check with your doctor.
- **Zinc** May make the antibiotic less effective. Take zinc supplements at least 2 hours after the drug.

Anticoagulants

Enoxaparin, warfarin, and other anticoagulants *(Blood thinners)*
Supplement Interactions:

- **Bromelain** Use with caution. Intensifies the blood-thinning effect of the medication. May lead to excessive bleeding.
- **Feverfew** Use with caution. Intensifies the blood-thinning effect of the medication. May lead to excessive bleeding.
- **Fish oils** Use with caution. Intensifies the blood-thinning effect of the medication. May eventually lead to internal or excessive bleeding.
- **Garlic** Consult your doctor before taking together. May intensify the blood-thinning effect of the medication.
- **Medicinal mushrooms** Consult your doctor. Reishi may intensify the blood-thinning effect of the medication.
- **Pau d'arco** Use with caution. Intensifies the blood-thinning effect of the medication. May lead to excessive bleeding.
- **Vitamin E** Consult your doctor before taking together. May intensify the blood-thinning effect of the medication.
- **Vitamin K** May counteract the effects of the medication.

Antidepressants

Prozac, all other antidepressants
Supplement Interactions:

- **Ephedra** Avoid taking within 14 days of using an MAO inhibitor.
- **5-HTP** Avoid taking within 4 weeks of using an MAO inhibitor. Check with your doctor before combining with conventional antidepressants; may cause anxiety, confusion, and other potentially serious side effects.
- **Ginseng (Panax)** Consult your doctor if you're taking an MAO inhibitor.
- **Kava** May cause excessive drowsiness when taken together.
- **Melatonin** Check with your doctor. Adverse drug reactions in people taking conventional antidepressants along with melatonin have been reported.

- **St. John's wort** Consult your doctor before adding this herb to conventional antidepressants. The combination may lead to serious adverse reactions.

Antihistamines

Antihistamines
Supplement Interactions:

- **5-HTP, GABA, Kava, Melatonin, and Valerian** Any of these may cause excessive drowsiness when taken with sedating antihistamines.

Cholesterol drugs

Atorvastatin, lovastatin, simvastatin, and other "statin" drugs
Supplement Interactions:

- **Iron** May make the medication less effective. Take iron supplements 2 hours before or after the drug.
- **Niacin** May cause muscle pain and inflammation. In severe cases, may lead to kidney failure. Stop taking these drugs together and consult your doctor if any muscle aches develop.
- **Red yeast rice** Do not take with cholesterol drugs; may lead to dangerous buildup of drug blood levels.

Cold remedies

OTC and prescription remedies containing ephedrine or pseudoephedrine
Supplement Interactions:

- **Ephedra** Do not take with these cold remedies because this herb contains the same active ingredient and may result in an overdose.
- **5-HTP** May cause anxiety, confusion, or other serious side effects if used with these cold remedies. Use with caution.

Diabetes drugs

Insulin and oral diabetes drugs
Supplement Interactions:

- **Alpha-lipoic acid** Long-term supplementation may require a change in insulin or diabetes medication dosage.
- **Cat's claw** Do not take with glipizide; adverse effects have been reported.
- **Chromium** Consult your doctor; may alter insulin or other drug requirements.
- **Dandelion** Use with caution; may intensify the blood sugar-lowering effect of glipizide.
- **Ephedra** Use with caution if you're taking diabetes drugs; can elevate blood sugar levels.

- **Ginseng (Panax)** Long-term supplementation may require a change in insulin or other diabetes medications.
- **Gymnema sylvestre** Check with your doctor. May require altering the dosage of insulin or other diabetes medications.
- **Siberian ginseng** Use with caution; may intensify the blood sugar-lowering effect of glipizide.

Diuretics

Amiloride, spironolactone, triamterene *(Potassium-sparing diuretics)*
Supplement Interactions:

- **Phosphorus** Consult your doctor before taking together. When used with phosphates containing potassium, may increase the risk of hyperkalemia (too much potassium in the blood), possibly leading to serious side effects.
- **Potassium** Do not take together. May increase the risk of hyperkalemia (too much potassium in the blood), possibly leading to serious side effects.

Bumetanide, ethacrynic acid, furosemide, torsemide *(Loop diuretics)*
Supplement Interactions:

- **Dandelion** May boost the diuretic effects of these drugs when taken in high doses.
- **Ephedra** When used to treat hypertension, furosemide's effects may be weakened if taken with ephedra.
- **Ginseng (Panax)** If you're taking furosemide, may intensify the blood pressure-lowering effects of the drug.
- **Glucosamine** Higher doses of the diuretic may be necessary.

Chlorothiazide, hydrochlorothiazide, indapamide *(Thiazide diuretics)*
Supplement Interactions:

- **Aloe vera** Overuse or misuse of aloe vera juice can cause loss of potassium (necessary for proper heart function) and intensify the potassium-depleting effects of the medication.
- **Calcium** Consult your doctor. May cause buildup of excessive, possibly toxic, calcium levels in the body, leading to kidney failure if taken together.
- **Dandelion** May boost the diuretic effects of these drugs when taken in high doses.
- **Ephedra** Do not take together. The effects of the drug may be reduced.
- **Glucosamine** Higher doses of the drug may be necessary.

● **Hawthorn** Consult your doctor. May intensify the diuretic's blood pressure-lowering effect.

● **Licorice** May lead to dangerously low levels of potassium in the body.

● **Potassium** If taking together, do not discontinue the thiazide diuretic suddenly. May cause hyperkalemia (too much potassium in the blood), possibly resulting in serious side effects.

● **Vitamin D** Consult your doctor. May cause buildup of excessive, possibly toxic, calcium levels in the body, resulting in kidney failure.

Heart/Blood pressure drugs

All antihypertensives

Supplement Interactions:

● **Black cohosh** May intensify the drug's blood pressure-lowering effect.

● **Ephedra** Do not take together. May cause a dangerous rise in blood pressure.

● **Garlic** Check with your doctor. May increase the potency of blood pressure medication.

● **Ginseng (Panax or Siberian)** Check with your doctor if you're using blood pressure medications.

● **Hawthorn** Consult your doctor. May intensify the drug's blood pressure-lowering effect. A lower dose of the medication may be warranted.

● **Licorice** May neutralize the medication's blood pressure-lowering effect.

Amlodipine, diltiazem, verapamil, and other calcium channel blockers

Supplement Interactions:

● **Ephedra** Do not take together.

● **Flavonoids** Do not take a citrus bioflavonoid preparation containing naringin (flavonoid present in grapefruit, but not oranges) when using a calcium channel blocker.

● **Hawthorn** Consult your doctor. May intensify the drug's blood pressure-lowering effect. A lower dose of the medication may be warranted.

Atenolol, metoprolol, propranolol, and other beta-blockers

Supplement Interactions:

● **Ephedra** Do not take together.

● **Hawthorn** Consult your doctor. May intensify the drug's blood pressure-lowering effect. A lower dose of the medication may be warranted.

● **Potassium** Consult your doctor before taking together. May increase

the risk of hyperkalemia (too much potassium in the blood), possibly leading to serious side effects.

Benazepril, enalapril, fosinopril, and other ACE inhibitors

Supplement Interactions:

● **Ephedra** Do not take together.

● **Hawthorn** Consult your doctor. May intensify the drug's blood pressure-lowering effect. A lower dose of the medication may be warranted.

● **Phosphorus** Do not take together. When used with phosphates containing potassium, may increase the risk of hyperkalemia (too much potassium in the blood), and lead to serious side effects.

● **Potassium** Do not take together. May increase the risk of hyperkalemia (too much potassium in the blood), and lead to serious side effects.

Digitoxin, digoxin (*Digitalis drugs, cardiac glycosides*)

Supplement Interactions:

● **Aloe vera** Overuse or misuse of aloe vera juice can cause loss of potassium (necessary for proper heart function) and may lead to toxicity from the medication.

● **Ephedra** Do not take together. Ephedra may interfere with the rate, rhythm, and force of the heartbeat and raise blood pressure.

● **Hawthorn** Consult your doctor. May intensify the drug's blood pressure-lowering effect. A lower dose of the medication may be warranted.

● **Licorice** May neutralize the medication's blood pressure-lowering effect.

● **Phosphorus** Consult your doctor before taking together. Using digitalis with phosphates containing potassium, may increase the risk of hyperkalemia (too much potassium in the blood), possibly leading to serious side effects.

● **Potassium** Consult your doctor before taking together. When used together, may increase the risk of hyperkalemia (too much potassium in the blood), possibly leading to serious side effects.

● **Siberian ginseng** Consult your doctor before using together. Increases medication levels.

Amyl nitrite, isosorbide mono- or dinitrate, nitroglycerin (*Nitrates*)

Supplement Interactions:

● **Ephedra** Do not take together. Ephedra may interfere with the rate, rhythm, and force of the heartbeat and raise blood pressure.

● **Hawthorn** Consult your doctor. May intensify the drug's blood pressure-lowering effect. A lower dose of the medication may be warranted.

Muscle relaxants

Carisoprodol, cyclobenzaprine, and other muscle relaxants

Supplement Interactions:

● **5-HTP, GABA, Kava, Melatonin, and Valerian** Any of these may cause excessive drowsiness when taken with muscle relaxants.

Narcotic pain relievers

Codeine, hydrocodone/acetaminophen, and other narcotic analgesics

Supplement Interactions:

● **5-HTP, GABA, Kava, Melatonin, and Valerian** Any of these may cause excessive drowsiness when taken with narcotic pain relievers.

Neurology drugs

Methylphenidate (Ritalin) and other nervous system stimulants

Supplement Interactions:

● **Ephedra** Do not take together. May result in overstimulation, causing nervousness, irritability, insomnia, and possible seizures or heart arrhythmias.

● **Flavonoids** Exercise caution when taking a citrus bioflavonoid preparation containing naringin (flavonoid present in grapefruit, but not oranges) with methylphenidate.

● **Ginseng (Panax)** Increases the risk of overstimulation and stomach upset.

NSAIDs

Etodolac, ibuprofen, ketoprofen, naproxen, and other nonsteroidal anti-inflammatory drugs

Supplement Interactions:

● **Betaine HCl** Do not take together; increases the risk of potentially serious stomach bleeding.

● **Phosphorus** Consult your doctor before taking together. When used with phosphates containing potassium, may increase the risk of hyperkalemia (too much potassium in the blood), possibly leading to serious side effects.

● **Potassium** Consult your doctor. When taken together, may increase the risk of hyperkalemia (too much potassium in the blood), possibly leading to serious side effects.

Aspirin

Supplement Interactions:

● **Betaine HCl** Do not take together; increases the risk of potentially serious stomach bleeding.

● **Feverfew** Intensifies the blood-thinning effect of long-term aspirin use. May lead to excessive bleeding.

● **Fish oils** Intensifies the blood-thinning effect of long-term aspirin use. May lead to internal or excessive bleeding.

● **Garlic** Consult your doctor. May increase the blood-thinning effect of long-term aspirin use.

● **Ginkgo biloba** Intensifies the blood-thinning effect of long-term aspirin use. May lead to excessive bleeding.

● **Medicinal mushrooms** Consult your doctor. Reishi may intensify the blood-thinning effect of long-term aspirin use.

● **Vitamin K** May counteract the blood-thinning effect of long-term aspirin use.

● **White willow bark** Do not take together because the two act similarly, increasing the risk of aspirin-related side effects, including stomach bleeding.

OB/GYN drugs

Conjugated estrogens, estrogen-progestin products, and other female hormones
Supplement Interactions:

● **Black cohosh** Consult your doctor. May interact adversely when taken together.

● **Cat's claw** Use with caution; may affect levels of female sex hormones.

● **Chasteberry** Should not be used by women taking hormone medications, including estrogen, because it affects hormone production.

● **Flavonoids** Exercise caution when taking a citrus bioflavonoid preparation containing naringin (flavonoid present in grapefruit, but not oranges) together with estrogens.

Oral contraceptives (combination estrogen-progestin products)
Supplement Interactions:

● **Black cohosh** Consult your doctor. May interact adversely when taken together.

● **Cat's claw** Use with caution; may affect levels of female sex hormones.

● **Chasteberry** Should not be used by women taking hormone medications, including estrogen, because it affects hormone production.

Parkinson's drugs

Levodopa
Supplement Interactions:

● **5-HTP** May cause anxiety, confusion, and other serious side effects when taken together; check with your doctor.

● **Vitamin B6** May prevent the medication from working properly.

Psychiatric drugs

Antipsychotics
Supplement Interactions:

● **Ginseng (Panax)** Check with your doctor if you're on antipsychotics.

● **Kava** May cause excessive drowsiness when taken together.

Buspirone *(Anti-anxiety drug)*
Supplement Interactions:

● **5-HTP** May cause anxiety, confusion, and other serious side effects when taken together; check with your doctor.

● **Kava** May cause excessive drowsiness when taken together.

Lithium *(Antimanic agent)*
Supplement Interactions:

● **5-HTP** May cause anxiety, confusion, and other serious side effects when taken together; check with your doctor.

● **Iodine** When used together, may increase the chance of side effects.

Sedatives/Tranquilizers

Sleep aids and other sedatives
Supplement Interactions:

● **Black cohosh, 5-HTP, GABA, Kava, Melatonin, and Valerian** Any of these may cause excessive drowsiness when taken with sedatives.

● **Gotu kola** Do not take together.

Seizure/Epilepsy drugs

Carbamazepine, gabapentin, phenytoin, and other anticonvulsants
Supplement Interactions:

● **Folic acid and Vitamin B6** Have been shown to interfere with some anticonvulsants when consumed in higher than recommended doses. Let your doctor know you are taking these B vitamins, and never exceed recommended doses.

Steroids

Beclomethasone, methylprednisolone, prednisone, and other oral corticosteroids
Supplement Interactions:

● **Aloe vera** Overuse or misuse of aloe vera juice can cause loss of potassium (necessary for proper heart function) and may lead to toxicity from the medication.

● **Betaine HCl** Do not take together.

● **Ginseng (Panax)** Use with caution. May interact when taken together.

● **Melatonin** Check with your doctor. May cause adverse interactions.

● **Phosphorus** Consult your doctor before taking together. Use of corticosteroids with phosphates containing sodium may increase the risk of swelling.

Thyroid drugs

Methimazole, propylthiouracil
Supplement Interactions:

● **Iodine** May decrease effectiveness of these and other antithyroid agents.

● **Kelp** Taking high doses could provide too much iodine and interfere with the actions of these medications.

Transplant drugs

Tacrolimus and other immunosuppressant drugs
Supplement Interactions:

● **Flavonoids** Do not take a citrus bioflavonoid preparation containing naringin (flavonoid present in grapefruit, but not oranges) when using an immunosuppressant.

● **Phosphorus** Consult your doctor before taking together. When used with phosphates containing potassium, may increase the risk of hyperkalemia (too much potassium in the blood), possibly leading to serious side effects.

other supplements

The following supplements are recommended for various ailments in this book, but are not individually profiled. A brief overview of each is provided, with its suggested uses and any warnings, side effects, and general comments.

agrimony A wildflower with yellow blossoms (*Agrimonia eupatoria*) commonly found on the grasslands of Europe.
Uses: Taken internally for indigestion, heartburn, and diarrhea; used topically for wound cleansing or sore, inflamed eyes.
Comments: May cause increased sensitivity to sunlight or aggravate constipation.

arnica A wild perennial with yellow daisylike blooms and oval leaves (*Arnica montana*) that grows in the mountains.
Uses: Applied topically as an ointment for bruises, aches, sprains, and strains.
Comments: Never take arnica internally or use on open wounds or broken skin.

blackberry/raspberry leaves Prickly stemmed bushes native to North America. The leaves are cultivated for medicinal purposes; the berries, for culinary use.
Uses: As a tea, treats diarrhea and menstrual cramps. Used in Europe to prevent miscarriage and treat morning sickness.
Comments: No serious side effects have been reported.

boswellia An extract of the gummy resin from a tall branching tree (*Boswellia serrata*) found in dry, hilly areas of India.
Uses: Reduces inflammation and helps build cartilage in people with arthritis.
Comments: Rare side effects include skin rash, nausea, and diarrhea.

bromelain A protein, or enzyme, that is derived from the pineapple plant.
Uses: Reduces inflammation, swelling, and pain from surgery, sports injuries, arthritis, and other causes.
Comments: Take between meals. Do not use if you have an ulcer.

butcher's broom A small, spiny, asparaguslike evergreen bush (*Ruscus aculeatus*) that is native to the Mediterranean region.
Uses: Applied topically or taken internally to reduce inflammation and shrink hemorrhoids and varicose veins.
Comments: No known side effects.

cactus grandiflorus A low-growing cactus with 8- to 12-inch white flowers that open only in the evening. Also called the night-blooming cereus.
Uses: Helps to stabilize the rhythm and rate of the heartbeat.
Comments: May cause mild diarrhea. Do not use if you are taking an MAO inhibitor or have high blood pressure.

calendula A common garden flower with orange or yellow blooms (*Calendula officinalis*). Also called the pot marigold.
Uses: Applied topically or used as a tea or vaginal suppository. Soothes skin inflammations, insect bites, cuts, and burns; heals ulcers; fights athlete's foot, nail fungus, and yeast infections.
Comments: Those allergic to daisylike flowers may be sensitive to calendula.

cascara sagrada A laxative herb that comes from the bark of the California buckthorn tree (*Rhamnus purshiana*), native to the western U.S.
Uses: Relieves constipation.
Comments: Use for no longer than one to two weeks. Can cause cramping; if this occurs, lower the dose. Avoid if you are pregnant or nursing, or if you have intestinal obstruction or inflammatory bowel disease.

charcoal, activated A highly absorbent substance used as an antidote for poisons.
Uses: Reduces flatulence; absorbs poisons.
Comments: Side effects include black, tarry stools and nausea. May interfere with the absorption of any drug taken within two hours of its administration. If mixing the powder in water, drink it with a straw to prevent staining of teeth. Also available in pill form.

chitosan A substance found mainly in the shells of shellfish. Binds fat molecules in the intestine, preventing their absorption.
Uses: Aids in weight reduction.
Comments: Take with meals. People with a shellfish allergy should not take chitosan.

chondroitin A molecular substance found in cartilage and the lining of blood vessels and the bladder.
Uses: May help to stem the degenerative progression of arthritis.
Comments: No known side effects with recommended doses. Taken commonly with glucosamine, a nutritional supplement.

creatine An amino acid-like nutritional supplement that is produced naturally by the liver, pancreas, and kidneys and found in muscle tissue.
Uses: Typically ingested as an odorless, colorless powder. Helps repair the microscopic tears in muscles following a strenuous workout or injury. May increase lean muscle mass.
Comments: High doses may cause weight gain; muscle cramps, pulls, and tears; stomach upset, dehydration, and diarrhea. Long-term studies, especially regarding high doses, have not been done.

eucalyptus oil An oil derived from an evergreen tree with yellowish leaves (*Eucalyptus globulus*) native to Australia.
Uses: Applied topically as a massage oil to soothe sore muscles; used as an inhalant and in cough drops to open sinuses and airways and relieve coughs and asthma.

Comments: Do not take the oil internally, except for the small amount found in cough drops or candies. Limit use to no more than a few days at a time.

eyebright A plant with red-tinged white or purple blossoms (*Euphrasia officinalis*) that resemble bloodshot eyes. Native to the grasslands of Europe.

Uses: As an eyewash, treats eye infections. Can also be taken as a tea or tincture.

Comments: May cause rash or nausea. Make sure eyewashes are sterile to prevent infections. Avoid using eyebright as a topically applied eye compress because of the possibility of bacterial infection.

false unicorn root A perennial with greenish white blooms (*Chamaelirium luteum*) found in the low, damp ground east of the Mississippi River.

Uses: Stimulates ovulation; treats infertility in women.

Comments: Large doses may cause nausea and vomiting. Do not use during menstruation or if you are pregnant or nursing. Commonly taken with chasteberry.

forskolin A small plant (*Coleus forskohlii*) in the mint family found on the dry mountain slopes of India, Nepal, Sri Lanka, and Thailand.

Uses: Used to counteract underactive thyroid. Sometimes used to treat asthma and heart disease.

Comments: Avoid if you have peptic ulcers or low blood pressure. Use with caution if you are taking any prescription medication, especially asthma or blood pressure drugs.

FOS Fructo-oligosaccharides are indigestible carbohydrates present in certain foods that promote the growth of so-called friendly intestinal bacteria.

Uses: Orally, helps relieve flatulence and irritable bowel syndrome. Vaginal suppositories may aid in treating yeast infections.

Comments: Often taken with acidophilus and bifidus. May cause diarrhea.

GABA Gamma-aminobutyric acid; an amino acid that acts as a neurotransmitter, boosting nerve signals in the brain.

Uses: Helps treat epilepsy and insomnia.

Comments: Too much GABA can cause numbness, tingling, or anxiety.

gamma-oryzanol An antioxidant extract of rice bran oil that appears to work on the part of the central nervous system that controls digestion.

Uses: Treats ulcers and heartburn by promoting healthy levels of digestive juices.

Comments: No known side effects.

garcinia cambogia A small pumpkin-shaped fruit from Southeast Asia.

Uses: May suppress appetite and aid dieting.

Comments: Contains hydroxycitric acid (HCA), a fruit extract similar to citric acid.

glutathione An amino acid-like substance produced by the liver and other cells.

Uses: Acts as a cell-protecting antioxidant; may help prevent cancer.

Comments: Take with food to minimize the chances of digestive upset.

gymnema sylvestre A climbing vine from the tropical forests of Africa and India. Also known as Gurmarbooti.

Uses: Enhances the body's uptake of blood sugar (glucose) in people with diabetes.

Comments: Use may require a change in dosage for insulin or diabetes medication.

horehound A perennial aromatic herb (*Marrubium vulgare*) in the mint family. Also known as white horehound.

Uses: May be included in cough drops or taken as a tea. Serves as an expectorant to treat coughs or asthma.

Comments: Do not use if you have heart disease. Large doses may disturb heart rhythm. Do not take if you are pregnant.

horse chestnut A tree (*Aesculus hippocastanum*) with red, yellow, or white flowers that produces fruits containing one to three knuckle-size seeds.

Uses: Helps reduce inflammation and swelling of varicose veins.

Comments: Don't take with aspirin or anticoagulants. People with liver or kidney disease, those with bleeding problems, and pregnant women should not take it.

kudzu A fast-growing, high-climbing vine (*Pueraria lobata*) native to China and Japan. Grows rampant in the southern U.S.

Uses: Reduces cravings for alcohol; may aid in the treatment of alcoholism.

Comments: No known side effects.

lavender oil An oil derived from an evergreen plant (*Lavandula officinalis*) native to the Mediterranean region.

Uses: Applied topically, treats skin inflammations, cuts, sunburn, earaches, insect bites, and sore muscles.

Comments: Do not take internally.

marshmallow A plant with pale pink flowers (*Althaea officinalis*) that grows primarily in marshes in many parts of Europe and the United States.

Uses: As a tea, aids digestion and soothes coughs, sore throat, ulcers, heartburn, and inflammatory bowel disease. Pills (combined with ginger) may relieve allergies.

Comments: When steeped in water, releases mucilage, a gel-like plant substance that coats the throat and larynx and soothes coughs.

melissa A plant with a lemony smell and white flowers (*Melissa officinalis*) native to southern Europe. Also called lemon balm.

Uses: Applied topically, relieves cold sores and shingles. As a tea, soothes upset stomach and diverticular disorders.

Comments: Do not use internally if you are pregnant or have thyroid problems.

muira puama A shrub (*Ptychopetalum olacoides*) native to the Amazon.

Uses: Treats impotence.

Comments: Also known as potency wood, it has a long folk history as an aphrodisiac.

mullein flower A woolly leafed plant with honey-scented yellow flowers (*Verbascum thapsus*) found in the U.S.

Uses: Applied topically, the oil helps relieve the pain and itching of earache; as a tea, soothes sore throat and relieves coughs.

Comments: Use only *Verbascum thapsus*.

NADH Nicotinamide adenine dinucleotide, a fairly new supplement related to the B vitamin niacin.

Uses: Acts as an antioxidant; raises levels of the brain chemical dopamine, helping to ease symptoms of Parkinson's disease.

Comments: Take on an empty stomach. High doses may cause restlessness.

oat extract Derived from the common grain. Also called *Avena sativa*.

Uses: Reduces cravings for cigarettes.

Comments: Used in India for centuries to treat opium addictions.

PABA Para-aminobenzoic acid, one of the B vitamins.

Uses: May prevent hair loss; soothes the intestine in inflammatory bowel disease.

Comments: Do not take with sulfa drugs. Rarely, high doses may cause liver damage.

parsley A plant *(Petroselinum sativum)* used worldwide as a culinary herb.

Uses: Improves bad breath.

Comments: No known side effects.

pygeum africanum An evergreen tree found in African forests.

Uses: Helps relieve prostate disorders.

Comments: May cause mild stomach upset.

red yeast rice A yeast *(Monascus purpureus)* fermented on rice containing the active ingredient lovastatin.

Uses: Inhibits the buildup of cholesterol deposits in the arteries.

Comments: Do not use if: you are taking any other cholesterol-lowering medications ("statin" drugs); you're pregnant; you have liver disease or a serious infection; you're recovering from major surgery; you drink more than two alcoholic beverages a day. Stop taking it if you experience any unexplained muscle pain, tenderness, or weakness, especially if these feelings are accompanied by flulike symptoms.

rosemary A small evergreen bush with aromatic, silvery green leaves and pale blue flowers *(Rosmarinus officinalis)* native to the Mediterranean region.

Uses: Applied topically as an oil to relieve pain and help reduce swelling.

Comments: Do not take oil internally.

SAM S-adenosylmethionine, a form of the amino acid methionine.

Uses: May help slow the degenerative progression of arthritis.

Comments: May cause mild stomach upset; should not be taken by people with manic depression (bipolar disorder).

sea cucumber A Chinese remedy derived from a marine animal related to starfish and sea urchins.

Uses: May help reduce pain and stiffness in arthritis sufferers.

Comments: Also provides vitamins A, thiamin (B_1), riboflavin (B_2), niacin (B_3), and C, as well as the minerals calcium, iron, magnesium, and zinc.

shepherd's purse A weed *(Capsella bursa-pastoris)* with leaves resembling the leather pouches once worn by European shepherds. Used medicinally as well as for culinary purposes.

Uses: Reduces heavy menstrual bleeding.

Comments: Do not take if you are pregnant. People with kidney stones should use with caution. Long-term or excessive use may interfere with medications for thyroid, heart, or blood pressure.

slippery elm A tree *(Ulmus rubra)* native to the moist woods of eastern Canada and eastern and central United States. The inner bark is used medicinally.

Uses: As a tea, aids digestion and soothes sore throat, heartburn, ulcers, inflammatory bowel disease, and diverticulitis.

Comments: Has mild laxative effects.

sodium bicarbonate Commonly known as baking soda.

Uses: Provides short-term relief from nicotine cravings.

Comments: Do not take with any other OTC medications containing sodium bicarbonate, such as Alka-Seltzer. Do not take with milk or milk products or if you have any sign of appendicitis (stomach pain, bloating, nausea, and vomiting). Be sure to account for the large amount of sodium in baking soda if you are on a salt-restricted diet. Baking soda interacts adversely with many different medications, including common antibiotics and pain relievers. Consult your doctor before taking it with other drugs or if you have heart, liver, or kidney disease, or any other medical condition.

sweet marjoram A strongly scented herb *(Origanum majorana)* grown in cold climates and used in cooking.

Uses: Applied topically to relieve pain and help reduce swelling.

Comments: Also used as a culinary herb.

turmeric A perennial plant in the ginger family with funnel-shaped flowers *(Curcuma longa)*. The active ingredient in turmeric is called curcumin. Long used in the traditional (Ayurvedic) medicine of India, and as a popular cooking spice.

Uses: When taken in combination with bromelain, enhances that supplement's anti-inflammatory effects and may help to relieve the pain of carpal tunnel syndrome. May have antiviral effects against HIV, the cause of AIDS.

Comments: Do not use if you have blood-clotting disorders or are pregnant, trying to conceive, or have fertility problems. Those over age 65 should use as low a dose as possible.

uva ursi A low-growing evergreen bush with red berries and flowers *(Arctostaphylos uva-ursi)* found in colder northern climates from Asia to the United States. Also called bearberry.

Uses: An infection fighter used in the treatment of urinary tract infections.

Comments: Do not take if you have kidney disease or are pregnant, or for more than one week at a time. Limit use of the herb to no more than five times a year. Do not combine uva ursi with substances that acidify the urine, such as vitamin C or cranberry (these are commonly used as well to treat urinary tract infections). May cause nausea, mild stomach upset, and a greenish discoloration of the urine.

vitamin B complex A combination supplement that provides a balanced blend of B vitamins: thiamin (B_1), riboflavin (B_2), niacin or niacinamide (B_3), pantothenic acid (B_5), vitamin B_6 (pyridoxine), vitamin B_{12}, biotin, folic acid, choline, inositol hexaniacinate, and PABA (para-aminobenzoic acid).

Uses: B vitamins maintain nerves, skin, hair, eyes, brain, intestine, and other organs.

Comments: Sometimes prescribed along with individual B vitamins to assure a proper vitamin balance. Older people are often deficient in B vitamins.

yellow dock An herb *(Rumex crispus)*, the roots of which are used to make iron-rich medicinal extracts.

Uses: Helps treat iron-deficiency anemia.

Comments: Doctor must determine cause of anemia before supplements are started.

glossary

ABSORPTION The uptake by the body of a supplement, drug, or other substance through the digestive tract, skin, or mucous membranes.

ACUPUNCTURE A therapy originating in China in which very thin needles are inserted into the skin at key points on the body to restore health and to balance the flow of energy, called *qi* (pronounced chee).

ACUTE Short, severe, nonchronic; designates an illness or condition, typically lasting no more than a week or two.

ALTERNATIVE MEDICINE Any of various approaches to healing, such as herbal therapies and acupuncture, that fall outside the domain of conventional mainstream medicine.

AMINO ACIDS Chemical substances, found in foods and produced in the body, which are used to build protein.

ANTIBIOTIC A drug that kills or inhibits infection-causing bacteria.

ANTICOAGULANT A drug (such as warfarin or aspirin) that deters blood clotting; often used by those at risk for heart attacks. Also known as a blood thinner.

ANTICONVULSANT A drug that prevents seizures; used to treat epilepsy.

ANTIFUNGAL A drug that combats athlete's foot or other infections caused by a fungus.

ANTI-INFLAMMATORY A drug or supplement that fights inflammation, a body response to injury or irritation, characterized by redness, heat, swelling, and pain.

ANTIOXIDANT A substance that protects cells from the damaging effects of highly reactive oxygen molecules called free radicals. Some antioxidants are made by the body; others, such as vitamins C and E, are obtained through diet or supplements.

ANTISEPTIC An infection-fighting herb, drug, or other substance.

ANTISPASMODIC A drug or supplement that prevents spasms or cramps in the digestive tract or elsewhere.

ATHEROSCLEROSIS The buildup of cholesterol and other substances in the artery walls ("hardening of the arteries"), leading to heart disease, angina, heart attack, stroke, intermittent claudication, and other ailments.

AUTOIMMUNE DISORDER An ailment, such as lupus or rheumatoid arthritis, in which the immune system mistakenly attacks the body's own healthy tissues.

AYURVEDA The traditional medicine of India, dating back thousands of years. It relies on herbs (such as boswellia and gymnema sylvestre), cleansing diets, meditation, and other forms of therapy.

BETA-BLOCKER A type of drug that affects the heart, blood vessels, and other areas; often prescribed to treat high blood pressure or angina.

BILE A fat-digesting substance produced in the liver, stored in the gallbladder, and then released into the intestine when needed.

BIOFEEDBACK A technique that uses visual and auditory cues to train people to recognize and gain control of involuntary body processes, thereby helping them control muscles, lower blood pressure, and relax.

BOTANICAL An herb or plant that has healing properties.

BOTANICAL NAME The scientific, or Latin, name of an herb or plant.

CAPILLARIES Tiny blood vessels that connect veins and arteries. In the capillaries oxygen and nutrients are transferred from the blood to the cells, and waste products are removed.

CARTILAGE A dense yet flexible tissue in the joints, spine, throat, ears, nose, and other areas. It is not as hard as bone, but it does provide protection and support.

CHOLESTEROL A fatlike substance that circulates in the blood and helps build cell membranes; high levels increase the risk of heart attack.

CHRONIC Persistent or long term; designates an illness or condition, often requiring months or years of treatment.

COENZYME A substance that acts in concert with enzymes to speed up chemical reactions in the body.

COLLAGEN A tough, fibrous protein that provides support throughout the body and helps form bones, cartilage, skin, joints, and other tissues.

COMMISSION E A special body of scientists, health professionals, and lay experts formed in Germany in 1978; studies the usefulness and safety of herbal remedies.

COMPLEX A term designating a mixture of vitamins, minerals, herbs, or other nutrients. Examples include vitamin B complex, liver (lipotropic) complex, and amino acid complex.

COMPRESS A soft cotton or flannel cloth or piece of gauze that has been soaked in an herbal tea or other healing substance, then folded and placed on the skin to help reduce inflammation and pain.

CONVENTIONAL MEDICINE Also known as allopathic medicine, the approach to healing most commonly practiced in the United States and other Western countries. A doctor diagnoses a problem and typically treats it with drugs or surgery.

DEMENTIA Loss of mental faculties as a result of Alzheimer's disease or other brain impairment.

DIABETIC NEUROPATHY Diabetes-related nerve damage producing loss of sensation, numbness, tingling, or burning; often occurs in the limbs.

DIURETIC A substance that draws water from the body and increases the total output of urine.

DOUCHE Herbal teas, acidophilus and water, or other substances that can be used to flush the vagina; may be recommended for infections.

ENDORPHINS Natural pain-reducing substances released by the pituitary gland, producing an effect similar to that of narcotic pain relievers.

ENTERIC COATING A protective covering that enables a pill to pass intact through the stomach into the small intestine, where the coating dissolves and the contents are absorbed.

ENZYME A protein that speeds up specific chemical reactions and processes in the body, such as digestion and energy production.

ESSENTIAL FATTY ACIDS (EFAs) The building blocks that the body uses to make fats. The body must get various kinds of EFAs through diet or supplements (such as fish oils and flaxseed oil) to assure proper health.

ESSENTIAL OIL A concentrated oil extracted from herbs or other plants.

ESTROGEN A female sex hormone, produced mainly in the ovaries, that helps regulate menstruation, reproduction, and other processes.

EXPECTORANT A substance that makes it easier to cough up mucus.

EXTRACT A pill, powder, tincture, or other form of an herb that contains a concentrated, and usually standard, amount of therapeutic ingredients.

FOOD AND DRUG ADMINISTRATION (FDA) The United States government agency that regulates and monitors the safety of food and drugs (but not supplements).

FREE RADICALS Highly reactive and unstable oxygen molecules, generated in the body, that can damage cells, leading to heart disease, cancer, and other ailments. Antioxidants help minimize free-radical damage.

GDU (GELATIN DIGESTING UNIT) A dosage measure for the pain- and inflammation-reducing supplement bromelain. Potencies of bromelain are based on GDUs or MCUs (milk clotting units). One GDU equals 1.5 MCU.

GRAM A metric measure of weight, sometimes used in dosages. There are 1,000 milligrams (mg) in 1 gram, and 28.35 grams in an ounce.

HDL CHOLESTEROL A protein in the blood that collects cholesterol from the body's tissues and returns it to the liver for reprocessing; also known as "good" cholesterol.

HEMOGLOBIN The oxygen-carrying component of red blood cells. Made of iron and protein, it transports oxygen from the lungs to the cells and transports carbon dioxide from the cells back to the lungs.

HERB A plant or plant part—the leaves, stems, roots, bark, buds, or flowers—all of which can be used for medicinal or other purposes (such as flavoring foods).

HOMOCYSTEINE An amino acid-like substance; high levels have been linked to heart disease.

HORMONE Any of various chemical messengers, produced by the adrenal, pituitary, thyroid, ovaries, testes, and other glands, that have far-reaching effects throughout the body. Hormones regulate everything from growth and tissue repair to metabolism, reproduction, blood pressure, as well as the body's response to stress.

HORMONE REPLACEMENT THERAPY (HRT) The use of supplemental estrogen and progesterone (in the form of progestin)—female sex hormones—to relieve the adverse effects of menopause. The therapy may also help prevent osteoporosis and heart disease.

IMMUNE RESPONSE The body's natural defense system against infectious microbes—including disease-causing bacteria and viruses—as well as cancer cells within the body itself.

INSULIN RESISTANCE A condition in which the body's cells do not respond adequately to the hormone insulin. It can lead to higher blood sugar (glucose) levels, increased insulin production by the pancreas, and possibly even to diabetes.

INTEGRATIVE MEDICINE An approach to healing that utilizes aspects of both conventional and alternative medicine. Also called complementary medicine.

INTERFERON Any of various virus-fighting proteins that are made by the body and that activate the immune response.

INTERMITTENT CLAUDICATION A condition caused by poor circulation in the legs (usually from atherosclerosis), characterized by painful calf cramps, often after walking or other exercise. Is relieved by rest.

INTERNATIONAL UNIT (IU) A standardized dose measure that provides a set amount of a specific supplement, such as vitamin A, D, or E.

JAUNDICE A symptom of hepatitis and other liver disorders marked by a yellow hue of the skin and eyes.

LDL CHOLESTEROL A protein in the blood containing high levels of cholesterol and triglycerides; also known as "bad" cholesterol.

LIPOTROPIC COMBINATION A "fat-digesting" blend of choline, inositol, methionine, milk thistle, and other nutrients used to promote the health of the liver. Also called liver complex.

MACROPHAGE A type of white blood cell that can surround and digest disease-causing bacteria and other foreign microbes.

MALAISE A general feeling of overall weakness or discomfort.

MCU (MILK CLOTTING UNIT) A dosage measure for the pain- and inflammation-reducing supplement bromelain. (See also GDU.)

MELANIN A black or dark brown pigment (color) that occurs naturally in the skin, hair, and eyes.

METABOLISM The cascading array of chemical reactions by which the body converts food into packets of energy that the body can use or store.

MICROGRAM (mcg) A metric measure of weight used in dosages. There are 1,000 mcg in 1 milligram (mg).

MILLIGRAM (mg) A metric measure of weight used in dosages. There are 1,000 mg in 1 gram.

MINERAL An inorganic substance found in the earth's crust that plays a crucial role in the human body for enzyme creation, regulation of heart rhythm, bone formation, digestion, and other metabolic processes.

MIXED AMINO ACIDS A balanced blend (complex) of amino acids, often taken in conjunction with individual amino acid supplements.

MONOAMINE OXIDASE (MAO) INHIBITOR A specific class of drugs used to treat depression. They have frequent interactions with various foods, drugs, and supplements.

MUCILAGE A gummy, gel-like plant substance that when ingested forms a protective layer in the throat, digestive tract, and other areas, suppressing coughs and irritation.

MUCOUS MEMBRANES The pink, shiny skinlike layers that line the lips, mouth, vagina, eyelids, and other cavities and passages in the body.

NEURALGIA Sharp, sometimes severe pain resulting from damage to a nerve and often affecting a specific area of the body, such as the face.

NEUROTRANSMITTER Any of various chemicals found in the brain and throughout the body that transmit signals among nerve cells.

NONSTEROIDAL ANTI-INFLAMMATORY DRUG (NSAID) A drug—such as aspirin, ibuprofen, or naproxen—that reduces pain and inflammation by blocking the production of prostaglandins (see also Prostaglandins).

NUTRITIONAL SUPPLEMENT A nutrient, synthesized in the lab or extracted from plants or animals, that is used medicinally.

OVER-THE-COUNTER (OTC) A drug that can be sold without a doctor's prescription.

PCOS (PROCYANIDOLIC OLIGOMERS) A group of antioxidant compounds, also called proanthocyanidins—found in pine bark, grape seed extract, green tea, red wine, and other substances—that may help protect against heart and vascular disease.

PERNICIOUS ANEMIA A rare but dangerous deficiency of vitamin B_{12} that can lead to low red blood cell counts and nervous system impairment.

PHYTOESTROGENS Estrogenlike compounds present in soy and other plants that may help treat symptoms of menopause, certain cancers, and other complaints.

PHYTOMEDICINES Therapeutic ingredients found in fruits, vegetables, grains, herbs, and other plants that may help protect against cancer, heart disease, and other ailments.

PLACEBO Also called a dummy pill, a substance that contains no medicinal ingredients. Often used in scientific studies as a control so its effects can be compared with those of the drug or supplement under study.

POULTICE A soft, moist substance spread between layers of cloth or gauze, and applied, usually heated, to the skin to help reduce pain.

PROBIOTICS "Friendly" bacteria, similar to those found in acidophilus supplements, that are normally present in the intestine and help to promote healthy digestion.

PROGESTERONE A female sex hormone, made by the ovaries, that helps regulate menstruation.

PROLACTIN A hormone, secreted by the pituitary, that promotes lactation.

PROSTAGLANDINS Hormonelike chemicals, occurring naturally in the body, that produce a wide range of effects, such as inducing inflammation, stimulating uterine contractions during labor, and protecting the lining of the stomach.

RECOMMENDED DIETARY ALLOWANCE (RDA) The daily amount of a vitamin or mineral needed by healthy individuals to meet the body's needs and prevent a deficiency. These guidelines are set by the Food and Nutrition Board of the National Academy of Sciences.

STANDARDIZED EXTRACT A concentrated form of an herb that contains a set (standardized) level of active ingredients. Standardization helps guarantee a consistent dosage strength, or potency, from one batch of herb to the next. Standardized extracts are available only for certain herbs, either as pills or tinctures, or in other forms.

STEROIDS A common designation for corticosteroids, inflammation-fighting drugs that are sometimes prescribed to treat allergic reactions, asthma, skin rashes, multiple sclerosis, lupus, and other ailments.

SUBLINGUAL Beneath the tongue. Some supplements, such as vitamin B_{12}, are formulated to dissolve in the mouth, providing quick absorption into the bloodstream without interference from stomach acids.

T'AI CHI An ancient Chinese method of exercise using precise movements and breathing techniques to promote balance, control, and relaxation.

TANNIN An astringent substance derived from plants that can contract blood vessels and body tissues.

TENS (TRANSCUTANEOUS ELECTRICAL NERVE STIMULATION) A method of relieving pain by sending painless electrical impulses from a machine to nerve endings through electrodes placed on the skin.

TESTOSTERONE The principal male sex hormone, produced in the testes, that induces changes at puberty and helps build strong muscles and bones. Women also make a small amount in their ovaries.

THERAPEUTIC DOSE The amount of a vitamin, mineral, herb, nutritional supplement, or drug needed to produce a desired healing effect (as opposed to the minimum amount needed to prevent a deficiency—such as the RDA, for example).

TINCTURE A liquid usually made by soaking a whole herb or its parts in a mixture of water and ethyl alcohol (such as vodka). The alcohol helps extract the herb's active components, concentrating and preserving them.

TONIC An herb (such as ginseng) or herbal blend that is used to "tone" the body or a specific organ, imparting added strength or vitality.

TRADITIONAL MEDICINE An approach to healing that relies on customs and knowledge passed from one generation to the next, often based on thousands of years of practice. Examples are Chinese medicine and Ayurveda (practiced in India).

TRIGLYCERIDE The main form of fat found in the body. High levels in the blood increase the likelihood of developing heart disease.

VITAMIN An organic substance that plays an essential role in regulating cell functions throughout the body. Most vitamins must be ingested, because the body cannot produce them.

WAFER A chewable tablet or cookie-like form of supplement. Often activated by saliva or used to bypass powerful stomach acids.

index

N

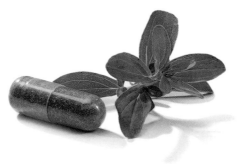